Gua sha
A Traditional Technique for Modern Practice

Illustrations by Peter Cox
Gua sha photographs by Arya Nielsen
Cover photograph, Thermogram, by Howard Sochurek (reproduced with permission from Corbis)
Thermogram showing a child sitting on a cold surface. Red reveals the warmest areas while blue-green shows the coolest. The child's body heat is conducted to the floor while the floor's cold is absorbed by the child. This image demonstrates a concept held by every traditional medicine in history, that environmental factors including temperature can impact the body and potentially influence function.

Content Strategist: *Claire Wilson*
Content Development Specialists: *Fiona Conn, Alison McMurdo*
Project Manager: *Julie Taylor*
Designer/Design Direction: *Miles Hitchen*
Illustration Manager: *Jennifer Rose*

Gua sha
A Traditional Technique for Modern Practice

2nd EDITION

Arya Nielsen PhD
Director, Acupuncture Fellowship for Inpatient Care
Senior Attending Acupuncturist
Beth Israel Medical Center's
Department of Integrative Medicine
New York, NY, USA

Foreword by

Ted J. Kaptchuk
Associate Professor of Medicine, Harvard Medical School
Director of the Harvard Program in Placebo Studies and the Therapeutic Encounter
Beth Israel Deaconess Medical Center
Harvard Medical School, Boston, Massachusetts, USA

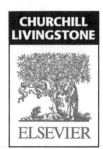

CHURCHILL LIVINGSTONE

ELSEVIER

Edinburgh London New York Oxford Philadelphia St Louis Sydney Toronto 2013

First edition 1995
Second edition 2013

ISBN 978 0 7020 3108 3

British Library Cataloguing in Publication Data
A catalogue record for this book is available from the British Library

Library of Congress Cataloging in Publication Data
A catalog record for this book is available from the Library of Congress

your source for books,
journals and multimedia
in the health sciences
www.elsevierhealth.com

Working together to grow
libraries in developing countries

www.elsevier.com | www.bookaid.org | www.sabre.org

ELSEVIER   BOOK AID
            International   Sabre Foundation

The
publisher's
policy is to use
paper manufactured
from sustainable forests

Printed in China

This work is dedicated to my mother
Apolonia Anastasia Jaskowiak Nielsen,
to my grandmothers Leona Dell Robey Nielsen
and Sophia Witt Jaskowiak, and to their mothers, and theirs;
all who care for me still in the medicine I learned at home.

Arya Nielsen, PhD

Dr Arya Nielsen is an American acupuncturist taught in the classical lineage of Dr James Tin Yau So and in practice for over 35 years. She graduated in the first class of the first acupuncture college in the United States in 1977. She is a practitioner, teacher, author, and researcher and is considered the Western authority on the traditional East Asian technique Gua sha. Dr Nielsen has a faculty appointment at a New York teaching hospital, Beth Israel Medical Center, where she treats patients and also directs the Acupuncture Fellowship for Inpatient Care through the Department of Integrative Medicine.

Ted J. Kaptchuk

Ted J. Kaptchuk is an Associate Professor of Medicine at Harvard Medical School, Boston, MA. He is Director of the Program in Placebo Studies and the Therapeutic Encounter at Beth Israel Deaconess Medical Center in Boston and the author of *The Web that has no Weaver*.

Contents

The plates will be found between pages xiv and 1

Foreword

Medical 'sedimentation' is a term that has been used to describe a process where a residue of the literate traditions of the past filters down to the lower classes, where they remain even after the erudite abandon them (Starr 1982). Gua sha, an East Asian healing technique that has been tagged with the label 'folk tradition' is an excellent example of this process where an important medical intervention is generally forsaken by elite practitioners and only continued by ordinary people in the absence of professionals and by practitioners of tradition when not in the company of the elite. The erudite do not like to have to depend on techniques that may appear simple and unsophisticated.

Arya Nielsen has taken this important technique and reversed the 'sedimentation' process. By using historical examinations of East Asian medical texts, cross-cultural historical documents, contemporary scholarly sources, interviews with living elder practitioners and her own keen clinical experience she has brought Gua sha to the center of Oriental medicine clinical practice. She has found a precious lost ring that might have gone down the drain of disuse.

Arya Nielsen has always been involved in movements to rescue potential valuable knowledge and methods from the inattention of neglect and fashion. When I first met Arya Nielsen in 1976 she had just notified an eminent conventional medical school that she was rejecting their admission acceptance to, instead, make a full-time commitment to learn acupuncture and Oriental medicine. Not many people knew much about acupuncture in those days; it was also discussed as a 'folk' tradition of the East. Her commitment and dedication to seeking what is valuable for patients has made Arya Nielsen an important teacher and leader of our profession. Her book is another example of not allowing prejudice, prestige, appearance, circumstances, or habit get in the way of something that can benefit patients.

This second edition has been seasoned by Dr Nielsen's additional years of scholarship and practice. She has added a literature review that locates Gua sha in the medical discourse of both East and West. Indeed, this therapy has a complex cross-cultural history. Further, Dr Nielsen has also gathered the latest scientific research that demonstrates the anti-inflammatory and hepatoprotective properties of Gua sha.

Dr Nielsen has done a tremendous service to bring to the attention of healthcare providers a low-tech practice that has many applications. Dr Nielsen continues to teach us that therapies developed over centuries using ordinary human sensory awareness can help to guide our research inquiry, our passion and compassion to respond to human suffering.

Ted J. Kaptchuk
2012

Starr P 1982 The social transformation of American medicine. Basic Books, New York. p. 47.

Much has changed since the 1995 edition of this Gua sha text. Traditional East Asian medicine has come of age as an engaged practice, an object of evidence-based and mechanism research, and the focus of study in dedicated schools, colleges and courses within universities and medical schools. Once an outlier or alternative to conventional medicine, it now leads efforts toward integrative and pluralistic care. Traditional East Asian practices, including Gua sha, are no longer isolated to the private setting but are merged in conventional clinics, hospitals and inpatient facilities.

It is good to acknowledge how far we have come. We have helped to create a regulated medical profession in the United States that did not exist forty years ago. This is no small feat given the political landscape of bias and resistance within medicine, and yet it could not have been accomplished without the support of physicians, researchers, academics, regulators and the public committed to sound options in healthcare.

We have established a safety record of 'relative risk'. That is, there is some risk with traditional East Asian medicine that is managed and greatly reduced with proper training, such that acupuncture therapies are one of the safest forms of medical intervention. We have established schools, a national board, qualifying exams that are psychometrically sound, and strong partnerships with medical, academic and regulating institutions.

My own journey is no longer defined by my acceptance to medical school (declined). I am now on faculty at a medical teaching hospital, Beth Israel Medical Center in New York City, where I also direct an Acupuncture Fellowship for Inpatient Care. My choice to study and practice traditional East Asian medicine came out of a sense that prevention is the best medicine, that physical medicine calls on a cognitive and somatic rapport that creates possibility where an informed and engaged patient is the best ally. This medicine was never meant to supplant modern medicine but to make it better, to respond to what are called 'gaps in care', to support patients who are getting care but continue to suffer.

Interest in the practice continues to mount but as a colleague recently noted: acupuncture therapy studies do little to guide or improve actual practice but continue to focus on whether acupuncture works at all. For example, acupuncture studies funded by the German Government mandated that needle insertion be used as a control. So while both real and control acupuncture treated back pain better than usual care alone, 'real' acupuncture performed only a bit better than what was situated as 'placebo'. Many researchers rebutted that, pointing out that needle insertion is not an inert control but

an active form of acupuncture comparable to styles that needle 'off-channel'. In other words, if a study compared two antibiotics and found one worked a bit better than the other, but both worked much better than no antibiotic, the conclusion would not be that 'antibiotics do not work'.

This may well be how acupuncture therapies persisted over 2000 years. You did not have to be that good to have 'some effect'. The better trained and more experienced the practitioner the better the effect. Moreover, some of the studies that showed a strong placebo effect with acupuncture also found that the placebo aspect may wear off over time, i.e. real acupuncture with proper frequency and dosage of treatment is therapeutic.

There has been sufficient study of acupuncture for headache and migraine prophylaxis, neck, back, and knee pain, and for pain, anxiety, nausea and vomiting in the perioperative period as well as during chemotherapy to culminate in systematic reviews that recommend acupuncture as a safe treatment for these disorders with few side-effects. And there is positive study for many other areas and conditions that together speak well for this medicine. As of this writing, acupuncture is reimbursable by national health insurance plans in Germany and England for specific conditions.

Research into the physiology of acupuncture therapies has advanced beyond the simple endorphin effect found decades ago. Discoveries of mechanical and chemical signaling within the connective tissue are now theorized to be the 'bed' of the channel system. Brain and neurochemical studies as well as research into acupuncture's ability to regulate the autonomic nervous system each add partial knowledge as pieces to a puzzle of how this medicine works and where and when it is most useful.

While I have had a hand in shaping the practice of traditional East Asian medicine in the United States, our success has in turn shaped my priorities. I was on the first State Board for Acupuncture in New York, involved in writing New York's regulations for professional practice, and was Board Chair for two of eight years served. Those regulations allowed for practice in New York and recognition soon followed that the practices themselves needed to be researched and represented in the West. For example, there were no studies concerning Gua sha and without quantitative measures it could not begin to be situated within the science of medicine.

I wanted to research the effects of Gua sha and so entered the Academy for a research doctorate. I matriculated in a doctoral program at Union Institute and University where I received my PhD in Philosophies of Medicine with a specialty in Integrative Clinical Science and Health Care.

During my doctoral study I was invited to the University of Duisburg–Essen in Germany to conduct laboratory research on Gua sha with Drs Andreas Michalsen and Gustav Dobos, who directed the Department of Integrative Medicine there as well as the Kliniken Essen, a 54-bed hospital where patients with chronic illnesses are treated with integrative therapies.

During this same period the Chinese-language database became accessible online. Now a thorough background and literature review could be done and was sorely needed to situate Gua sha in medical discourse. Together these circumstances clarified a need for revising *Gua Sha, a Traditional Technique for Modern Practice*. This is more than a freshening of the existing text, though some areas have stood the test of time and remain essential. It was time to advance Gua sha from a curious technique that amazes providers and patients with its curative effect while instilling trepidation in others because of the 'look' of the transitory therapeutic petechiae. It was time to fix on Gua sha with a scientific gaze and interpret what can be known, to inform practitioners and patients alike. Such a project is no longer contained in a book on theory and practice but must include evidence in addition to background and personal/archival experience.

A revised chapter on history illuminates the homogeneity of early Western medicine and traditional East Asian medicine in the application of Gua sha for the treatment of cholera. The history and theory of Hippocratic medicine connecting bloodletting with the evolution of acupuncture provides a new context for the link between Hippocrates and how his name would have been pronounced in early Chinese: 'Chih-Po' (oddly similar to the famous physician whose discourse with the Yellow Emperor is recorded as the oldest Chinese medical text). A tracing of the lineage of Dr So, the doctor from Hong Kong who taught me Gua sha, sheds light on classical practice as distinct from traditional Chinese medicine (TCM) theory that has been represented as orthodoxy from China.

Chapter 2 presents the evidence relating to Gua sha; a thorough literature review gives a current picture of medical discourse on Gua sha that until now has not benefited from such an endeavor. I find literature reviews to be extraordinarily satisfying; they set what is 'known' and become the basis for situating research inquiry. While the Chinese language database has only been available relatively recently, it is also important to note that the Chinese-language database includes articles about traditional medicine only since 1984. An abundance of the Chinese-language articles are case series with more recent randomized trials. While randomized trials remain the watermark of proof in the West, Chinese-language discourse on care and technique in the form of case series articles is worth considering in its own right. It establishes a record of use, a record of safety and lays the foundation for therapeutic relevance that can guide clinical trials.

I spent a year analysing over 600 articles in Chinese, finding over 500 to be relevant medically. I translated and organized publication types of articles in tables to provide an overview of how Gua sha has been and is being used in China.

Gua sha's register in the Western medical database is also detailed. Western medicine's first regard for Gua sha was in response to the Vietnamese version 'cao gio' as practiced by Southeast Asians who came to the States after the Vietnam War. Cao gio is described as abuse/pseudo-abuse, a religious or cultural ritual to be discouraged and pitied. Some East Asian immigrants were persecuted for using Gua sha/cao gio; a conflation of those incidents was rendered in the feature film *The Gua Sha Treatment*, the most popular film in China in 2001, representing intercultural misunderstanding and yet a turning tide. Science now helps us to appreciate Gua sha, like acupuncture, while its persistence over time is a credit to those engaged with it because it seemed to work.

How Gua sha works, the research into the physiology of Gua sha, is taken up in Chapter 3, including my team's first biomechanism study that demonstrates a 400% increase in surface microperfusion measured by laser Doppler scanning. How Gua sha may fit into the new connective tissue models of healing is discussed. Researchers at Harvard/Mass General have demonstrated an upregulation of heme oxygenase-1 (HO-1) that may well inform the anti-inflammatory and hepatoprotectant effect of Gua sha that is worth exploring in the treatment of hepatitis.

For the student of traditional East Asian medicine, this text explains 'sha syndrome', the quintessentiality of the 'organ' San Jiao, the theory of kinds of illness and appropriate response, including explicit instructions on how to apply Gua sha and how to speak about it to patients and other providers. Gua sha can be used immediately in practice with impressive results because it moves 'blood stasis', a feature of illness associated with protracted symptoms including pain. Gua sha breaks the cycle of stasis that acupuncture cannot address.

Those familiar with classical Tongue observation will find a surprising application discussed in Chapter 7, where immediate and significant Tongue changes as a direct result of Gua sha advance understanding of both Gua sha and Tongue diagnosis. Tongue observation goes beyond a quick fix on status and becomes a way to assess the depth and direction of a disorder via a person's response to Gua sha.

How to treat specific disorders detailed in Chapter 8 is based on classical 'diagnosis': what is the location, quality and mutability of a problem; what happens when I touch the problem, interact with it? There are additional new cases in Chapter 9 to support the application of Gua sha in common and also severe illness.

This revised edition is meant to be a resource for practitioners, researchers and scholars alike. It is my hope that my efforts make this material accessible. Writing is incredibly demanding, time-consuming and isolating. A writer has to have a certain passion for their project in addition to the pleasure of its culmination, which is this moment now: the privilege of offering it to you.

With respect

Arya Nielsen PhD
2012

I am indebted to Dr James Tin Yao So for his syncretic adaptation of the Cheng Dan'an lineage of classical Chinese medicine: 'to use what works'; and for his dedication to practice and teaching that led to the first acupuncture school in the US in Boston in 1976.

To Ted Kaptchuk: visionary, teacher, writer and friend, for the many hours of discursive articulation: to 'eliminate unnecessary suffering'.

I am grateful to Deborah Rose who encouraged me to act on my desire to study acupuncture while I mulled my acceptance to Tuft's medical school. I am grateful that I had the good fortune to be in the first class of the first acupuncture school in the US, the New England School of Acupuncture. For their part in creating that first program, Arnie Freeman, Steve Breeker; and to Jim Donovan MD, who hosted Dr So at his clinic in Newton Centre where I interned.

I am so grateful to those colleagues who encouraged and were part of my journey into Gua sha research: Drs Helene Langevin, Gustav Dobos, Andreas Michalsen, Nicola Knoblauch, and Ben Kligler. And to Drs Ken Kwong and Phoebe Chan, who are moving Gua sha research into new realms.

I am indebted to the New England School of Acupuncture (NESA) for permission to access the Chinese-language database through the Kelly library through which I was able to conduct a literature review of Gua sha in Chinese. I am also grateful to Miya Cao PhD, for her assistance with sticky translation points and access to full texts not available through Chinese Asia on Demand (CAOD). Thanks to Marsha Handel, Beth Israel Medical Center's Integrative Medicine's Informatics librarian, for her careful reading of several chapters.

To the acupuncture schools and programs where I have been on faculty or invited to teach over the last 35 years: Tri-State College of Acupuncture in New York (Mark Seem), New England School of Acupuncture, now in Newton, MA, and the Pacific College of Oriental Medicine (Belinda Anderson; Jack Miller); the Anglo–Dutch Institute of Oriental Medicine in Holland, and Annemarie Hemken, whose invitation opened Europe to me: the Rothenburg Kongress (Gerd Ohmstede and Velia Wortman), the First TCM Hospital Kötzting; (Christoph Blass, Erich Wehr, and Stephen Hager), and the University of Duisburg–Essen at the Kliniken Essen (Gustav Dobos and Andreas Michalsen) all in Germany; the Acupuncture College at York, England (Hugh MacPherson), the Switzerland TCM Group (Regula Engetschwiler), the Scandinavian Kongress in Denmark (Marion Nielsen Joos), the Akupunkture Akademiet in Aarhus and Copenhagen, Denmark, (Camilla Gliemann and Jan Nørmark), the Maryland Acupuncture Society (MAS), the American Organization for Bodywork Therapies of Asia (AOBTA), the American Medical Student Association (AMSA), the FASCIA Conference at Harvard in 2007, the International Research Congress on Integrative Medicine & Health, 2012, and to Dr Woodson Merrell and Beth Israel Medical Center's Department of Integrative Medicine, whose commitment to integrative medicine in general, and support of my work in particular, is tantamount to my continued success. For the opportunity to present at Department Grand Rounds in the Hospital, to the faculty and Residents at Family Medicine, to the integrative medicine physician fellows and acupuncture fellows: each venue, each seminar has afforded me the opportunity to hone a teaching of traditional East Asian medicine and Gua sha that made it better. To every single student whose interest and questions helped me to be a better teacher.

Who I am and to what I commit have been shaped by my family and I want to acknowledge them and hope that my work reflects well on their hopes for me. I acknowledge my father Arthur Alonzo Nielsen, who grew up in rural Wisconsin wanting to be a forest preservationist but whose life was forever changed by the battles of WWII. His courage and contribution led me to see the world as a place I could change, in which I had a place, and to which I had responsibilities. My father was a leader.

To my mother, Apolonia Anastasia Jaskowiak, who provided me with a faith that nature heals. The tenth of thirteen children, my mom used to say: we had no idea we were poor; we were happy with each other and what we had. Her words remind me now of the Buddha's notion of the second arrow. The first arrow is what has happened to you; the second arrow is what you tell yourself about it. Apolonia had an amazing ability to be positive and identify with the good in others. My mother was a healer.

And I want to acknowledge my siblings: Gregory, Patricia (Carlson) and David Arthur are each a leader and healer in their own right and I love them. And to the next generation, my nephews and nieces: Greg, Polly, Jeannie, and Jeff Nielsen; Lindsay, Matt and Caitlin Carlson, and Kara Nielsen. Most of them have experienced Gua sha even as children and are now interested in how to do it as young adults and that is gratifying.

I am grateful to my editors Alison McMurdo, Fiona Conn, Marcela Holmes and Julie Taylor for their detailed and extremely patient care of this project. And foremost to Claire Wilson who oversaw this revision from start to finish: thank you.

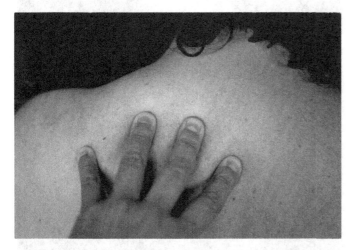

Plate 1 • Pressing palpation. The provider palpates the surface to discover not only painful or tight areas but to examine the color and response of the flesh

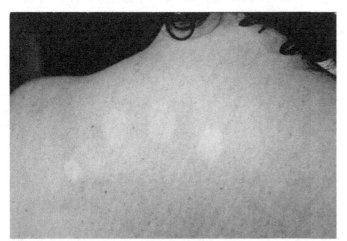

Plate 2 • Blanching from pressing palpation that is slow to fade indicates sha stasis in the surface tissue

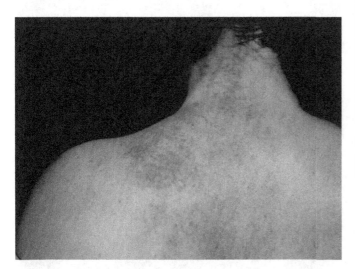

Plate 3 • Sha has been raised on the patient palpated in Plates 1 and 2. Most sha is a variation of red, with other colors signaling aspects of stasis

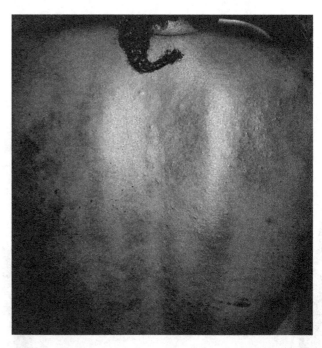

Plate 4 • Sha for a person of color appears as petechiae that redden the skin.

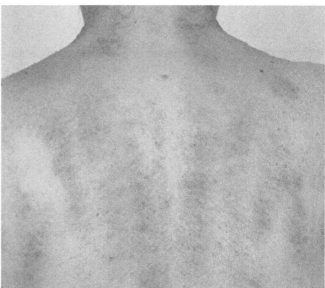

Plate 5 • Two-day-old sha shows the effect of sha fading; the yellow tinge to the hyperpigmentation is indicative of bilirubin and biliverdin in the tissue.

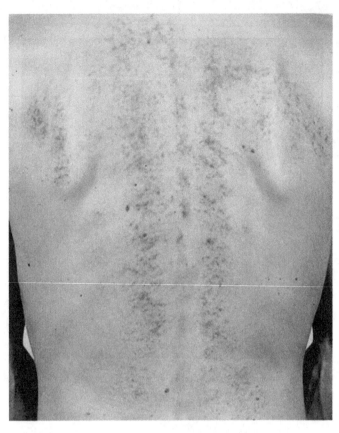

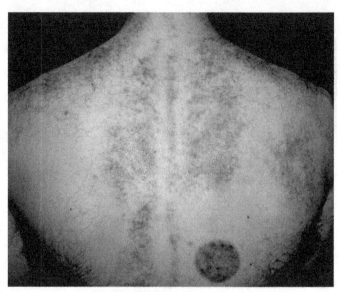

Plate 7 • Blue sha may relate to cold, Liver Qi constraint or Heart problems retarding the circulation of blood. Dark round-shaped area at bottom right is from over-cupping done by a student a few days prior to Gua sha.

Plate 6 • Pale sparse sha: may associate with blood deficiency (or may be from incomplete expression of sha by poor technique)

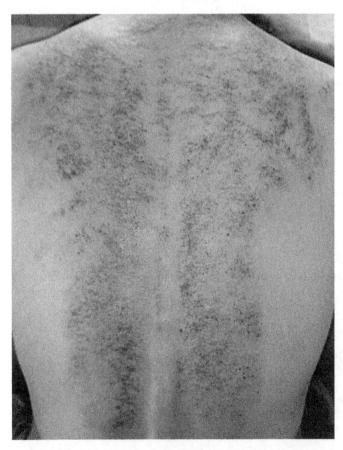

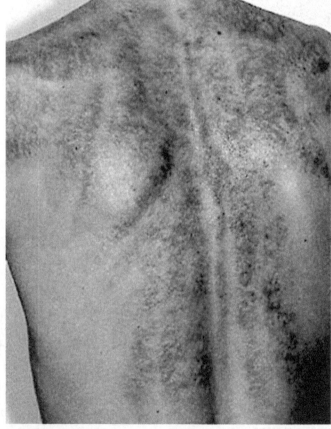

Plate 8 • Gua sha to entire back. (For a case of chillphobia, knee pain and swelling associated with deficient Yang see Chapter 9)

Plate 9 • Dark red sha, purple or black sha reflects more intense stasis or Heat within longer-standing blood stasis

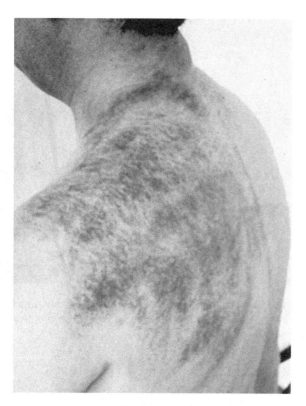

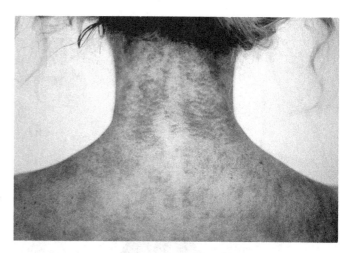

Plate 11 • Gua sha to neck and shoulder for tension pain: Xu Deficiency condition. (For case see Chapter 9).

Plate 10 • Brown sha appearing here at the neck area may be associated with Yin deficiency. Gua sha was applied to the neck and shoulder for treatment of pain and constriction from whiplash. This subject also had hyperglycemia but refused diabetic medication.

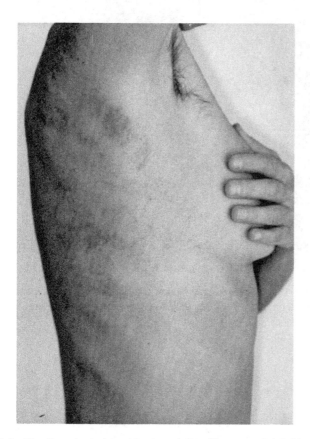

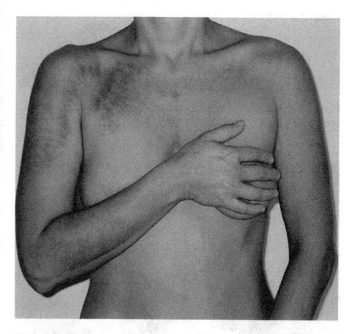

Plate 13 • Gua sha to chest and arm. (For case of deltoid-pectoralis pain see Chapter 9)

Plate 12 • Gua sha to lateral back and ribs. (For case of deltoid-pectoralis pain see Chapter 9)

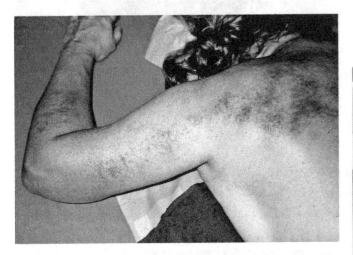

Plate 14 • Gua sha to upper back, shoulder, upper arm and forearm for fibromyalgia

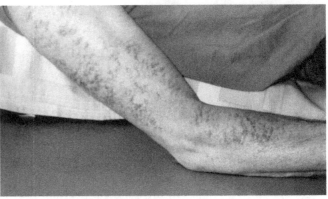

Plate 15 • Gua sha to the arm for tennis elbow. Gua sha was first applied to the upper back, shoulder and neck. (For case of tennis elbow see Chapter 9)

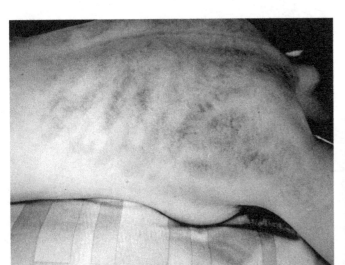

Plate 16 • Gua sha to back, upper back and ribs. (For case of fibrocystic breast normala see Chapter 9)

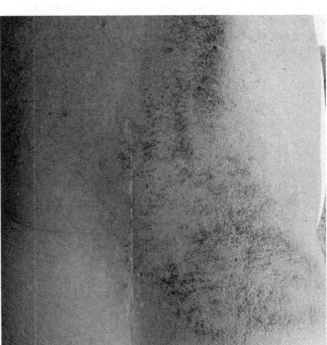

Plate 17 • Gua sha to lower back and buttock in the treatment of a knee problem. (For case of knee Bi syndrome (arthritis) see Chapter 9)

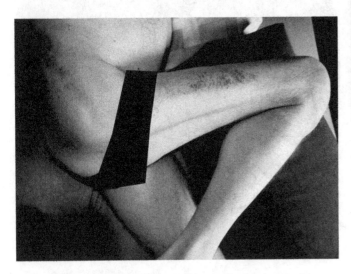

Plate 18 • Gua sha to buttocks and leg for the treatment of sciatica.

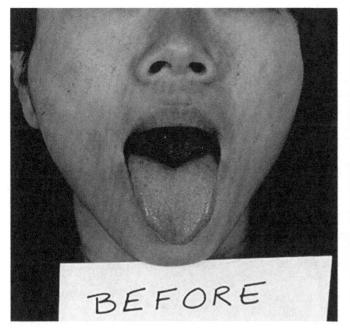

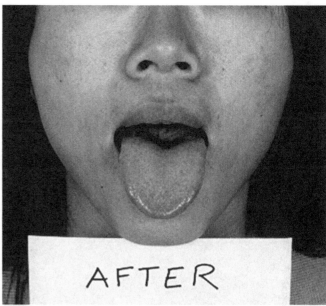

Plate 19 • Subject 1 was experiencing fatigue and early onset upper respiratory symptoms. The 'before Tongue' shows redness concentrated at the front and sides of the Tongue

Plate 20 • Immediately after Gua sha the Tongue is less red with residual Heat at the front end corresponding to sinus inflammation. Tongue coat is slightly increased. Notice after Gua sha the face is also paler with some appearance of Heat still at nasi anni. With Gua sha clearing Heat, the underlying Blood deficiency is more apparent.

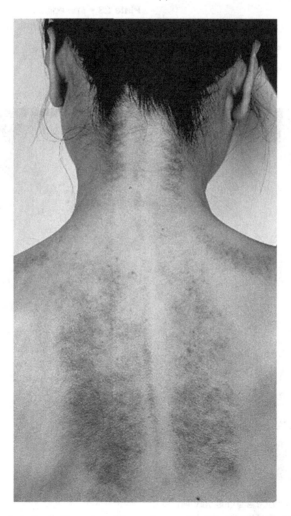

Plate 21 • Note the sha is bright red and similar to the color of the redness of the 'before Tongue' (Plate 19). This Gua sha was performed in a student seminar: even with a beginner's technique where some areas were missed, Gua sha had a significant effect on the Tongue

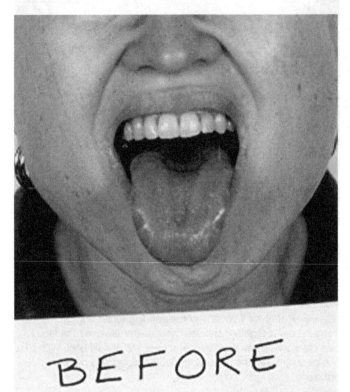

BEFORE

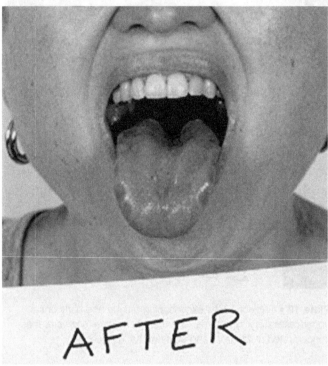

AFTER

Plate 23 • Immediately after Gua sha on Subject 2, her Tongue, lips and face are less red, with resumption of very slight coat. Heat has been vented

Plate 22 • Gua sha vents Heat. Subject 2's Tongue is very red, with redness and scalloping at the sides. Subject 2's sha (Plate 24) is similar to the color of her 'before' Tongue

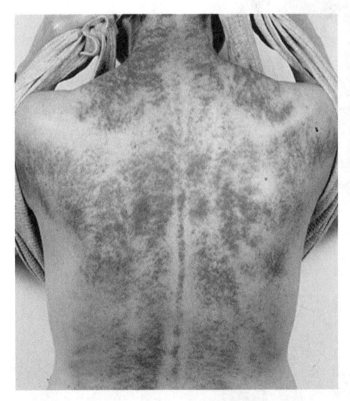

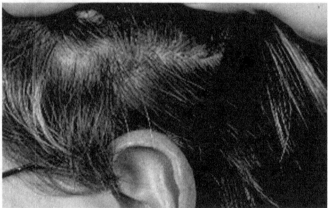

Plate 25 • For subject 2's migraine and cluster headaches Gua sha is applied to the upper back, neck and shoulders and then to the scalp at the site of the fixed pain. For Gua sha at the scalp, expose the area to be treated and press-stroke across the exposed area, here left to right.

Plate 24 • Sha, Subject 2. Note the color of the sha is very similar to the color of the 'before Tongue', Plate 22. Also the sha is excessively ecchymotic, indicating the student who performed Gua sha here may have over-stroked the subject (Chapter 6)

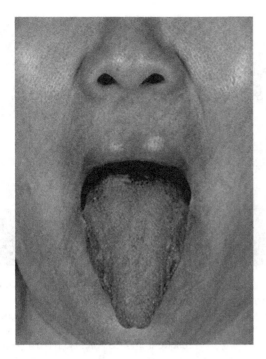

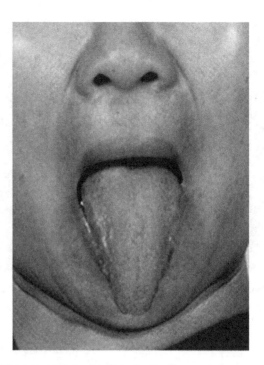

Plate 26 • The 'before Tongue' of Subject 3 is purple–red with concentrated redness at front end and sides; the coat is concentrated on back right portion

Plate 27 • Immediately after Gua sha the Tongue is less purple, less red, with a thicker coat overall. The coat at the back right portion is thicker, pasty and less rooted. Note the face and lips and nasi anni are less red after Gua sha

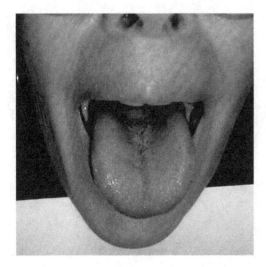

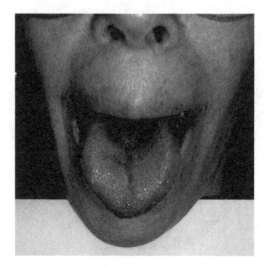

Plate 28 • Before Gua sha the Tongue is pale peachy. The more concentrated peachy color at the front and sides represents Heat (a kind of redness) within blood Deficiency associated with the peachy color

Plate 29 • Immediately after Gua sha the peachy areas of the Tongue are darker, almost red, with appearance of points that are often associated with concentration of Heat; the coat is slightly increased, especially on the right. The face is a bit 'redder' as well. Heat appears to increase here, further clarifying deficiency of Blood/Yin

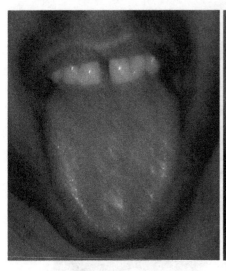

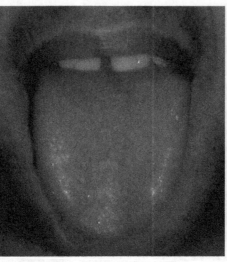

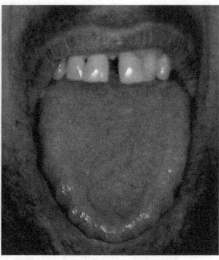

Plate 30 • The 'before Tongue', while blurry, is recognizably blue, fluted and redder at the front

Plate 31 • Immediately after Gua sha the blue of Plate 27 has almost completely resolved. The front end of the Tongue is less red, less fluted. The 'Shen' of the Tongue has brightened

Plate 32 • Shows the Tongue from Plate 30 and 31 two weeks later. The Tongue is fluted with red scalloped front rim. The progression demonstrates that Tongue blueness can resolve from Gua sha, and remain resolved

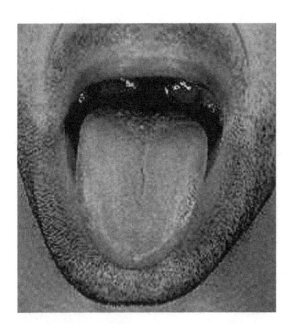

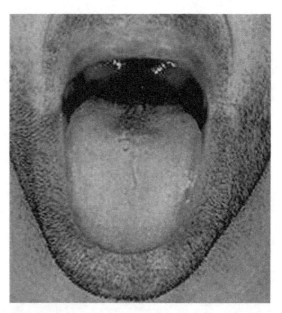

Plate 33 • The 'before Tongue' is red, with red fluted sides and a Stomach crack

Plate 34 • Immediately after Gua sha the Tongue is slightly less red, it is less fluted with an increase in coat throughout. As Gua sha circulates fluids the Stomach crack is less pronounced. However, because of the general lack of fluids/dehydration the coat has increased. In fact, this subject had gotten little sleep and was dehydrated

Gua sha and the history of traditional medicine, West and East

1

I wish I could make a petechial fever; in other words I wish I could produce upon the skin that state of counteraction existing when petechial spots are formed.

(Boerhave (1668–1738) quoted in Epps (1832))

CHAPTER CONTENTS

Counteraction medicine: the crisis is the cure

Although Western historians refer to Hippocrates (459–377 BC) as the father of medicine, this is as accurate as the assertion that Columbus discovered America. American Indians had, of course, discovered the continent and themselves. Furthermore, Viking ships were known to have visited the Americas long before Columbus, as evidenced by the dating of mollusk fossils that are thought to have hitched a ride by attaching themselves to the ships.

The bulk of medical knowledge collected and practiced by Hippocrates was Egyptian in origin, not Greek. Egyptian physicians taught in Greece, Persia and Arabia. Atkinson (1956) notes that the principles of the Hippocratic Oath date back to the Egyptian Ebers Papyrus, written in 1553 BC. The Ebers Papyrus is one of the oldest, most complete and unspoiled books in existence. It verifies that Egyptian medical and surgical knowledge was as advanced at the time of its writing as it was 1500 years later during the time of Galen.

Medical education in Greek society passed from father to son. Hippocrates' own grandfather studied with an Egyptian. What distinguished Hippocrates as a practitioner of the medicine of his day was his bedside observations and the recording of his patients' symptoms and treatments that make up the Hippocratic Canon: 'The intention of the physician should be called to the position of the patient in bed, to the nature of his expectoration, and to the character of his breathing' (Atkinson 1956). Scholars do not think the Hippocratic Canon was written by one person, but rather, constructed over time by many authors following principles attributed to Hippocrates. As in Greece, so in China. Ch'i Po, the legendary physician whose conversations with Emperor Huang Di were recorded in the *Huang Di Nei Ching Su Wen* (2nd century BC), states in chapter 5:

... by observing the external symptoms one gathers knowledge about internal disturbances. One should watch beyond the ordinary limits ... one should observe minute and trifling things as if they were of normal size, and when they are thus treated they cannot become dangerous.

(Veith 1966)

In *Celestial Lancets*, Lu Gwei-djen and Joseph Needham (1980) note that the Chinese medical classics, the *Nei Ching* and early Han texts of the 2nd and 1st centuries BC, correspond in large measure with the Hippocratic Corpus. The *Nei Ching* (~ 200 BC) is a record of a constructed conversation between the Yellow Emperor Huang ti and his physician, Ch'i Po. Nigel Wiseman (personal communication, 2000) has noted that in early Chinese, a mono- and disyllabic language, the name 'Hippocrates' (~ 400 BC), would have been pronounced as 'chee-po', or the softer 'hee-po', which is remarkably akin to the name of the *Nei Ching* physician 'Ch'i Po'. This correspondence was noted in 1685 by Willem ten Rhijne (1647–1700). According to Baldry (1989), ten Rhijne is credited as the first person to give the modern Western world a detailed account of Chinese acupuncture and moxibustion.

The shared understanding of ancient medical traditions will be considered below. Their very correspondence indicates common origins, collaboration or profound synchronicity. If exchange of medical ideas among ancient cultures cannot be dated, it can be assumed to have coincided with trade of goods. With traffic of goods came traffic of diseases and epidemics, and the opportunity for trade in notions and materials of medicine.

In *Plagues and Peoples*, McNeill (1989) contends that when travel from China and India to the Mediterranean became regularly organized and routine, a homogenization of the germ pool occurred. From the study of disease and epidemic patterns, he believes that something approximating this did, in

fact, occur, beginning in the 1st century AD. Chinese silk was exchanged by traders from these ancient civilizations and their route of trade is well documented along the famous Silk Road.

The Silk Road

Chinese silk was traded via the Silk Road (see Figure 1.1) long before the Christian Era. According to *The Silk Road on Land and Sea* (China Pictorial Publications 1989), the Silk Road was the artery for the exchange of commerce, technology and culture, and was a significant influence on the development of the great civilizations of China, India, Egypt, Persia, Arabia, Greece and Rome:

> Inscriptions on bones and tortoise shells of the Shang Dynasty (c. 16th–11th century BC) bear the characters for 'silkworm', 'mulberry', 'silk' and 'silk fabric'. In the Book of Isaiah in the Old Testament, which was written between 740–701 BC, the Chinese are referred to as 'Sinim' (silk men) and the Chinese silk is mentioned in the Book of Ezekiel.
>
> One Roman poet wrote that Chinese silk yarn was finer than a spider's threads. Julius Caesar (100–44 BC) is said to have appeared in the theater dressed in a toga of Chinese silk, and his garment became the focus of attention as an unprecedented luxury, so that from then on aristocratic families considered it an honor to wear Chinese silk.

Agents did not necessarily travel the Silk Road end-to-end but transported goods to exchange at markets in towns or oases along the route. Various groups or tribes, the Scythians for example, demanded compensation for passage of goods (Wood 2002). When Anxi (Iran) tried to control the silk trade by obstructing the overland route, this necessitated a route by sea. As *The Silk Road on Land and Sea* explains: 'In 166CE[AD],

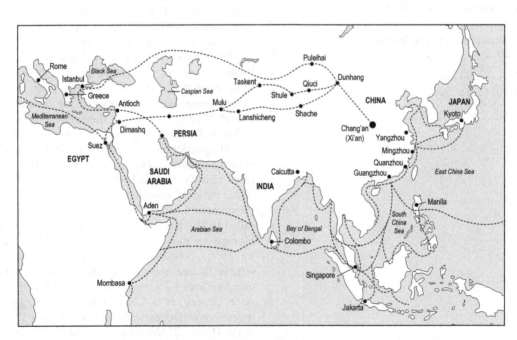

Figure 1.1 • The Silk Road crossed land and sea connecting ancient civilizations including Egypt, Rome, Greece and China.

Roman Emperor Marcus Aurelius succeeded in dispatching an envoy to China via Rinan (Vietnam) with ivory, rhinoceros horns, and hawksbill tortoises, initiating direct trade between Rome and China'.

The most recent archeological studies suggest that the silk trading trade across Eurasia started even earlier than was previously thought. Strands of silk known to have been Chinese in origin were found in the hair of an Egyptian mummy dated 1000 BC. The mummy was found at a burial ground of the King's workers at Thebes. These findings give greater credibility to previous reports of silk fabrics being excavated from 7th century BC German sites and 5th century BC burial sites in Greece. When this discovery was first reported in the *New York Times*, Wilford (1993) wrote:

> Caravans headed east with gold, woolens, ivory, amber, and glass. From China the camels were laden with furs, ceramics and lacquer, as well as silk. By the first century BC the Romans could not get enough of this commodity, which to them was synonymous with China. The Romans had learned of the Chinese from the Greeks, who called them 'Seres' and the Latin word for silk became 'serica'.

McNeill (1989) sees striking similarities in Roman and Chinese history. He postulates that the similar religious and political trends were cultural accommodations of similar disease trends, which reflected homogenization of infections from repeated trade contact.

Scythians and other nomadic peoples ranged widely across Eurasia and had fairly extensive contact with both Greek and Chinese cultures. Hippocrates noted in his text *Airs, Waters and Places* that the Scythians, cauterized and let blood. Moreover, Scythian bloodletting presupposed ties between remote parts of the body similar to the perceptions of the Greeks and Chinese (Kuriyama 1999).

An idea beyond the scope of this book, it nonetheless corroborates a connection between the two civilizations. Their medical approach suggests communication and a synchronous perception of and response to illness.

Hippocrates, Galen and Ch'i Po: humoral medicine

Galen (AD 129–200) was one of the most famous physicians in Rome during the reign of Marcus Aurelius, who established direct trade with China. A Greek, Galen followed the methods of medicine passed from Greece, known as Hippocratic. The four elements of Fire, Water, Earth and Air combined to form the four body humors: blood, phlegm, yellow and black bile. Galen spoke of *pneuma*, translated as 'air' or 'breath', having many of the same qualities that the Chinese attribute to Qi. Lu Gwei-djen and Needham (1980) and Epler (1980) have translated Qi as pneuma.

Hippocratic medicine held that sickness resulted when one of the humors became impure, out of place or out of balance. Restorative treatment, or apotherapy, aimed at removing or diminishing the offending humor by purging, bleeding, vomiting, blistering, urinating, salivating or sweating. Note that almost all of these forms of evacuation occur naturally. A

deficient humor would be restored by diet or herbs and drugs. Drugs, herbs and food were classified according to their Warm, Cold, Moist, or Dry qualities. For example, pepper was a warming herb that countered Cold; cucumber was a cooling herb that countered Heat. The similarities to Chinese dyadic classification are striking. Did the Chinese acquire this 'methodology' from the Greeks? Is the *Nei Ching* a volume of Hippocratic method where Huang ti recorded a hypothetical conversation with a heavenly Hippocrates (Ch'i Po) as suggested above, or did the ancient Greeks acquire it '... from China where it is very widespread ... and known since the earliest time' (Kleinman et al. 1975)? The introduction of a technology or paradigm might be dated if from new contact or from trade between areas and peoples that had little or no previous contact. However, multidirectional contact and trade within and across Eurasia dates to antiquity. While the origins are obscured, the similarities are clear, as in the case of bloodletting that is also critical to the origins of acupuncture and Gua sha.

Bloodletting as a restorative treatment and origin of acupuncture

Although bloodletting was practiced by every ancient culture, no one knows its precise origin. Neither Hippocrates nor any of the early Greek physicians spoke of bloodletting as a novel technique. According to Garrison (1913) it had been in general use in Egypt, Assyria and Scythia before being introduced to Greece. He states, 'The earliest Egyptian representation of bloodletting dates to BC 2500.'

Pliny's fable credits the Egyptians with learning to open a vein from watching the clumsy hippopotamus wound itself against the reeds. Others speculate on the extrapolation of therapeutic bloodletting from the natural process of menstruation. The humoral view considered menstruation as a hygienic and prophylactic method of depletion or diminishing of residue. More recently, the evolutionary biologist Margie Profet (Angier 1993) theorized that menstruation may be an adaptive event designed to rid the body of bacteria and foreign matter that may have gained entrance through sexual activity. Though presented as new and radical, this theory actually coincides with the ancient humoral view of bloodletting.

According to Haller (1981), Hippocrates explained that therapeutic bloodletting derived from the natural and spontaneous occurrence of 'critical hemorrhages' that preceded the crisis stage in acute disease. Herein lies Hippocrates' strategy of close observation. Scrutiny of disease progression allowed the induction of an artificial crisis to hasten the resolution of disease, diminishing the patient's discomfort and risk.

Galen wrote that the principal indication for bloodletting was to eliminate 'residues' or to prevent them from accumulating (Brain 1986). These residues or 'excesses' were known to cause fever and disease. Seasonal bloodletting was used preventively in Egypt, Greece, Rome and China. Ancients prescribed bloodletting in most cases of fever to reduce the body's heat. According to Epler (1980) there are indications that bloodletting was being used in China from the mid-second millennium as a mechanical release of malevolent spirits that

3

were thought to cause disease. This use of bloodletting was common to all early or primitive cultures. In 1975, unedited medical texts were recovered from a Western Han dynasty tomb sealed in 165 BC. Presumed to be written in 220–200 BC, the Han tomb's texts contain the earliest detailed picture of the vascular system found in Chinese medical literature. Each of these texts consists of a list of vessels and a related disease syndrome. The vessels contain both Blood and Qi. Epler (1980) compares the Han tomb medical texts to the dated editions of the *Su Wen*, and the later *Ling Shu*, tracing the progression of medical thought in China. These early texts regarded Qi as substantive, whose material was also let when blood was extravasated.

In the *Su Wen*, bloodletting was indicated at specific sites and applied for fever, as in ancient Greece and Rome. The principle was similar to the Greek or Roman idea of 'excess of blood' or 'residue' promoting fever. However, Chinese medicine specified sites according to vessel theory, a point of departure from other ancients.

Acupuncture evolves from bloodletting

Vessels or meridians were organic structures filled with Blood as fluid and Qi as material substance. Diseases were identified with a particular vessel that contained the noxious element. Notions of pathogenicity evolved from 'invasion of a malevolent spirit' to 'penetration of atmospheric factors' as a form of Qi. The disease-causing agent was thought to enter the vessel and become lodged in the blood of the vessel. Removing blood from the vessel removed the cause of the illness.

Pain and other visible symptoms, like redness and warmth, were used to locate the vessel involved. Bloodletting was applied to the site of pain or to the vessel 'whose course coincides with the site of pain'. In early Western medicine these were vertical 'zones'. Blood was let at sites local to the problem and distally along the zone or channel (Nielsen 1996). The ancients would have observed an effect from needling even when blood could not be persuaded from a site, for example, in situations of deficiency or low blood pressure, and recognized that this effect, even without blood being let, was an expression of Qi. Epler (1980) argues that the technique for needling Qi, local and distal, is similar to and probably derived from these early techniques for bloodletting. Epler deduces that acupuncture likely evolved from bloodletting therapy. Needling without the intention of letting blood also marks a profound change in the notion and potency of Qi.

The Han tomb texts (thought to be written around 200 BC and buried around 165 BC) record the poking of points to draw blood and apply cautery; the *Nei Jing* indicates a transition from bloodletting to acupuncture needling. The first Chinese text devoted to acupuncture did not appear until the 1st century BC. The *Shih-chi* (90 BC) is the biography of physician Ch'un-yü I, and chronicles his case histories from the years 167–154 BC (Epler 1980, 365; Unschuld 1985, 94). In this account of Ch'un-yü's practice, needling is used to affect the Qi; bleeding a point is mentioned only in terms that it should be prevented (Nielsen 2007).

What happened to bloodletting?

Bloodletting techniques in China departed from the excessive venesection of early Western medicine as practiced in Europe and the United States. Bloodletting in Chinese medicine was limited to a small needle stick, where drops of blood were allowed to seep until the blood color changed from dark to light (typically three to five drops), indicating that the pathogen residing in and congesting the blood was evacuated (Epler 1980). Blood was let from a specific site associated with the diseased vessel, additionally observing color and hue of the skin. As stated above, needling was eventually applied to affect the Qi, not always to let blood.

In the West, bloodletting became venesection or phlebotomy, which actually cuts into a vein. This became a technique of amount and of repetition, devoid of theory beyond 'the more the better'. Patients were bled until they fainted, or feigned fainting (Kluger 1978). This continued in the West into the mid-19th century (Haller 1986). Bacteriology hailed a shift in view from humors to microbes, the perception that inflammations were caused by specific microorganisms, which could not be flushed out of the body through bloodletting alone. Castiglione (1941) notes that the emergence of a few useful drugs such as quinine, codeine and salicin downgraded the role of bloodletting.

Although there were schools of thought that deplored bloodletting, some physicians continued to adhere to the principles of Hippocratic medicine, and bloodletting experienced a renaissance beginning in the 1890s in Germany; viewed in terms of red blood cells, bone marrow stimulation and therapeutic depletion of iron (Risse 1979), with research continuing today. Bloodletting may be therapeutic because it reduces the level of iron in the blood, which invading bacteria need in trace amounts (Kluger 1978; Podolsky 1982). Bacteria need even more iron at higher temperatures, as in fever. For rare diseases like hematochromatosis, where there is a toxic level of iron that the body cannot filter without causing severe liver damage, bloodletting is the only therapy.

Bloodletting and leech therapy have become the focus of more recent research. Leeches have been used in hospitals to relieve blood congestion in serious bruising, to drain and recirculate the blood in reattached appendages (Halton 1984). Michalsen et al. (2003) have found leech therapy to be effective for pain and mobility in knee osteoarthritis for a period of 3 to 6 months following one treatment; some patients experienced relief for up to a year. Sequential bloodletting has been supported in research for severe ulcerative colitis (Premehand et al. 2004), sepsis (Fortenberry and Paden 2006), and diabetes (Mascitelli and Pezzetta 2007). The German eigenbluttherapie, also known as autologous blood therapy or autohaematotherapy, involves the application or infusion of a person's own blood; it continues to be used and studied (Courivaud et al. 2005; Dixon et al. 2003; Pfeiffer et al. 1998). Gua sha and baguan, cupping, may be considered a kind of autologous blood therapy in that extravasated blood cells are resorbed and that resorption is metabolically significant as detailed in Chapter 3.

Bloodletting has been a part of every culture's medicine (Haller 1981). Hippocrates thought the 'cause of disease should be sought in nature, the cure due to nature'. The Chinese saw humans as a microcosm of nature, whose internal Qi was in resonance with the Qi of the cosmos. Lu Gwei-Djen and Needham (1980) note that these two systems of medicine currently and historically share the same two principles of treatment:

- direct attack of pathogens;
- strengthening resistance to disease, *vis medicatrix naturae.*

'Strongly imbedded in Western medicine from the time of Hippocrates and Galen onward', according to Lu Gwei-Djen and Needham the 'strengthen resistance' approach dominated Western medicine until the last century. Western medicine has furthered the science of 'attack the pathogen', cultivating therapies, both surgical and pharmaceutical, that combat disease on the microscopic plane. Chinese medicine has cultivated therapies, physical and herbal, that strengthen or counter body function, thereby changing the course of disease. Prior to this departure in emphasis, humoral therapies, including bloodletting, were the bulk of world traditional medicine and were collectively known as methods of counteraction, summarily: allopathy.

Theory of counteraction

In the West it was considered a maxim of medicine, articulated by John Hunter but dating to the Hippocratic Corpus, that 'No two diseased actions, affecting the general constitution, can go on at the same time, for any considerable period in the same system'. Epps (1832) explains:

> A patient is troubled with wheezing, difficulty of breathing, cough, mucous expectoration, incapacity to lie in a horizontal position when an attack of the gout supervenes, and all their symptoms pass away. The gout subsides, the other symptoms return. Asthma itself has been removed by the attack of a fit of the gout and has returned when the gout passed off. How often are severe affections of Lungs relieved by discharge of Blood from piles. 'A woman who vomits blood is cured if her monthly term issue' (Hippocrates).

The new disease action in the body was said to 'counteract' the original. A more recently documented example: a patient with refractory asthma had a significant improvement of airway symptoms after developing jaundice secondary to acute jaundice hepatitis B. However, when his bilirubin level decreased to 4 mg/100 ml, the asthma exacerbated again (Ohrui et al. 2003; Xia et al. 2008). (A direct relationship with the upregulation of heme oxygenase-1 (HO-1) from Gua sha producing bilirubin is discussed in Chapter 3). A disease or condition that is interrupted or subdued by another disease or condition qualified as natural counteraction. Reports of accidental counteraction, resulting in relief of longstanding conditions, supported the notion that 'inducing an artificial crisis would hasten the resolution of disease', Haller (1981). John Epps (1832) cites a case of an artificial crisis altering a longstanding condition:

> There was the case of an epileptic boy who fell on a red hot poker which burnt his body, a sore was produced and discharge took place. As long as the discharge continued the boy was not troubled with fits. The action, connected with the formation of the matter discharged, relieved the diseased action causing the fits; hence their cessation.

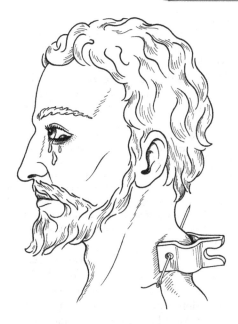

Figure 1.2 • A seton is the early Western medicine counteractive technique closest to acupuncture. Here the skin was pinched at the back of the neck and a fiber or hair was threaded into the flesh. The subsequent surface infection, although mild, counteracted a deeper infection, in this case, a chronic running eye sore.

To imitate this process 'setons' and 'issues' were applied to create an infected discharge, thus counteracting the original inflammation (Brockbank 1954). A running sore was made deliberately by threading strands of twine, silk or other material through the skin. The strands would be left there indefinitely (see Figure 1.2). If a heavier material was used it was called an 'issue'. Cantharides (Spanish fly), blister beetles and other agents were applied at the body surface to cause violent inflammations and rashes.

Acupuncture, A Comprehensive Text (O'Connor and Bensky 1981) describes a procedure similar to application of a seton, called 'threading, embedding sutures, and loop-tying of points'. Surgical gut is introduced at subcutaneous locations corresponding to acupuncture loci to provide prolonged therapeutic stimulation. Studies have shown such a technique to improve muscle nutrition and metabolism, to increase blood flow, leukocyte and neutrophil cell count and build muscle and nerve fibers. Seton or catgut-embedding has been studied in the treatment of epigastric pain (Zhang 2003), chronic gastritis (Zhan et al. 2007), duodenal and peptic ulcer (Fan 2001; Liu et al. 2007), irritable bowel syndrome (Hong et al. 2011), ulcerative colitis (Li et al. 2006; Xiao 2001) obesity and insulin resistance (Chen et al. 2007; Wang et al. 2009), angina pectoris (Li 2003) and hypomenorrhea (Jin and Jin 2008). The normal reaction to this procedure is aseptic inflammation, i.e. redness, swelling, pain and fever, possibly with a milky exudite. This may have been the closest early Western medical practice came to a kind of acupuncture therapy, where intentional penetration and perturbation of the surface tissue was used to produce a therapeutic effect. Gilles (1895) records these techniques as counterirritation, stating:

If there be an inflammation deep down in the tissues, let us by counterirritation start one on the surface. We shall 'destroy' the deeper action, and we have in place of it a superficial inflammation which we can deal with easily.

Broussais (1772–1838), a surgeon to the French army, was known to be the most sanguinary physician in history (Castiglione 1941), and is quoted by Gilles (1895) as saying:

> The theory of disease took irritation to be at the bottom of every morbid condition, and held that this irritation always resulted in an increased flow of blood to the part. This was inflammation, and the seemingly reasonable way to act in such a case was, if possible, prevent that flow of Blood and that inflammation. An External irritant would serve this purpose. It would determine the flow of Blood outwards and away from the diseased direction in which it might be going. It would stop the inflammation. This is called counterirritant.

Counterirritation is, by Galenic definition, a derivation technique. Derivation involved the diversion of blood from an affected part to an adjacent one. Revulsive techniques concerned the diversion of blood from an affected part to a distant one (Brain 1986). Most bloodletting techniques were revulsive, in that blood was let from a part of the body distal to the inflammation. Local bloodletting, cupping and frictioning were considered derivations, with secondary revulsive effects. Haller (1981) notes:

> The choice of bleeding technique depended in great measure on the type, duration, and obstinacy of the disease. Light affections yielded easily with simple applications such as frictioning, warm fomentations, leeches (sanguisuction) or cups, while more serious diseases demanded a greater evacuation of blood with free sanguine depletion (opening a vein or artery).

Granville (1841) reports another view of counteraction as the directing of fluids. He states:

> Where a force has been used to direct fluids to a particular region of the body, with a view to relieve another region of the body labouring under disease. We have affected that object by merely changing the location of those fluids.

This is an image evocative of the San Jiao in Chinese medicine. Expulsion of fluids at the surface, as in the perspiration associated with resolution of a fever, was a natural counteraction. Epps (1832) explains:

> In cold and hot stages, difficulty of breathing, severe pain in the head, weight at the pit of the stomach, oppression at the precordia are present. All pass away at the occurrence of perspiration; and what is this perspiration but a counteraction set up upon the skin, and thus relieving the internal disease.

Sudorifics (agents causing sweat) counter a deeper inflammation by mimicking the natural movement of fluids to the surface. Gua sha is a counteractive method similar to frictioning, the purpose of which, it could be said, is to induce an artificial crisis, hastening the resolution of disease by countering the internal inflammation.

Frictioning

Tripsis and *anatripsis* are Greek terms meaning 'to rub' or 'friction'. Anatriptology was the scientific consideration of the remedial use of friction. In Latin, *frictio*, from *fricare*, means to move along a surface with pressure, to rub, grate, chafe, stress or irritate. In Sanskrit the word is *bhrinanti*, meaning 'they injure'. The apotherapy of frictioning or rubbing was considered a derivative technique if done locally and revulsive if done distally to an inflamed or diseased part.

Hippocrates specified four types of frictioning as counteractive therapy. Galen expanded this to six different kinds of friction. Kaim (1756) reports that 'Friction has the power of loosening, binding, augmenting, and diminishing'. All friction excites heat. These kinds of rubbing could be applied by hands alone, or with oils, aromatic spirits, or soft or rough linen invested with aroma, fumes or liquids the purpose of which was to penetrate. Jackson (1806) reports that *iatralyptes* was the title, derived from Greek, for a physician who healed by anointing with oil. In the West, as in China, the type of friction applied was determined by the time of year as well as the condition of the patient. Kaim (1756) states:

> … certainly a man … endures a more vehement and longer massage in winter … because friction reactivates the perspiration which has been impeded throughout the winter cold … and moves whatever had begun to stagnate in the vessels beneath the skin, and brings together the freest movement of humors through the vessels: but in summer, due to the motion of the fluids which is augmented through friction, a massage makes the skin, which is exposed everywhere, to perspire more, and deprives the blood of its more subtle elements.

Jackson (1806) writes in support of frictioning in his doctoral dissertation, drawing on its use in China:

> It is a remedy of an old date … and has been used not only in restoration, but also in preservation of health. In some nations particularly in China, it has become as necessary a part of their daily habits as the use of bath or razor; an old gentleman is waited on by his iatralyptes as regularly as he is with us by his barber. The effects of this process are astonishing; that he who before its commencement was languid, dull and inactive is rendered by it sprightly, animated and nimble. Hippocrates himself was said to have written a treatise on it. The effects are similar to currying a horse.

Frictioning and Gua sha as a treatment for cholera

It is thought that cholera was endemic to the lower Ganges of India and was spread by Hindu pilgrims. Outbreaks periodically reached China by trade ships. Those who contract cholera and do not die of the disease are thought to carry immunity for about 6 months. Thus, without proper public sanitary measures to stem contagion an epidemic of cholera can ravage a population repeatedly over time. McNeill (1989) reports that 'When cholera penetrated China early in the 19th century, the Chinese did not regard it as a new disease'. It is likely the Chinese knew that cholera was spread by water contamination; outbreaks were attributed to a noxious or evil element in the water.

The Chinese character for sha is translated as 'reddish elevated, millet-like skin rashes' (Ou Ming 1988). Weiger (1965) and Mathews (1931) translate sha as cholera, or sometimes malaria. The ideogram for sha is the radical for sickness joined by the radical for sand (see Figure 4.1). Reduced, the latter radical for sand is 'that which appears when water decreases' or 'sediment, gravel or sand deposed by water' (Weiger 1965). Cholera very quickly dehydrates its victims. It is characterized by diarrhea, vomiting, cramps, suppression of urine and collapse. McNeill (1989) states that 'Radical dehydration meant that a victim shrank into a wizened caricature of his former self within a few hours, while ruptured capillaries discolored the skin, turning it black and blue'.

The petechial or ecchymotic stage of cholera is naturally occuring sha. The petechiae and ecchymosis appear 'when water resides', that is, when there is severe dehydration.

Gua sha was used in Asia to treat cholera (Zhao et al. 2008), cholera-like disorders and basically any disorder involving fever or pain, unless contraindicated, for example, by open wounds, hemorrhage, sunburn, etc. In his book *Treatment of Disease with Acupuncture, Vol II*, James Tin Yao So (1987) prescribes Gua sha for cholera-like disorder, where there is vomiting, diarrhea and 'unrelieved pain in the entire abdomen, with cold hands, arms, legs, and feet'.

Likewise, rigorous frictioning was applied in cases of cholera in the West (Jackson 1806):

> Several symptoms connected with cholera are … dependent upon an affection of the nervous system, occasioned by or connected with a congestion of Blood. There is great internal heat at the pit of the stomach, excessive coldness at the surface: Excite counteraction at the surface. We relieve the internal congestion. Warmth is the counteragent.

Western frictioning and Eastern Gua sha, as counteractive therapies to cholera, induce a crisis to cure the disease. Both relieve inflammation and congestion of blood internally by counteraction at the surface. Both warm. Gua sha may be said to preempt the ruptured capillaries that mark advanced cases of cholera. Likewise, Kaim (1756) notes with frictioning '… nor is it unusual that the part vexed by friction, begins to be red, to swell, to be warm, indeed by a clear sign, the humors with greater swiftness … flow in by the law of health'.

Counteraction continues to be utilized by traditional East Asian medicine because it is consistent with the traditional perception of the body. In Western medicine, physical methods used to counteract or counterirritate have been abandoned or dissociated from the counteractive paradigm.

The term allopathy is often mistakenly applied to conventional medicine to distinguish it from traditional medical practices. But allopathy was a term introduced by Hahnemann, the father of homeopathy, to distinguish ordinary counteractive practice, the use of opposites to cure, from homeopathy's use of 'similars' to cure. Traditional East Asian medicine is allopathic.

Western physicians were confronted by acupuncture and Gua sha in the 1970s when immigrants from Asia and Southeast Asia came to the United States. Paul Wolpe (1985) documents Western doctors' efforts to exert a cultural authority over these practices, in hopes of keeping acupuncture from becoming a regulated profession that could be practiced without a medical degree. On a conscious level, many US and European physicians perceived forms of traditional East Asian medicine as an antiquated oral tradition.

However, the lack of curiosity or scientific analysis by the medical establishment into traditional East Asian practices perhaps expressed an unconscious bias against counteractive methods that had been ridiculed in favor of modernity in the West. How Gua sha is reported in the Western literature then and now is reviewed in Chapter 2.

Gua sha as classical practice: the lineage of Dr James Tin Yau So

In July of 1971, New York Times reporter James Reston traveled to Peking to cover Henry Kissinger's involvement in President Richard Nixon's initiative to 'bring down the bamboo curtain'. While there, Reston required an emergency appendectomy and his postsurgical pain was treated successfully with acupuncture and moxibustion. This he detailed in a front-page article that brought acupuncture and Chinese medicine to the forefront of American minds (Reston 1971).

While acupuncture and Gua sha are likely to have been used for decades in the US by Asian immigrants as part of their domestic care, it was first formally taught by Dr James Tin Yau So at the New England School of Acupuncture (NESA) in 1976. Founded in 1975 by Dr So, Arnie Frieman and Steven Breeker, NESA was the first acupuncture school in the United States to have State approval to confer a diploma in acupuncture. Dr So was the principal and founding instructor and is considered to be the Father of American Acupuncture. Several months into NESA's inaugural program, Ted Kaptchuk, having completed his study in Macau, joined the faculty of acupuncture doctors from England, China and Japan, together with Western physicians who taught at the school, notably Jim Donovan who hosted Dr So at his clinic in Newton Centre, MA.

Before his acupuncture career, Dr So was a preacher. When Japan invaded China and the church where Dr So preached was closed he turned his attention to the study of acupuncture. Dr So studied with Tsang Tien Chi from 1937–1939, and soon after opened his own clinic in Hong Kong where he treated patients until he came to the US in 1973. Dr So opened the Hong Kong College of Chinese Acupuncture in 1941. During his years of teaching in Hong Kong he graduated over 500 students, who went on to practice in the tradition of Dr So, Tsang Tien Chi and Cheng Dan'an.

Dr So compiled his first book on acupuncture in 1946, which was published in Chinese in 1960 and printed in sections in English by NESA in 1977 as part of the school's course of study. He later supervised the publication of his work by Paradigm Publications: *The Book of Acupuncture Points* and *Treatment of Disease with Acupuncture*, comprise volumes I and II of *A Complete Course in Acupuncture*. The texts are almost an exact reproduction of the material printed by NESA, with a few changes, probably in response to the atmosphere of the 1980s, during which acupuncture gained some notoriety that risked legal scrutiny. For example, Dr So taught that Gua sha was a treatment for cholera; in fact, 'cholera' is one translation of the word 'sha' (as discussed above). However, in Dr So's recommendation of Gua sha as a treatment for cholera, the word 'cholera' was changed to 'cholera-like disorder' in the Paradigm text. The change most likely relates to the fact that according to Western medical practice, cholera is considered to only be treatable with antibiotics and intravenous (IV) fluid support. Therefore, even though Gua sha was/is a treatment for cholera, to say so would appear to either challenge or ignore Western medicine, something Dr So and his editors would have avoided.

Tsang Tien Chi

The story of Dr So's teacher Tsang Tien Chi is interesting and helps to situate acupuncture in the context of his time. Tsang was a high school teacher who lost his mother to dropsy, a son to dysentery, another to severe vomiting and diarrhea, none being successfully treated by the available Western medicine and Chinese herbal medicine. Tsang himself experienced ill health: he had breathing difficulties associated with asthma as well as 'external piles', neither of which were responsive to surgery, medicine or herbs.

In 1930, a friend of Tsang's from Shanghai told him that acupuncture might cure him and that there was a famous teacher who had opened a school in Shanghai. Tsang quit his job, sold his property and went to Shanghai to study acupuncture with Cheng Dan'an. Tsang returned to South China and in 1934 and opened the College of Scientific Acupuncture in Canton where Dr So studied.

Cheng Dan'an

Cheng Dan'an (Ching Tan An), 1899–1957, is central to the story of the modernization of acupuncture in China. As mentioned above, the first Chinese text devoted to acupuncture appeared in 90 BC and chronicled Ch'un-yü I's case histories between 167 and 154 BC (Epler 1980, 365; Unschuld 1985, 94). Over the course of 2000 years, acupuncture practice waxed and waned throughout the different regions of China. During this time it was not organized in an overarching homogenous system (Farquhar 1994). That acupuncture experienced at least one decline in favor of oral medicine is described by Hsü Ta-Ch'un (1757, 244):

> … people in high antiquity valued the method of needling. However, learning the doctrine of needling is difficult, while it is easy (to use) prescriptions and drugs. Also, patients enjoy taking drugs, but they suffer from the needles. Hence, in later times the (use of) prescriptions and drugs flourished widely while no one spoke of the method of needling anymore.

Dr So mentions that before 1930 acupuncture was not widely practiced in the south of China. In Canton there was only one well-known acupuncturist, a Buddhist monk. However, traditional herbal medicine and Western medicine were prevalent (So 1985, vi).

It was Cheng Dan'an who established a school of acupuncture in Shanghai in 1930, differentiating modern disease categories using traditional Chinese classifications. By so doing, Cheng reified the linguistics and paradigm of traditional medicine as a tool of perception and response, much as it had been

in the scholarly archive of the classics and *vis-à-vis* the oral disseminations of this medical tradition. Wu Ming translated a text by Cheng (1996), *Acupuncture and Moxibustion Formulas & Treatments*. Reviews of that text have suggested Cheng to be one of the architects of modern traditional Chinese medicine (TCM) acupuncture (Deadman 1996). Others argue that Cheng represents engaged classical practice that stands in sharp contrast to the theoretical preoccupations of TCM texts in English.

Tin Yau So

As stated above, Dr So was the principal and founding instructor of the first acupuncture school in the United States and is considered to be the Father of American Acupuncture. Dr So's work is described as 'classical' not only because it was based on his careful reading of the classics but also because of his lineage's style of practice. In contrast with TCM practice, this kind of classical acupuncture is best described as a bidirectional interaction, where sessions were characterized by precise palpation and location of points and active needling for de qi response, then withdrawal. Needles were retained at some points and not others. Practice in this tradition involved strong cutaneous interventions in addition to acupuncture, such as bloodletting, Gua sha, cupping, plum blossom needling and direct moxibustion. Theirs was a measured but strong counteractive intervention of the 'flesh' and not an ethereal dance with 'energy'.

Equally important, their treatment interaction also assessed immediate changes within the session that were tantamount to an evolving 'diagnosis', for 'how to think about' and respond to a problem. The ability to contextualize immediate changes with the innate waxing and waning of a disease/condition represented an active and volatile diagnostic process, not a diagnosis in the Western sense (Nielsen 1999). 'Diagnosis' itself was never the central aim, as it is represented by modern TCM; it is the clinical interaction and the ability to shift a problem that engages in that moment a transformation for the patient in the experience and perception of their condition, upon which is built a reformation of the 'habitual' nature of a problem.

This was Chinese acupuncture practice as Dr So taught it; he would not have known to call his practice 'classical'. It was only when TCM texts, with their emphasis on theory in a bifurcation of theory and practice, appeared and were used by schools in the West, did the work of Dr So stand in contrast.

During the 1980s, the use of published texts from China led to Chinese medicine as a theoretical paradigm being valued over classical practice that was interpreted as mere point prescriptions. Classical practice was misrepresented as narrow, repetitive and pat. It was not at all the case that Dr So taught restrictive point prescriptions, but rather offered points that must always be considered for a problem, with additional points to be added depending on symptoms and palpation, and response. TCM texts, in turn, listed points in simple acupuncture formulae to be repeated, confounding the TCM claim of innovation based on sound diagnosis. The People's Republic of China (PRC) represented acupuncture as an overarching homogenous system based in the theory of diagnosable patterns of disharmony and organ pathology. Even NESA, for a time, renounced the teachings of Dr So, and, except for a picture in the library, held Dr So in a degree of disregard.

Today there is renewed interest in syncretic classical practice, as is evidenced by the translation of Cheng Dan'an's work in 1996, the colloquium tributes to Dr So's work sponsored by NESA (2002) and the work of Heiner Fruehauf, founder of the School of Classical Chinese Medicine at the National College of Natural Medicine in Portland, Oregon, as well as my own. The pendulum has swung away from the reductionism of TCM toward a reexamination of classical practice *vis-à-vis* reading of classical texts. Some consider this to be misguided, that is, to search for classical practice by reading classical texts, particularly when these texts are read without any knowledge or understanding of historical terminology or context. Historically, training in traditional East Asian medicine was always based in practice: 'we take practice to be our guide' (Farquhar 1994), with apprenticeship, case studies and experience valued over didactics based in theory, the latter being the norm in the West. While Dr So left us textbooks, his *oeuvre* is the preservation and continuation of the classics in praxis.

It is not clear if Dr So learned Gua sha from Tsang. When I asked where he learned Gua sha, Dr So replied with uncharacteristic impatience, 'Where to learn? Everyone knows!' It is the case that Dr So visited Pentecostal groups throughout Southeast Asia, where it is likely that his experience with Gua sha was fortified.

So's emphasis on Gua sha, although not explicit in his texts, was clear to those who attended his lectures or clinic. As the first female intern for Dr So at his clinic in Newton Centre, I can testify to the importance of Gua sha in his practice. He checked every patient for sha stasis by palpation. If a patient had sha, Gua sha was applied by one of us, his interns. Gua sha was used almost as often as acupuncture and more often than moxibustion. Dr So did not use cupping and did not teach it during his term at NESA because he thought Gua sha was more effective, easier to use over a larger area and did not risk burning a patient (fire-cupping).

We were unaware then that during this same period of the late 1970s and 1980s the first articles about Gua sha as cao gio/coining appeared in Western medical journals and for the next 30 years Gua sha/cao gio/coining was situated in a negative register of 'abuse/not abuse'; it was considered, at best, an unfortunate practice among immigrants based in cultural and/or religious beliefs (Nielsen 2009). Now randomized controlled trials and biomechanism studies establish Gua sha in a positive and therapeutically relevant register in the West. Chapter 2 includes a review of the literature on Gua sha from the Western medical database as well as the Chinese-language database. Chapter 3 details the current science of the biology of Gua sha.

References

Angier, N., 1993. Radical new view of the role of menstruation. New York Times: Science Times, September 21.

Atkinson, D., 1956. Magic, Myth, and Medicine. New World Publishing, New York.

Baldry, P., 1989. Acupuncture, Trigger Points and Musculoskeletal Pain. Churchill Livingstone, Edinburgh.

Brain, P., 1986. Galen on Bloodletting. Cambridge University Press, Cambridge.

Brockbank, W., 1954. Ancient therapeutic arts. In: Fitzpatrick Lectures, Royal College of Physicians. Heinemann Medical Books, London.

Castiglione, A., 1941. A History of Medicine. Krumbhaar E B (trans and ed). Alfred Knopf, New York.

Chen, F., Wu, S., Zhang Y., 2007. [Effect of acupoint catgut embedding on TNF-alpha and insulin resistance in simple obesity patients.]. Zhen Ci Yan Jiu 32 (1) 49–52.

Cheng, Dan'an, Wu, M., trans. 1996. Acupuncture & Moxibustion Formulas & Treatments. Blue Poppy Press, Boudler, CO, pp. 278.

China Pictorial Publications, 1989. The Silk Road on Land and Sea. China Pictorial Publishing Company; Distributed by China International Book Trading Corp, Beijing.

Courivaud, D., Segard, M., Darras, S., et al., 2005. Topical haemotherapy as treatment for necrotic angiodermatitis: A pilot study. Ann Dermatol Venereol 132 (no. 3), 225–229.

Deadman, P., 1996. Review: Acupuncture & Moxibustion Formulas and Treatments. Journal of Chinese Medicine 51, 45–46.

Dixon, A., Riesberg, A., Weinbrenner, S., et al., 2003 *Complementary and Alternative Medicine in the UK and Germany: Research and Evidence on Supply and Demand*. Anglo-German Foundation for the Study of Industrial Society/Deutsch-Britische Stiftung Fur das Studium der Industriegesellschaft. Reinhard Busse site editor: Available at www.mig.tu-berlin.de/files/2003.publications/2003.dickson_CAM.report.2003.pdf. Accessed March 2, 2007.

Epler, D.C., 1980. Bloodletting in early Chinese medicine and its relation to the origin of acupuncture. Bulletin of the History of Medicine 54, 337–367.

Epps, J., 1832. Counteraction, Viewed as a Means of Cure with Remarks on the Use of the Issue. Renshaw and Rush, London.

Fan, Z., 2001. Observation on 105 Cases of Duodenal Bulbar Ulcer Treated by Combined Therapy of Catgut Embedding and Chinese Drugs. J. Tradit. Chin. Med 21 (2), 111–115.

Farquhar, J., 1994. Knowing Practice. The Clinical Encounter of Chinese Medicine. Westview Press, Boulder CO.

Fortenberry, J.D., Paden, M.L., 2006. Extracorporeal Therapies in the Treatment of Sepsis: Experience and Promise. Semin Pediatr Infect Dis 17 (no. 2), 72–79.

Garrison, F., 1913. History of bloodletting. New York Medical Journal 971, 432–437, 498–501.

Gilles, C., 1895. The Theory and Practice of Counter Irritation. Macmillan and Company, London.

Granville, A., 1841. Counterirritation, Its Principles and Practice Illustrated by 100 Cases. Carey and Hart, Philadelphia.

Haller, J., 1981. American Medicine in Transition 1840–1910. University of Illinois Press, Urbana.

Haller, J., 1986. Decline of bloodletting: a study in 19th century ratiocinations. Southern Medical Journal 79, 469–474.

Halton, C., 1984. New use for an old treatment: modern medicine is successfully employing leeches in microsurgery. Paradise Magazine, June 17.

Hong, Z.-M., Wang, Z.-L., Chen, X.-J., 2011. [Therapeutic effect of acupoint catgut embedding on irritable bowel syndrome of diarrhea type.]. Zhongguo Zhen Jiu 31 (4), 311–313.

Hsü Ta-Ch'un, 1757; Paul Unschuld, trans. Forgotten Traditions of Ancient Chinese Medicine (I-HsüehYüan Liu Lun). Paradigm Publications, Brookline, MA 1990.

Jackson, H., 1806. On efficacy of certain external applications. Inaugural Dissertation printed in Medical Theses, University of Pennsylvania, T W Bradford, Philadelphia.

Jin, H.-F., Jin, Y.-B., 2008. [Treatment of hypomenorrhea by acupoint catgut embedding]. Zhongguo Zhen Jiu 28 (12), 891–893.

Kaim, S., 1756. Dissertatio inauguralis medica de frictionibus. Chipok R 1994 (trans). Kaliwodian Press, University of Vienna.

Kleinman, A., Kunstadter, P., Alexander, E., et al., 1975. Medicine in Chinese cultures. Comparative studies of health care in Chinese and other societies. US Department of Health Education, and Welfare, Washington DC. Dhew Publication No. (NIH) 75–653.

Kluger, M., 1978. History of bloodletting. Natural History 87, 78–83.

Kuriyama, S., 1999. The Expressiveness of the Body and the Divergens of Greek and Chinese Medicine. Zone Books, New York.

Li, H.-J., Li, G.-P., Li, H.-Y., 2006. [Clinical observation on acupoint catgut embedding therapy for treatment of ulcerative colitis.]. Zhongguo Zhen Jiu 26 (4), 261–263.

Li, Z., 2003. Clinical observation in 46 cases of angina pectoris treated by the catgut-embedding therapy. J. Tradit. Chin. Med 23 (3), 199–200.

Liu, W., Yuan, H., Wang, B., et al., 2007. Gua sha with point catgut implantation TCM treatment of 100 cases of peptic ulcer. Modern Journal of Integrated Traditional Chinese and Western Medicine 16 (12), 1610–1611.

Lu, Gwei-djen, Needham, J., 1980. Celestial Lancets. A History and Rationale of Acupuncture and Moxibustion. Cambridge University Press, Cambridge.

Mascitelli, L., Pezzetta, F., 2007. Reduction of body iron stores and the prevention of type 2 diabetes. Am J Med 120 (no. 10), e13, author reply e15.

Mathews, R.H., 1931. Mathews' Chinese-English Dictionary. Harvard University Press, Cambridge, MA.

McNeill, W., 1989. Plagues and Peoples. Anchor Press, New York.

Michalsen, A., Klotz, S., Ludtke, R., et al., 2003. Effectiveness of leech therapy in osteoarthritis of the knee: A randomized,

controlled trial. Ann. Intern. Med 139 (no. 9), Nov 4, 724–730.

Nielsen, A., 1996. Gua Sha as Counteraction: The Crisis is the Cure. J Chinese Med 50 (January), 5–12.

Nielsen, A., 1999. Why we do not diagnose in Chinese Medicine. Anglo-Dutch Institute for Oriental Medicine Journal Jan.

Nielsen, A., 2007. 'Gua sha' and the Scientific Gaze: Original Research on an Ancient Therapy in a Call for Discourse in Philosophies of Medicine [doctoral dissertation]. Union Institute & University.

Nielsen, A., 2009. Gua sha research and the language of integrative medicine. J Bodyw Mov Ther 13 (1), 63–72.

Ohrui, T., Yasuda, H., Yamaya, M., et al., 2003. Transient relief of asthma symptoms during jaundice; a possible beneficial role of bilirubin. Tohoku J Exp Med 199, 193–196.

O'Connor, J., Bensky, D. (trans), 1981. Acupuncture: A Comprehensive Text. Shanghai College of Traditional Chinese Medicine, Shanghai.

Ou Ming (Ed.), 1988. Chinese–English Dictionary of Traditional Chinese Medicine. Guandang Science and Technology Publishing House, Hong Kong.

Pfeiffer, K.A., Sillem, M., Daniel, V., et al., 1998. Activated autologous blood therapy in recurrent spontaneous abortion–results of a pilot study. Hum. Reprod 13, 491–497.

Podolsky, D., 1982. The Human Body. Skin: the Human Fabric. US News Books, Washington DC.

Premehand, P., Takeuchi, K., Bjarnason, I., 2004. Selective bloodletting for severe ulcerative colitis. Scand J Gastroenterol 39 (no. 5), 416–417.

Reston, J., 1971. Now, let me tell you about my appendectomy in Peking. New York Times, July 26. New York, NY.

Risse, G., 1979. The renaissance of bloodletting: a chapter in modern therapeutics. Journal of the History of Medicine XXXI (1), 3–22

So, J.T.Y., 1985. The Book of Acupuncture Points. Paradigm Publications, Brookline, MA.

So, J.T.Y., 1987. Treatment of Disease with Acupuncture. Paradigm Publications, Brookline, MA.

Unschuld, P.U., 1985. Medicine in China, a History of Ideas. Univ Cal Press, Berkley.

Veith, I., 1966. Huang Ti Nei Ching Su Wen (The Yellow Emperor's Classic of Internal Medicine). University of California Press, Berkeley, CA.

Wang, H.-Q., Ge, B.-H., Dong, G.-R., 2009. [Observation on therapeutic effect of catgut implantation at acupoint on simple obesity of different syndrome types]. Zhongguo Zhen Jiu 29 (3) (March), 192–196.

Weiger, L., 1965. Chinese Characters, Their Origin, Etymology, History, Classification and Signification: A Thorough Study from Chinese Documents. Dover, New York.

Wilford, J., 1993. New finds suggest even earlier trade on fabled silk road. New York Times: Science Times, March 16.

Wiseman, N., 2000. Personal communication. Nigel Wiseman PhD, linguist, School of Traditional Chinese Medicine, Chang Gung University, Taiwan.

Wolpe, P.R., 1985. The Maintenance of Professional Authority: Acupuncture and the American Physician. Soc Problem 32 (5) (June), 409–424.

Wood, F., 2002. The Silk Road: Two Thousand Years in the Heart of Asia. University of California Press, Berkeley, CA.

Xia, Z.W., Zhong, W.W., Meyrowitz, J.S., et al., 2008. The role of heme oxygenase-1 in T cell-mediated immunity: the all encompassing enzyme. Curr Pharm Des 14 (5), 454–464.

Xiao, G., 2001. Catgut Point-embedding Therapy in Treatment of 76 cases of Ulcerative Colitis. J. Tradit. Chin. Med 21 (12), 116–117.

Zhan, Q.-Y., Cha, H.-P., Zhou, L.-M., 2007. Observations on Clinical Efficacy of Point Zhongwan Catgut Embedding for Treating Chronic Gastritis. Shanghai Journal of Acupuncture and Moxibustion 26 (5), 3–4.

Zhang, X., 2003. 60 cases of treatment of epigastric pain with Gua sha combined with catgut embedding. Henan Trad Chin Med 23 (3), 21.

Zhao, M.-L., Li, X.-Q., Zhang, Y., 2008. Ancient fever diagnosis and differential diagnosis. Chinese J of Basic Med in Trad Chinese Med 11, 859–861.

Suggested reading

Epler, D.C., 1980. Bloodletting in early Chinese medicine and its relation to the origin of acupuncture. Bulletin of the History of Medicine 54, 337–367.

Anne F., 1997. The Spirit Catches You and You Fall Down. Straus and Giroux, New York, Farrar.

Farquhar, J., 1994. Knowing Practice. The Clinical Encounter of Chinese Medicine. Westview Press, Boulder CO.

Kuriyama, S., 1999. The Expressiveness of the Body and the Divergence of Greek and Chinese Medicine. Zone Books, New York.

So, J.T.Y., 1987. Treatment of Disease with Acupuncture. Paradigm Publications, Brookline, MA.

Wolpe, P.R., 1985. The Maintenance of Professional Authority: Acupuncture and the American Physician. Soc Problem 32 (5), 409–424.

Evidence for Gua sha: A review of Chinese and Western literature

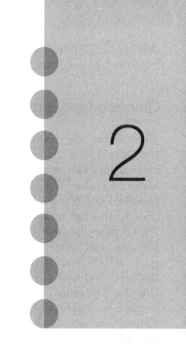

2

Context

Traditional indigenous medicine, like traditional diets, evolved over time out of direct human sensory awareness (Kaptchuk 2002), interaction with and cultivation of the environment, with familial, community and literary transmission of knowledge. The health benefits of traditional diets, like the Mediterranean diet, for example, are supported but not discovered by science. Research confirms benefit somewhat after the fact. So too with medicine, if our ancestors had had to wait for science to discover how to treat a fever, none or few of us would likely be here.

Also known as *cao gio* (Vietnam), *kerik* (Indonesia), *khoud lam* (Laos), *ga sal* (Cambodia), coining or scraping (Nielsen 2007), Gua sha has been used for centuries in Asia (Tsai et al. 2008; So 1987), in Asian immigrant communities (Craig 2002; Fadiman 1997; Hautman 1987; Van Nguyen and Pivar 2004) and by acupuncturists and practitioners of traditional East Asian medicine worldwide (Kaptchuk 2002; Nielsen 1995; Wang and Yang 2009; Zhang and Hao 2000). A 2009 review of articles published between 1994 and 2007 in Chinese found Gua sha to be commonly applied in departments of internal medicine, surgery, gynecology, pediatrics and orthopedics (Wang and Yang 2009). With the expansion of traditional East Asian medicine, Gua sha has been used over a broad geographic area and by millions of people (Braun et al. 2011).

English-language database

A review of articles from the Western database will be considered in three groups: the first includes the early articles (1975–2007), that situate Gua sha/cao gio/coining as an 'unfortunate cultural or religious phenomenon'; the second more recent articles are evidence-based supporting the therapeutic effect of Gua sha. The third are biomechanism studies, and these are discussed in Chapter 3 on the physiology of Gua sha with those from the Chinese language.

Chinese-language database

The Chinese-language database on traditional medicine dates from the 1980s and has steadily expanded as traditional medical practice has been formalized in China and has advanced in the West. The earliest articles on Gua sha were published in 1994, but it is likely that articles were published prior to this but are not available online. A 2005 search of the Chinese database (1984–2004) yielded 120 articles on Gua sha; one quarter of those treated neck pain (Nielsen et al. 2007). The 2011 literature search detailed in this chapter found over 500 clinically relevant articles related to Gua sha. The range of conditions treated by Gua sha reflects its place in traditional East Asian medicine. A review of the Chinese-language database also establishes a record of both use and safety, while providing a foundation for therapeutic relevance that can inform clinical options and direct future research.

Search methodology

The English-language search was done on Ovid Medline and Pubmed, searching the keywords 'Gua sha', 'Guasha', 'cao gio', 'coining' and 'scraping'. Articles in the Western medical literature (1975–2007) identify Gua sha, cao gio, or coining as a superfluous and even dangerous attempt by Asians to care for their cultural rather than physical health (Nielsen 2009). More recent articles support the therapeutic relevance of Gua sha and are discussed below and in Chapter 3.

The Chinese language search was done through China/Asia on Demand (CAOD), formerly China Online (COJ) via special access through the New England School of Acupuncture Kelly Library. Search terms included 'Gua sha', 'Guasha', '刮痧', 'scraping', and 'gua zuo liao fa': '刮痧疗法'.

The search was repeated and updated over the period of a year and yielded over 600 articles related to Gua sha. These results were cross-checked and combined with the 2004 search (1984–2004) conducted through Beijing TCM-Online Co. Ltd., through the China Academy of Traditional Chinese Medicine (Nielsen et al. 2007; Nielsen 2009). Articles were downloaded and translated by the author with the support of translation software and consultation with Chinese doctors.

English database 1975–2007: biased terms and unrelated complications

From the literature it is clear that the most significant and consistent complication relating to Gua sha is the *misdiagnosis* of sha petechiae by other providers who are naïve to Gua sha's operation and appearance. Inaccurate medical terminology used to describe Gua sha reflects this ignorance and subsequent bias. Traditional East Asian medicine was misconstrued as an oral tradition when it came to the attention of Western

doctors in the 1970s as they cared for immigrants from Southeast Asia after the Vietnam War. The loss of the Vietnam War by the most powerful armed force in the world and the divisions that the War created in the US could certainly have had an impact on conventional medical providers' view of Southeast Asian practices.

Gua sha is misconceived, with terms such as 'dermabrasion', 'pseudo-battery', 'child abuse' and 'dermatitis' appearing in the literature. 'Complications' reported in the Western literature for cao gio/coining include: burns, renal contusion and hematuria, brain bleed, camphor intoxication and toxicity, and misdiagnosis as hematoma, factitial dermatitis, strangulation, torture and child abuse. A careful look at each case report of complication reveals startling errors and misconceptions that have gone unchallenged until recently (Nielsen 2009).

'Complications': burns, renal contusion, brain bleed and camphor toxicity

A case of burn injury reportedly caused by Gua sha was, in fact, related to fire cupping (Amshel and Caruso 2000). Yet burns continue to be erroneously cited as a risk of Gua sha when there is absolutely no risk of burns with this technique (D'Allessandro and D'Allesandro 2005; Rampini et al. 2002; Sullivan and Trahan 2007). Microhematuria from unverified renal contusion were reported in an infant treated with Gua sha/cao gio without ruling out the microhematuria as a possible side-effect of the febrile illness for which the child was being treated (Longmire and Broom 1987).

The most egregious misreport concerned an unconscious patient who was brought to an emergency department where doctors interpreted her brain bleed as having been caused by 'painful' cao gio. However, it is unclear how she was able to communicate that the cao gio was so painful (that it theoretically caused her blood pressure to spike) given that she was unconscious (Ponder and Lehman 1994). Moreover, the patient did not present with, nor had ever had, high blood pressure. The physicians who treated her were so alarmed by the sha ecchymosis that they listed cao gio as causative rather than coincidental to her existing brain bleed (Nielsen 2009).

Reports of camphor intoxication or toxicity relating to Gua sha have stemmed from the use of camphor liniments (with or without Gua sha treatment) where the product used had a toxic concentration of camphor exceeding limits now prescribed by law in the West (Aliye et al. 2000; Rampini et al. 2002; Seigel and Wason 1986).

Table 2.1 lists all the terms and 'complications' that appear in the Western literature starting in the 1970s relating to this technique.

In fact, Gua sha is not a form of battery, trauma, injury, abuse, or even pseudo-battery or pseudo-abuse. Furthermore, Gua sha is not suitably described by terms such as dermabrasion, bruising, burns, factitial dermatitis, pseudo-factitial dermatitis, pseudo-bleeding, nummular erythema, purpura, cutaneous stigmata or hematoma. Yet these terms were accepted at peer review, have been published, and continue to be cited, thus affirming Gua sha in a negative register of abuse/not abuse, battery/pseudo-battery, dermatological disease/not disease.

Table 2.1 Some terms and 'complications' used to describe Gua sha/cao gio/coining in Western medical literature (1975–2007), with definitions, comments on their misapplication, and the articles in which the terms are used (Nielsen, 2009)

Terms	Definitions	Comments	Articles using terms*
Battery trauma, injury, abuse, torture, and strangulation	To injure; cause bodily harm	Gua sha does not injure or harm a patient. Red ecchymosis is 'mistaken' for bruising	Ashworth (1993); Bays (2001); David et al. (1986); Davis (2000); de Luna et al. (2003); Halder et al. (2002); Halder and Nootheti (2003); Heyman (2005); Hoffman (2005); Hulewicz (1994); Keller and Apthorp (1977); Levin and Levin (1982); Look and Look (1997); Mevorah et al. (2003); Morrone et al. (2003); Mudd and Findlay 2004; Ngo-Metzer et al. (2003); Rampini et al. (2002); Shah and Fried (2006); Stauffer et al. (2003); Tuncez et al. (2005); Walsh et al. (2004); Westby (2007); Willgerodt and Killien (2004); Wong et al. (1999); Yoo and Tausk (2004)
Pseudo-battery, pseudo-abuse	False, fraudulent or 'pretend' battery or abuse	Reinforces traditional medicine as 'pseudo' medicine. Does not clarify that harm is not inflicted	Anh (1976); Du (1980); Gellis and Feingold (1976); Kaplan (1986); Primosch and Young (1980); Rosenblat and Hong (1989); Saulsbury and Hayden (1985); Yeatman et al. (1976)
Dermabrasion	A painful technique for removing scars or tattoos where the surface of the skin is removed by abrasion: sanding or wire brushing. Skin is red, raw and takes several weeks to months to heal	The skin remains in tact with Gua sha. There is no abrasion; the ecchymosis fade completely in 2–4 days	Golden and Duster (1977); Kemp (1985); Dinulos and Graham (1999); Davis (2000)
Bruising	Trauma, injury or blow that causes bleeding from damage to capillaries and vessels. Takes weeks to months to heal and/or completely disappear	There is no injury with Gua sha. Seeping from capillaries is initial and transient with ecchymosis fading in days	Campbell and Sartori (2003); Graham and Chitnarong (1997); Hefner et al. (1997); Hulewicz (1994); Kemp (1985); Mevorah et al. (2003), citing Hulewicz (1994); D'Allesandro and D'Allesandro (2005); Roberts (1988); Scales et al. (1999)
Burns	Injury to the skin caused by heat	Gua sha does not involve heating the skin in any way but has been confused with fire cupping	Amshel and Caruso (2000); D'Allesandro and D'Allesandro (2005); Rampini et al. (2002); Sullivan and Trahan (2007)
Dermatitis	Inflammation of the skin, typically referring to eczema	Sha does not represent inflammation of the skin in terms of rash or eczema. Sha petechiae are transitory and fade in days	Silfen and Wyre (1981)
Factitial dermatitis	A primary psychiatric symptom: skin lesions or skin disorders created by or perpetuated by manipulation of the skin surface (Habif, 2004)	Sha is not true dermatitis and is not factitial, in that Gua sha is most often applied by someone other than oneself	Silfen and Wyre (1981)
Pseudo-factitial dermatitis	Skin condition that can lead the clinician to an erroneous diagnosis of factitial dermatitis. Author explains pseudo-factitial dermatitis does not exist	Here sha is responsible for 'leading the clinician to an erroneous diagnosis'	Lachapelle et al. (1994)
Pseudo-bleeding	'Fake bleeding'; a term intended to eliminate bleeding as cause or comorbidity	Clarifies sha does not represent blood thinning, low platelets or vascular problem	Overbosch et al. (1984)

Continued

13

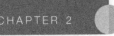
Table 2.1 Some terms and 'complications' used to describe Gua sha/cao gio/coining in Western medical literature (1975–2007), with definitions, comments on their misapplication, and the articles in which the terms are used (Nielsen, 2009)—cont'd

Terms	Definitions	Comments	Articles using terms*
Nummular erythema	Coin-shaped red lesions	This term confuses Gua sha with cupping, which results in nummular ecchymosis	Campbell and Sartori (2003)
Purpura	A condition characterized by hemorrhages in the skin and mucous membranes that result in the appearance of purplish spots or patches of 2 to 10 mm. May be secondary to platelet or coagulation dysfunction or vascular defect	Incorrect histological definition of sha	Leung (1986); Leung and Chan (2001); Ponder and Lehman (1994); Primack and Person (1985)
Cutaneous stigmata	Mark on the skin of infamy, disgrace or reproach, indicative of a history of disease or abnormality	Sha appearance associated with disgrace, disease or reproach per bias. Associates Gua sha with suffering	Buchwald et al. (1992)
Hematoma	Localized swelling filled with blood resulting from a break in a blood vessel	Sha marks are not the size of hematomas	Ponder and Lehman (1994); Zuijlmans and Winterberg (1996)
Linear petechiae and ecchymosis	Small crimson, purple, red, or livid spots on the skin due to extravasation of blood. Ecchymoses indicates passage of blood into subcutaneous tissue marked by discoloration	Most accurate medical terminology to describe sha, though sha is not related to the morbidities typically associated with petechiae or ecchymosis	Crutchfield and Bisig (1995); Dinulos and Graham (1999a); Lederman and Keystone (2002); Leung (1986); Leung and Chan (2001); Nielsen (1995); Roberts (1988)

*The full references for the articles cited are given in Appendix D.

The negative register that has contextualized Gua sha with alarm can itself be corrected by simply identifying Gua sha in specific terms, such as: therapeutic blood extravasation resulting in transient petechiae, maculae and ecchymosis. Or simply: sha represents 'transient therapeutic petechiae'.

Definition

Gua sha

A traditional East Asian medicine healing technique that applies instrument-assisted unidirectional 'press-stroking' of a lubricated area of body surface to intentionally create transitory therapeutic petechiae representing extravasation of blood in the subcutis.

Chinese-language database 1984–2011

Over 600 articles were found in Chinese with over 500 of clinical relevance. The articles were sorted according to the kind of report or study for Gua sha alone or in combination for particular conditions, illnesses or disease. Table 2.2 gives an overview of the literature, listing the number of articles that have been grouped as kinds of studies, evaluated here as evidence for the use of Gua sha from the Chinese-language database (the two English randomized trials are included). Each group of articles together with the relevant citations are listed in Tables 2.3–2.10 in Appendix D. Articles relating to research into the biomechanism of Gua sha are considered in Chapter 3.

Gua sha alone: descriptive clinical recommendations for specific conditions (121 articles)

Standards of practice in Western medicine are intended to be based on evidence from clinical trials. Traditional East Asian medicine practice is based on an archive of experience, expressed in case descriptions and treatment recommendations recorded through history in texts as well as in the present-day peer-reviewed journals. The following sets of discursive articles provide an indication of how Gua sha is used clinically: what Chinese medicine doctors want other providers to know about their use of Gua sha. Only in the last few decades have modern research techniques been applied to traditional East Asian medical modalities to qualify their use in the modern clinical setting.

Table 2.2 Overview of the literature

Table and number of articles*	Kind of article or study
Table 2.3 121 articles	Gua sha alone: descriptive clinical recommendations for specific conditions
Table 2.4 62 articles	Gua sha combined with other modalities: descriptive clinical recommendations for specific conditions
Table 2.5 100 articles	Case series: Gua sha alone for specific conditions
Table 2.6 106 articles	Case series: Gua sha paired with another modality for specific conditions
Table 2.7 38 articles	Case series: Gua sha in combination with two or more other modalities for specific conditions
Table 2.8 12 articles	Gua sha n = 1 case studies (9 Chinese, 2 English, 1 German)
Table 2.9 55 articles	Clinical trials: comparative, controlled, and/or randomized controlled (53 Chinese, 2 English)
Table 2.10 5 articles	Gua sha reviews

*Tables 2.3–2.10 are located in Appendix D.

Table 2.3 (see Appendix D) lists the articles that discuss the use of Gua sha alone in treating specific conditions. Of the 121 articles in this group, 15 describe the use of Gua sha in the treatment of 'sha syndrome', a main feature being fever. Several more articles discuss the historical application of Gua sha for fever, including fever related to cholera. The term 'sha', translated as 'red millet-sized rash', i.e. petechiae, is also translated as cholera (see Chapters 1 and 5). According to Dr James Tin Yau So Gua sha was historically used to treat cholera and cholera-like disorders (So 1987) and is similar to the technique of frictioning used in early Western medicine to treat cholera (Jackson 1806). These articles also point to the importance of Gua sha and its historical use in fevers associated with serious life-threatening illness.

Gua sha alone is also recommended for respiratory infection, cough, throat infection and mastitis, as well as autoimmune disorders such as rheumatoid arthritis and lupus. Another important area of clinic application of Gua sha alone is that of musculoskeletal problems, including neck pain, frozen shoulder (periarthritis), tennis elbow, lumbar disc herniation and soft tissue injury, as well as for facial paralysis, head and face neuralgia and postherpetic neuralgia.

Other indications include skin problems, cardiovascular problems, pediatric diarrhea, digestive problems, stress, insomnia, chronic fatigue, athletic fatigue and 'sub-health'. Gua sha alone is also considered to have a positive role in health maintenance and self-care, promoting vitality, and even beauty.

In addition, there are articles in this group discussing proper and comfortable application of Gua sha, Gua sha tools and oils, and how Gua sha is a form of natural medicine that improves clinical outcome and cost effectiveness. Gua sha has been formally incorporated into public health policy in China (Wu 2010).

Gua sha combined with other modalities: descriptive clinical recommendations for specific conditions (62 articles)

Real-life clinical practice frequently combines modalities. Table 2.4 (see Appendix D) lists articles that discuss combination therapies for a similar series of problems as covered by the articles on Gua sha alone (discussed above), ranging from acute infections, such as influenza, respiratory illness and conjunctivitis, to intractable diseases. Again, there are indications for musculoskeletal and neurological conditions, both acute and chronic, paralysis, postherpetic neuralgia, neck, shoulder, back and knee conditions, as well for self-care and support for sub-health. Authors describe the therapeutic effect of Gua sha combined with acupuncture and electroacupuncture, cupping, point injection, bloodletting, moxibustion, massage, traction, manual reduction methods, tai chi, qi gong, herbal medicine, Western medicine and counseling.

Case series: Gua sha alone for specific conditions (100 articles)

Table 2.5 (see Appendix D) lists articles where authors applied Gua sha for a number of patients with a specific problem called a case series. There are 15 articles and over 1000 patients with a cervical condition treated with Gua sha alone, and 10 articles of over 700 shoulder periarthritis patients treated with Gua sha. Over 500 patients with back pain, including lumbar disc herniation and ankylosing spondylitis, are described as well as patients with complicated pain syndromes involving multiple body sites.

There are case series for headache, migraine, facial paralysis, fever, influenza, adult and pediatric respiratory infection, sinusitis, bronchitis, pneumonia, and asthma – both for acute episodes and for prevention – and for pediatric enuresis. Gua sha is described in cases series of breast disease, mastitis, and hyperplasia, as well as for dysmenorrhea and recovery from induced abortion.

Gua sha is applied in cases of acute and chronic hepatitis, for hypertension, insomnia, neurasthenia, skin problems, such as eczema, chloasma, shingles and postherpetic neuralgia, and eye problems, including stye and trachoma. Gua sha is also described for postsurgical adhesions with intestinal obstruction.

Finally, Gua sha has a special role in acute situations of thermal dysregulation that resonate with its therapeutic role in fever. Gua sha is especially effective for heat stroke, sunstroke, and also for patients who are cold or have an aversion to cold. The full list with citations are found in Appendix D.

Case series: Gua sha paired with another modality for specific conditions (106 articles)

In this set of case series articles Gua sha is paired with another modality in the treatment of a specific condition. Gua sha is paired with one of the following: acupuncture, electroacupuncture, ear acupuncture and ear acupressure, massage, manual reduction, traction, TDP irradiation, cupping, point embedding, moxibustion, and herbal medicines (applied externally, taken orally or through enema). Gua sha is also used in combination with Western medication or supplements.

A similar spectrum of conditions as covered in the articles on case series for Gua sha alone is described in this set of papers. Gua sha and acupuncture are combined for neck, shoulder and back problems, as well as sciatica, ankle injuries, knee osteoarthritis, rheumatoid arthritis and general arthralgia. There are case series of Gua sha with acupuncture for pediatric and adult facial paralysis, cerebral palsy, and occipital and trigeminal neuralgia. Gua sha and acupuncture case series are given for juvenile chronic sinusitis and student 'sub-health'. There are also case series of Gua sha with ear pressure (seeds or magnets) for attention-deficit disorder (ADD).

Gua sha is combined with herbal medicine for hypothyroidism, stomach cramps, acne, hepatitis, and ulcerative colitis, and for other conditions where it has been described as effective alone. Gua sha is used with catgut point embedding for epigastralgia. Gua sha is paired with massage for headache, migraine, respiratory problems, neck, shoulder and back conditions, as well as other musculoskeletal conditions. In addition to conditions for which Gua sha is applied alone, Gua sha and cupping are used for acute and chronic gastroenteritis and gastrointestinal (GI) dysfunction, as well as influenza and neurodermatitis.

Gua sha is paired in this group of articles with Western medication in the treatment of prostatitis, insomnia in cancer patients, trachoma and chronic hepatitis B.

For the full list of case series articles of Gua sha paired with one other modality see Table 2.6 (Appendix D).

Case series: Gua sha combined with two or more other modalities for specific conditions (38 articles)

Table 2.7 (see Appendix D) lists 38 case series articles of Gua sha combined with two or more modalities, including acupuncture, massage, cupping, herbs, bloodletting, pressure points, exercise (including tai chi, aerobics, rehab or physical therapy), laser treatment, plasters, transcutaneous electrical nerve stimulation (TENS), traction, point injections, herbal medicine, dietary changes, moxibustion and ear pressure. The conditions listed are reported to be responsive to these combined modalities. Case series range from as few as 15 cases of cervical spondylosis treated by Gua sha, acupuncture and massage to one study of 1000 patients treated for rheumatism with Gua sha, acupuncture, cupping and massage. Food addiction, fibrositis and pseudo-myopia are conditions not seen in previous articles above.

Gua sha *n* = 1 case studies (12 articles: 9 Chinese, 2 English, 1 German)

Table 2.8 (see Appendix D) lists nine individual case studies published in Chinese, one case published in German and two in English. The breast engorgement/mastitis case led to a

randomized trial for the same condition (Chiu et al. 2008; Chiu et al. 2010) that qualified for peer-reviewed publication in a Western journal. The case by Chan et al. (2011) of Gua sha for chronic active hepatitis B, and their study of Gua sha in inactive chronic hepatitis B and healthy controls relates to the physiology of Gua sha and the role of heme oxygenase-1 (HO-1) (Chan et al. 2012) and are discussed in Chapter 3.

Clinical trials: comparative, controlled, and/or randomized controlled (55 articles: 53 Chinese, 2 English)

Table 2.9 (see Appendix D) lists comparative controlled trials for Gua sha alone or with one or more other modalities for specific conditions. The first column lists which modalities were compared in the study arms. The second column lists the total number of participants/the number in the active arm/the number in the control arm(s). A question mark indicates where an aspect of methodology was unstated or unclear.

There are 11 trials related to neck pain or neck conditions, three related to shoulder periarthritis, four related to back or low back pain, five related to breast problems, and four related to sleep or insomnia.

Clinical problems appearing in this group of papers that are discussed in previous articles and case series include: pediatric indigestion, diarrhea, prevention and treatment of pediatric influenza, obesity, insomnia, respiratory infection and pain. Some interesting new conditions are included in this list of articles, such as insomnia in chronic obstructive pulmonary disease (COPD) patients, and cases of diabetes, lobular breast hyperplasia, peptic ulcer, intractable hiccup, stroke sequelae, different types of obesity, recurrent respiratory infection, ascites related to liver cirrhosis, pain from internal injury, and intestinal obstruction after stomach cancer surgery. Table 2.9 (see Appendix D) provides a summary of comparative, controlled, and/or randomized controlled articles.

Almost all trials reported positive results. In the treatment of peptic ulcer, Gua sha and embedded catgut, a technique known in early Western medicine as 'seton', was no better than oral tagamet but reduced the relapse rate by half (Liu et al. 2007). Many of the 'randomized trials' compared Gua sha as an addition to other treatments, for example Gua sha plus interferon versus interferon alone for chronic hepatitis B, Gua sha plus herbs versus herbs alone for acute mastitis, or Gua sha and point injection versus point injection alone for cervical spondylosis. Others made uneven comparisons without a clear usual care control, such as Gua sha, herbs and point injection versus pain medication and warming for shoulder myofascitis, or Gua sha and cupping versus acupuncture and herbs for stroke sequelae.

Vickers et al. (1998), and more recently He et al. (2011), have discussed the tendency of some countries, the latter specifically cites China, to report only positive results or for results to be inaccurate due to poor randomization, control or concealment. Dr He's group reports that the quality of Chinese-journal acupuncture randomized controlled trials (RCTs) was higher than that of Chinese RCTs of drug interventions. However, they assert that while the quality of RCTs in China has improved over time, all RCTs covering all types of diseases were generally poor. He et al. (2011) did not specifically include any of the Gua sha RCTs in their review, but it can be assumed that they suffer from similar problems. Still, while the methodology of studies done in China is the focus of ongoing discussion, one can make several deductions from these trials of Gua sha. The number of articles and spectrum of conditions treated can be taken as a kind of evidence of the therapeutic effect of Gua sha that can and should inform high-quality research trials in the future, as is the case with Braun et al. (2011) and Chiu et al. (2010).

Research on Gua sha physiology

Research into the biomechanism of Gua sha is discussed in Chapter 3 (see Table 3.1).

Reviews (5 articles: 4 Chinese, 1 English)

There are four Chinese-language articles described as reviews of Gua sha (Liang and Yuan 2009; Luo 2008; Wang et al. 2006; Wang and Yang 2009). One English-language article (Lee et al. 2010) reviewed Chinese-language research on Gua sha for pain as of 2009, stating that while several trials showed positive results, the body of research suffered from methodological flaws, discussed above. The details of all of the review articles are given in Table 2.10 (see Appendix D). Each of these reviews was limited in scope and did not include a complete list of citations.

Popular culture (32 articles, 2 feature films)

The most popular feature film in China in 2001 was *The Gua Sha Treatment*. This film was shot in the United States and portrays the experience of a Chinese professional couple living in St Louis. Their young son is treated with Gua sha by a visiting grandparent. His sniffles resolve but a series of unrelated mishaps land him in an emergency room for a cut on his head where a Western provider misinterprets the sha petechiae as a sign of abuse. The child is removed from the home by social services and the family is traumatized. An eventual court hearing clears the parents and all ends well.

The film presents a conflation of more than a few stories of the persecution of immigrant families for their use of Gua sha in the home. Many of the early articles on Gua sha in the Western medical literature associated Gua sha with a risk of its sequelae appearing as abuse (Nielsen et al. 2007; Nielsen 2009; see Table 2.1). Two articles in Chinese discuss that Gua sha is misunderstood as abuse in the West (Hu 2002; Xu 2008). Thirty-two articles in Chinese (not cited here) analyze the film in terms of the conscious and unconscious cultural challenges that Chinese immigrants face living in America, as well as the challenge that Chinese medicine experiences in its globalization.

Other articles from the Chinese database discussing Gua sha for self-care and beauty (aesthetic medicine in the West) were included above if published in relevant clinical journals.

Finally, Gua sha (cao gio) appeared in one other American feature film, *The Three Seasons*, a postwar Vietnam story starring Harvey Keitel. One of the film's themes involves a prostitute who feels incapable of responding to love from a true, if poor, bicycle taxi driver. In one intimate scene, he applies cao gio ('Gua sha' in Vietnamese) to her back with slow intentional movements. The implication is that the technique will remove the 'stain' fixed on her body from the touch of her johns – the memory and constant reminder of her prostitution work that disenables her from feeling true loving touch. (In traditional East Asian medicine, memory is held in the Blood and Gua sha is thought to heal the pain of dissociated or painful memories.) Unfortunately, for an audience unfamiliar with Gua sha/cao gio, the shock detracts from the insight of another way in which Gua sha 'heals'.

Summary: the significance of a collective literature review

There are over 500 articles on Gua sha from the Chinese database that have been included for this analysis (see Table 2.2), including 175 discursive papers, 246 case series articles and 53 randomized or comparative trials, all focusing wholly or in part on Gua sha as treatment for pain and functional problems as well as acute, chronic and infectious illnesses. Thirty-two articles deal with the cultural challenges involved in Western misperceptions of Chinese medicine *vis-à-vis* Gua sha, as portrayed in a major feature film that was a hit in China. There are two case studies and two randomized controlled trials published in Western journals.

The spectrum of conditions treated and the number of studies indicates Gua sha is widely used in clinical practice and is a focus of discourse and research in China and increasingly in the West. While the methodology of randomized trials in China needs to be improved to establish a clear quantitative register for Gua sha, the number of articles and breadth of conditions covered are significant enough to demonstrate a record of its use and safety.

Discursive articles and case series versus randomized trials?

This body of literature suggests that descriptive articles and case series have a larger role in traditional East Asian medicine than they do in Western medical discourse where practice aspires to depend solely on evidence from randomized trials. Traditional systems of medicine did not come out of the laboratory or modern study, but are based in original forms of care: the first medical traditions of human beings. Like dietary traditions that are also based in ordinary human sensory experience (Kaptchuk 2002), healing 'practices' were transmitted by text and direct teaching or mentorship 'in the kitchen'. The health and longevity benefits of, say, the Mediterranean diet are supported by modern research. But the tradition itself coalesced over time and from a human sensory relationship with food, family and the environment.

Indigenous medicine developed in the same manner, out of a human sensory relationship with health, illness and what was available in the environment to treat. If our ancestors had waited for modern science to tell them how to treat a fever, none or few of us would be here. A review of the existing literature for Gua sha in the Chinese and English language database expands our knowledge of its therapeutic relevance and can focus future study. Several areas warrant further discussion.

Neck pain, mastitis

Many conditions can be followed through the different article types (above), but the use of Gua sha for three conditions in particular can be seen to evolve through the literature: neck pain, mastitis and hepatitis are responsive to Gua sha in descriptive articles, case series and comparative trials in Chinese. Now, recent randomized trials in Western peer-reviewed journals document that Gua sha is effective in treating neck pain (Braun et al. 2011) and breast engorgement (Chiu et al. 2010). Gua sha is among other viable options for neck pain, including acupuncture (Trinh et al. 2006) and manipulation/mobilization (Gross et al. 2010), but mastitis/breast engorgement has few options documented by Western literature (Mangesi and Dowswell 2010). Because antibiotics may be prescribed in breast engorgement/mastitis, and because nursing mothers may want to avoid antibiotic therapy if possible, Gua sha becomes an important treatment option.

Hepatitis

There are five articles and two randomized trials in Chinese using Gua sha for hepatitis. Gua sha has been shown to increase HO-1 (Kwong et al. 2009), which is discussed as the hepatoprotective mechanism by Chan et al. (2011) for a case study where a patient with active chronic hepatitis B experienced a reduction in liver enzymes after one Gua sha treatment. Chan et al. (2012) examine the effect of Gua sha on liver function in normal subjects and subjects with inactive chronic hepatitis B. They establish that Gua sha provides benefit to an inflamed liver (Chan et al. 2011) but does not cause any significant change in liver function in healthy subjects whose immune response is working (see Chapter 3). They were also able to discount the hepatoprotectant effect of Gua sha as placebo since subjects are unaware of their liver status and are not able to manipulate 'liver status' response via expectation. These studies point to the need for a larger trial to establish to what degree and at what dosage Gua sha may be hepatoprotective in patients with active hepatitis, alcoholic liver disease and non alcoholic steatoheptaitis, fatty liver disease. Since therapies to manage chronic hepatitis are limited, Gua sha may be an important option to fill this gap in care.

Gaps in care: shingles, COPD, asthma

Manual therapies like Gua sha may become essential clinical options particularly for what are called 'gaps in care', i.e. when patients cannot or prefer not to take medicines for a problem, or when those medicines fail or are not available. Gua sha may serve to fill a 'gap in care' for several other conditions where current interventions may benefit from the addition of Gua sha. Herpes zoster (shingles) can be followed by debilitating postherpetic neuralgia (PHN). Observational evidence shows that Gua sha is effective in treating and preventing PHN and may be applied along the affected dermatome as soon as lesions have healed well enough (Nielsen 2005). While Gua sha may not experience widespread use to prevent PHN before larger trials are done, knowledge of Gua sha as an option may be important to clinicians, particularly for patients who continue to suffer from PHN weeks and months after their lesions have healed, an indication that PHN may never resolve unless Gua sha can be applied in a timely fashion.

Ability to breathe is positively affected by Gua sha in asthma, bronchitis, emphysema and COPD. While a combination of therapies is necessary to treat and manage these conditions, the addition of Gua sha is greatly appreciated by the patients who live with these disorders. Applied in an inpatient setting at Beth Israel Medical Center in New York, Gua sha has been used to stabilize acute asthma and immediately raise blood oxygen levels in patients with COPD (anecdotal evidence). The anti-inflammatory biomechanism of Gua sha is discussed in Chapter 3.

Gua sha can be of use in any chronic condition. Often physical care is overlooked in conditions that appear to have no cure, where the prospect of no cure translates to no hope of feeling better resulting in no inquiry into what may be engaged to feel better. 'Sha' blood stasis is common in chronic conditions and addressing this stasis relieves pain, anxiety, depression, insomnia and inflammation, and improves outlook, mobility, digestion and immunity.

Conclusion

This categorical review can assist Eastern and Western providers in developing research trials to clarify the therapeutic role of Gua sha. For clinicians and patients this review demonstrates Gua sha is a safe method of intervention that should be considered in a holistic integrative approach, particularly where other options have been exhausted.

Tables 2.3–2.10 are located in Appendix D, as are all of the references cited in this analysis.

References

Aliye, U.C., Bishop, W., Sanders, K., 2000. Camphor hepatotoxicity. South Med J 93, 596–598.

Amshel, C.E., Caruso, D.M., 2000. Vietnamese "coining": a burn case report and literature review. J Burn Care Rehabil 21 (2) (Mar-Apr), 112–114.

Braun, M., Schwickert, M., Nielsen, A., et al., 2011 January 28. Effectiveness of traditional chinese "Gua sha" therapy in patients with chronic neck pain; a randomized controlled trial. Pain Med 12 (3) (Mar), 362–369.

Chan, S., Yuen, J., Gohel, M., et al., 2011. Guasha-induced hepatoprotection in chronic active hepatitis B: A case study. Clin Chim Acta 412, 1686–1688.

Chan, S., Yuen, J., Gohel, M., et al., 2012. Does Gua sha offer hepatoprotective effect to chronic inactive Hepatitis B carriers? A built-in design to control subject expectation. J Altern Complem Med in press.

Chiu, C.-Y., Chang, C.-Y., Gau, M.-L. 2008. [An experience applying Gua-sha to help a parturient women with breast fullness]. Hu Li Za Zhi 55 (1) (February), 105–110.

Chiu, J.-Y., Gau, M.-L., Kuo, S.-Y., et al., 2010. Effects of Gua-sha therapy on breast engorgement: a randomized controlled trial. J Nurs Res 18 (1) (March), 1–10.

Craig, D., 2002. Familiar Medicine: Everyday Health Knowledge & Practice in Today's Vietnam. University of Hawaii Press, Honolulu, HI.

D'Allesandro, D.M., D'Allesandro, M.P., 2005. What Are Some of the Presentations for Child Abuse and Neglect? In: PediatricEducation.Org. A Pediatric Digital Library and Learning Collaborative. June 6; Jan 22, 2006.

Fadiman, A., 1997. The Spirit Catches You and You Fall Down. Farrar, Straus and Giroux, New York.

Gross, A., Miller, J., D'Sylva, J., et al., 2010. Manipulation or mobilization for neck pain: a Cochrane Review. Man Ther 15 (4) (August), 315–333.

Hautman, M.A., 1987. Self-care responses to respiratory illnesses among Vietnamese. West J Nurs Res 9 (2) (May), 223–243.

He, J., Du, L., Liu, G., et al., 2011. Quality Assessment of Reporting of Randomization, Allocation Concealment, and Blinding in Traditional Chinese Medicine RCTs: A Review of 3159 RCTs identified from 260 Systematic Reviews. Trials 12 (1) (May 13), 122.

Hu, M., 2002. Why is the United States selling Chinese medicine in the food store? – Talk about China and the West (drug food) and cultural exchanges. Food and Health 6, 4–6.

Jackson, H., 1806. On the efficacy of certain external applications. PhD Dissertation. University of Pennsylvania: Medical Theses, TW Bradford, Philadelphia. New York Medical College Library Rare Books Room.

Kaptchuk, T.J., 2002. Acupuncture: theory, efficacy, and practice. Annals of Internal Medicine 136 (5) (March 5), 374–383.

Kwong, K.K., Kloetzer, L., Wong, K.K., et al., 2009. Bioluminescence imaging of heme oxygenase-1 upregulation in the Gua sha procedure. J Vis Exp 30 (August 28), 1385.

Lee, M.S., Choi, T.-Y., Kim, J.-K., et al., 2010. Using 'Gua sha' to treat musculoskeletal pain: A systematic review of controlled clinical trials. Chinese Medicine 5 (5) (January), 1–5.

Liang, W., Yuan, B., 2009. Progress in Gua sha clinical research. China's Naturopathy 2, 65–66.

Liu, W., Yuan, H., Wang, B., et al., 2007. Gua sha with point catgut implantation TCM treatment of 100 cases of peptic ulcer. Modern Journal of Integrated Traditional Chinese and Western Medicine 16 (12), 1610–1611.

Longmire, A., Broom, L., 1987. Vietnamese coin rubbing. Ann Emerg Med 16 (5) (May), 602.

Luo, L.-N., 2008. Gua sha therapy research. Guiding Journal of Traditional Chinese Medicine and Pharmacology 4, 84–85.

Mangesi, L., Dowswell, T., 2010. Treatments for breast engorgement during lactation. Cochrane Database Syst Rev 006946.

Mevorah, B., Orion, E., Matz, H., et al., 2003. Cutaneous side effects of alternative therapy. Dermatologic Therapy 160 (27), 141.

Nielsen, A., 1995. Gua sha: A Traditional Technique for Modern Practice. Churchill Livingstone, Edinburgh.

Nielsen, A., 2005. Postherpetic neuralgia in the left buttock after a case of shingles. Explore (NY) 1 (1) (January), 74.

Nielsen, A., Knoblauch, N.T.M., Dobos, G.J., et al., 2007. The effect of Gua sha treatment on the microcirculation of surface tissue: a pilot study in healthy subjects. Explore (NY) 3 (5) (October), 456–466.

Nielsen, A., 2007. 'Gua sha' and the Scientific Gaze: Original Research on an Ancient Therapy in a Call for Discourse in Philosophies of Medicine [doctoral dissertation]. Union Institute & University.

Nielsen, A., 2009. Gua sha research and the language of integrative medicine. J Bodyw Mov Ther 13 (1) (January), 63–72.

Ponder, A., Lehman, L.B., 1994. 'Coining' and 'coning': an unusual complication of unconventional medicine. Neurology 44, 774–775.

Rampini, S., Schneemann, M., Rentsch, K., et al., 2002. Camphor intoxication after cao gio (coin rubbing). JAMA 288 (12) (Sept 25), 1471.

Seigel, E., Wason, S., 1986. Camphor toxicity. Pediatr Clin North Am 332, 375–379.

So, J.T.Y., 1987. Treatment of Disease with Acupuncture. Paradigm Pub, Brookline, MA.

Sullivan, T.M., Trahan, A., 2007. Coining. *Creighton University Medical Center, Complementary and Alternative Medicine* (website), Available at: http://altmed.creighton.edu/coining/complications.htm.

Trinh, K., Graham, N., Gross, A., et al., 2006. Acupuncture for neck disorders. Cochrane Database Syst Rev 3 (1–2), 004870.

Tsai, P.-S., Lee, P.-H., Wang, M.-Y., 2008. Demographics, training, and practice patterns of practitioners of folk medicine. J Altern Complement Med 14 (10), 1243–1248.

Tuncez, F., Bagci, Y., Kurtipek, G.S., et al., 2005. Skin trauma due to cultural practices: cupping and coin rubbing. London; P04.30. 14th Congress of the European Academy of Dermatology and Venereology.

Van Nguyen, Q., Pivar, M., 2004. Fourth Uncle in the Mountain. A Memoir of a Barefoot Doctor in Vietnam. St Martin's Press, New York.

Vickers, A., Goyal, N., Harland, R., et al., 1998. Do certain countries produce only positive results? A systematic review of controlled trials. Control Clin Trials 19 (26), 159–166.

Wang, L., Dang, H., Xu, L., et al., 2006. Analysis of efficacy of Gua sha scraping therapy. China's Naturopathy 14 (6), 55.

Wang, Y.-Y., Yang, J.-S., 2009. [Study and prospects for clinical diseases treated with Gua sha therapy]. Chinese Acupuncture & Moxibustion (Zhongguo Zhen Jiu) 29 (2) (February), 167–171.

Wu, J., 2010. Gua sha therapy exotic supplements. Jiangxi J Trad Chinese Med 4, 70–71.

Xu, L., 2008. Gua sha, left behind people's health prescription. Home Medicine 22, 36.

Zhang, X., Hao, W., 2000. Holographic Meridian Scraping Therapy. Foreign Language Press, Beijing.

Suggested reading and viewing

Film: Xiaolong, Z., Byers, M., 2000. *The Gua Sha Treatment*, Tony Leung, Zhu Xu, Liang Jiahui, Jian Wenli. 110 minutes. (www.yesasia.com)

Film: Bui, T., Bui, T., 1999 *The Three Seasons*. Nguyen Ngoc Hiep, Don Duong, Nguyen Huu Duoc, Zoe Bui, Tran Manh Cuong, Harvey Keitel, Hoang Phat Trieu. October Films USA. 104 minutes.

Fadiman, A., 1997. The Spirit Catches You and You Fall Down: a Hmong child, her American doctors, and the collision of two cultures. Farrar Straus and Giroux, New York.

Nielsen, A., 2009. Gua sha research and the language of integrative medicine. Journal of Bodywork and Movement Therapy 13 (1) (January), 63–72.

Van Nguyen, Q., Pivar, M., 2004. Fourth Uncle in the Mountain. A Memoir of a Barefoot Doctor in Vietnam. St Martin's Press, New York.

Physiology of Gua sha: Western biomodels and East Asian functional perspective

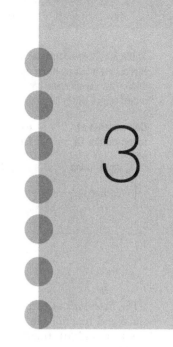

3

Introduction: how does touch or treatment at the body surface affect the body interior?

When I was young in practice I was called to a crisis situation. A man with severe back pain, unable to walk, was brought to his chiropractor's office on a stretcher. The chiropractor called me to see if there was anything acupuncture could do.

My first thought in any 'can't move' or 'frozen' condition is 'sha'. If he had sha I knew I could help him. I needled and applied Gua sha. The patient rose from the table, able to move. Now his chiropractor could adjust him and the adjustment would hold. The patient was stunned by this immediate shift in his condition as he had had massage without result. How did this press-stroking and raising of petechiae on the surface unlock the muscles deep in his back? An exploration of modern research and discourse will help illuminate what traditional East Asian medicine has 'known' for centuries. For some researchers it is the latter that has helped illuminate the former.

Anatomy of Qi

It is common to reduce East Asian's fundamental concept of Qi to 'Qi is energy', since energy seems to best describe the 'seemingly invisible transmission of effect'. Yet Qi is in fact substance as well as function, and the internal organs are not merely functional spheres of influence but substance influencing substance. In his introduction to *The Nan Ching*, Paul Unschuld (1986) agrees. He states:

> The core Chinese concept of Ch'i bears no resemblance to the Western concept of 'energy' (regardless of whether the latter is borrowed from the physical sciences or from colloquial usage).

Table 3.1 The ideogram for Qi depicts vapor rising from cooking rice. Hippocratic medicine had a similar concept dating from 300 BC (Unschuld 1985, 72): 'vapors rising from (digesting) food'. Early Greeks also assumed a heat source within the body

Components of ideogram for Qi	Ideogram for Qi	Equivalent in Hippocratic medicine
气 Vapor Rising 米 Cooking rice	氣 Qi	φῦσαι ἔχ τ(ι)ν πεοιττωιιὰτ(ι)ν Greek: 'vapors rising from (digesting) food'

The *Essentials of Chinese Acupuncture* describes Qi as substance and function. In *Celestial Lancets*, Lu Gwei-djen and Needham (1980) translate Qi as matter–energy. Maciocia (1989) refers to Qi as material and non-material. Although many other English-language articles and texts on Chinese medicine talk of Qi as energy (Porket 1974, Mann 1977, Schatz et al. 1978), it is a departure from a basic understanding of Yin and Yang.

The material body is the vessel (Yin) that holds and by that holding, affords Qi function, or activity (Yang). Qi reduced to 'energy' eclipses its substantive form. This is consistent with a modern tendency to prefer 'doing' to 'being'. The Chinese character for Qi implies both its material and non-material nature, as seen in Table 3.1 (also see Figure 4.1).

Cou Li: lining

In Chinese anatomy, the Biao is the surface, skin and body hair. Just below the skin is the Cou Li, or Li: the lining that covers and lines the body, but is not the skin itself. Cou Li is also translated as pores: that function of the lining that allows entry and exit. The Cou Li, or lining, is where the 'three Qi steam' or where the channels lie, providing an ancient basis for the conductive physiology, attributed to connective tissue by some modern scientists. The *Jinkui Yaolue Fanglun* (1987) or *Synopsis of Prescriptions of the Golden Chamber*, first published in 220 AD, states:

> In case pathogenic factors have invaded the Channels and Collaterals, medical treatment should be given in time to stop the transmission of pathogenic factors into the Viscera and Bowels. If there is heaviness and uneasiness in the extremities, daoyin, tui na, acupuncture and gaomo therapies should be practiced to clear the nine orifices … In this way, one can maintain good health and prevent the intrusion of pathogenetic factors through 'Cou li'.

The 'Li' will be discussed again in Chapter 4 as it relates to the San Jiao.

The Qi moves vertically in channels called Jing vessels. Jing vessels are the main rivers that 'pass through' (Epler 1980). Qi moves horizontally in channels called Lo vessels. Lo means 'to connect', here connecting the large vessels to one another and

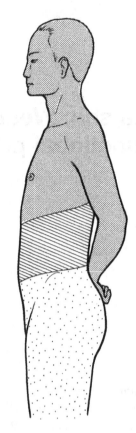

Upper Jiao
Disorders affecting the head, neck, chest, Heart, Lungs and upper extremities.

Middle Jiao
Disorders affecting the Stomach, Spleen, Liver, Gall Bladder and trunk

Lower Jiao
Disorders affecting the Kidneys, Bladder, Intestines, genitals, reproductive system, pelvic region and lower extremities.

Figure 3.1 • The Upper, Middle and Lower Jiaos representing the horizontal emanation of Qi (also see Figures 6.1 and 6.2)

to deeper tissue and organs. Horizontal movement of Qi in the Lo vessels is refered to as the 'Path of Qi' (O'Connor and Bensky 1981) (see Figure 3.1). The pathways are themselves recognized as substantive and based in the body's 'Li' or lining; they are associated with aspects of the connective tissue network.

Path of Qi

As shown in Figure 3.1, the horizontal emanation via the Path of Qi delineates the three Jiaos. Points on the trunk of the body, the ventral Mu points and the dorsal Shu points, express disharmony and afford direct access to the Organs (see Figures 6.3 and 6.4). Disease in one part of the Path can be treated by manipulating points elsewhere in the same segment of the Path, including the extremities, head and limbs (O'Connor and Bensky 1981). The Path of Qi:

* in the head indicates the relationship between the brain and face;
* in the chest suggests a connection among the upper back, neck, chest and upper limbs;
* in the abdomen relates the lumbar–sacral region, lower abdomen and lower limbs.

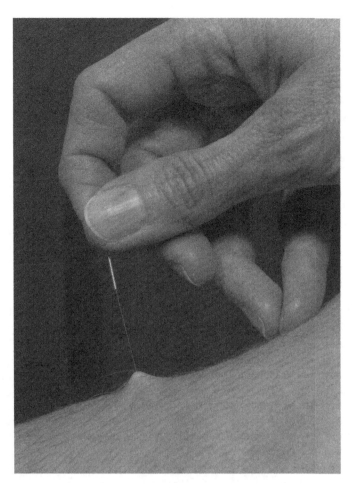

Figure 3.2 • Tenting of the skin observed during needle grasp
An acupuncture needle was inserted in the forearm of a human
volunteer. After insertion, the needle was rotated until needle grasp
was observed. Pulling back on the needle resulted in visible tenting
of the skin, an indication of whorling and grasping in the connective
tissue. From Langevin et al. (2001a) *FASEB J*, with permission

The Path of Qi accounts for the ability of surface techniques,
like acupuncture and Gua sha, to directly affect the tissues and
Internal Organs within a segment.

The vertical channels, Path of Qi (horizontal channels) and
movement of Blood are the context for the penetration of the
therapeutic effect of traditional East Asian medicine (TEAM).
In past models of Western anatomy, the nervous system
accounted for sensory perception at the body surface. However,
it is not the nervous system alone that accounts for referred pain,
what Ida Rolf (1977) calls 'congestion or malfunction of an
internal organ felt as a limited spot of pain, sometimes quite
intense under surface pressure, at a point very distant from the
organ'. In TEAM it is the channels at the Cou Li, or lining, that
mediate this phenomenon. Some modern theoretical models
relate aspects of this mediation to connective tissue. For example,
acupuncture's needle grasp, part of the 'de qi' response, results
in visible 'tenting' that has been related to connective tissue
response (Langevin et al. 2001a) (see Figure 3.2).

The fascial connection: connective tissue of Western anatomy and the ancient channel system

There are several varieties of connective tissue: blood, connective tissue proper, supporting tissues of cartilage, and bone. It
is connective tissue proper that we want to examine.

> Every muscle down to every muscle cell, every nerve down to
> every single axon, every organ as well as every vessel is ensheathed
> by connective tissue. Connective tissue is a continuous network of
> structure that binds tissues into their organ shape, supplies them
> with vessels and ducts and properly fastens the organs within the
> body cavity as well as binding organs to each other.
>
> (Schleip et al. 2012)

In forming the walls of blood and lymph vessels, connective
tissue surrounds and anchors the vessels within muscle, bone
or organ tissue. Each individual cell is wrapped in moist, fibrous
connective tissue. The individual as a whole is wrapped in a
large envelope of connective tissue just under the skin. Connective tissue is a *contiguous* fabric, from this large envelope
of subcutaneous fascia to the sheathing of each cell. If all other
tissue were removed, connective tissue would sustain the
structure of the human form.

Formerly viewed as the inert material covering the bodies
'valuable stuff', connective tissue is now regarded as a full-
fledged organ, 'one of the largest and most extensive organs in
the body' and the focus of intensive research and discourse
(see www.fascia.com). Connective tissue supports, connects,
contains and transmits (Juhan 1987).

Fascia supports and connects

Connective tissue is able to support not only by holding cells,
vessels and organs in relationship to each other and to the
whole body, but by its fluid nature it supports the entire body
structurally. The fluid medium of connective tissue is banded
in shape-giving compartments where the hydrostatic pressure
within the containers aids the weight-bearing capability of the
skeleton (Juhan 1987).

Connective tissue, muscles and bones theoretically provide
structural *tensegrity*. A concept promoted by Buckminster
Fuller, it contends that part of the body's structural strength
may come not from the stacking of solid parts but from the
integrity of tensional force: the balanced tension and proper
angles between the 'beams, cables and wires' of bones, muscles
and mesh (Juhan 1987). Tensegrity also explains how a pull or
injury in one part of the body may cause tension disruption
and pain far from the original site, via the network of angled
'guide wires'.

Fascia contains and transmits

Connective tissue is filled with ground substance, a clear fluid
the viscosity of which varies depending on the tissue it surrounds and serves. Ground substance is the fluid medium that

conducts all intercellular fluids. Nutrients, hormones and plasma are carried from blood vessels to cells through ground substance; cellular waste is carried from cells to blood and lymph vessels through the same connective fluid. If viscosity alters, that is, if 'sticking' of this fluid occurs due to stress, trauma or disuse, there results a compromise in the passage of gases, nutrients, waste, hormones, and immune cells between the capillaries and tissues they irrigate.

Besides fluid, ground substance also contains fibroblast cells and collagen fibrils. Collagen comprises up to 40% of all the protein in the body (Juhan 1987). The collagen molecule that makes up a collagen fibril is the longest molecule ever isolated (Juhan 1987). Collagen fibrils are hollow and require 10,000 times their own weight in order to be stretched.

Fibroblasts produce both the ground substance and collagen. A fibroblast may migrate anywhere in the body and produce collagen in a fibril arrangement that is signaled by the site. A more fluid ground substance with fewer fibrils conducts easily and serves metabolic function. More fiber and less fluid are found in connective tissue that holds organ and nerve cells. Fascia that holds muscle, tendon or ligament has even more fiber and less fluid.

The compartments of connective tissue influence the spread of toxins, infections, disease and tumors, implicating connective tissue in immunity. The fibrous walls, as well as chemicals in the fluid ground substance, prevent spread of agents from one site to a nearby one. If the integrity of the connective tissue is compromised, its immune function declines. For example, cortisone released during periods of stress reduces the number and size of fibroblasts and has been shown 'to facilitate the spread of infection from a previously localized area' (Juhan 1987).

Loose non-dense connective tissue: a 'body-wide signaling network'?

Subcutaneous fascia

Subcutaneous fascia is the connective tissue under the skin that completely surrounds the individual in two layers known as superficial fascia and deep fascia, which adhere to each other. The mediator of bodywork stimulation and therapeutic effect may be this subcutaneous fascia.

Superficial fascia

Superficial fascia divides into a top and bottom layer. Figure 4.2 represents the layers of loose non-dense connective tissue and their relevant East Asian counterparts. The top layer of superficial fascia is the fatty layer, which constitutes the main fatty tissue of the outer surface of the body and fascia lining the organs. The fatty layer or adipose tissue acts as an insulator, helping to maintain a constant body temperature. Adipose tissue is also metabolically active: it stores fat as fuel for metabolic function and releases it in response stimuli. This corresponds to the Eastern concept of the greasy layer, where the ancient Chinese Wei or Protective Qi circulates.

The deep layer of the superficial fascia lies immediately over the 'deep fascia' and is less dense than deep fascia (see Figure 4.2). Arteries, veins, nerves, lymph vessels and nodes run through this bottom layer of the superficial fascia rather than between layers. These vessels become surrounded by the fascia they penetrate and are thereby connected and held in place.

Deep fascia

Just below and adherent to the superficial fascia is the deep fascia. It covers most of the muscles, all the large blood vessels, all the large nerves, the deep lymphatics and nodes and certain glands. Besides covering, it also *invests* these structures. The term 'invest' means that a layer of this fascia, when traced in any direction (e.g. vertically or transversely), on meeting any one of the structures mentioned above splits into laminae that surround the structure and then reunite (Gallaudet 1931). A layer of this fascia may also split to enclose a potential space. Finally a layer may meet several superimposed strata of other structures (muscles, viscera, etc.) in which case it splits into as many layers as may be necessary to invest each stratum.

There is not a cell or space that connective tissue does not integrate. A global physiological role for the 'lining', or connective tissue, was suggested over 2000 years ago by the traditional East Asian channel system. In Langevin's (2006) words, 'Recent evidence suggests that a correspondence may exist between the network of meridians and the body-wide network formed by connective tissue.'

Connective tissue, channels and electrical impedance

Researchers in the 1970s conjectured that the highly ordered, crystalline arrangement of collagen would confer it with various semiconductive properties. Early studies that suggested a decreased impedance and increased conductivity associated with acupuncture channels and points were flawed, and a 2008 review of studies called into question the concept that points or meridians are electrically distinguishable (Ahn et al. 2008). Recent study showed that tissue impedance is lower along the Pericardium channel but not the Spleen channel compared to controls (Ahn et al. 2005), but more importantly that collagenous bands identified by ultrasound echogenicity are significantly associated with lower electrical impedance and may account for reduced impedances previously reported at acupuncture meridians (Ahn et al. 2010).

Connective tissue model

The most current model of manual therapeutic effect focuses on unspecialized, 'loose', non-dense connective tissue. This tissue is intimately associated with all other tissues, including organ systems and hypothetically forms a 'body-wide signaling network' (Langevin 2006). This anatomical network of connective tissue corresponds with functional aspects of the 'Cou Li' or 'Li' lining discussed in the earliest medical texts of

Chinese medicine as the expressed location of the meridians/channels regulated by the San Jiao, discussed below.

Some connective tissue models hypothesize that electrical, cellular and tissue remodeling signals in the connective tissue are responsive to mechanical forces (Schleip et al. 2012). These generate dynamic evolving patterns that interact with one another, i.e. that influence, and are influenced by, function that is normal, pathological (Langevin et al. 2001a,b; Langevin 2006) and, by inference, responsive to manual intervention. As can be seen from Figures 3.3 and 3.4, the needle grasp and fibril winding more strongly associated with unidirectional rotation of acupuncture needling propagates response within the connective tissue matrix. *In vitro* experiments of tissue winding showed that tissue alignment increased as the depth of insertion increased (Julias et al. 2008).

Iatridis et al. (2003) suggest that 'loose connective tissues may function to transmit mechanical signals to and from the abundant fibroblasts, immune, vascular, and neural cells present within tissues'. Table 3.2 sets out suggested physiological effects of acupuncture in Western terms, which may also contextualize other forms of bodywork (Langevin and Yandow 2002).

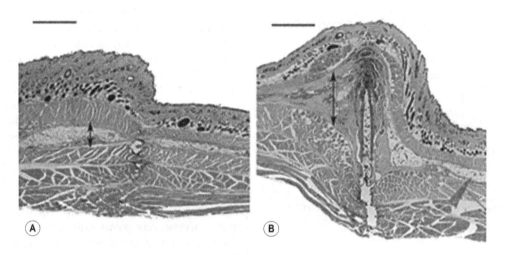

Figure 3.3 • Evidence of connective tissue response to acupuncture needle rotation • Rat abdominal wall tissue histology. An acupuncture needle was inserted into the abdominal wall of live anesthetized rats, followed by no rotation **A**, or unidirectional rotation **B**. Immediately after needling, the animal was killed, tissues were formalin-fixed, sectioned roughly parallel to the needle track (labeled with ink), and stained with hematoxylin/eosin. Abdominal wall layers include dermis, subcutaneous muscle, subcutaneous tissue (arrow), and abdominal wall muscle. Marked thickening of subcutaneous tissue is seen with needle rotation. Scale bars: 1 mm. From Langevin et al. (2002) *FASEB J*, with permission

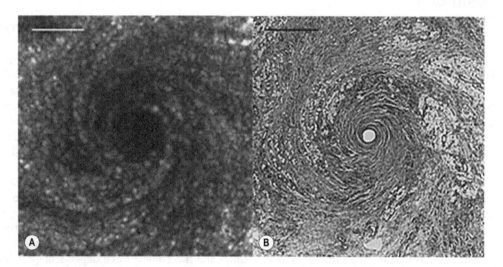

Figure 3.4 • Unidirectional acupuncture needle rotation pulling on the collagen fibers • The mechanical signal is transduced to local fibroblasts producing immediate effect of whorling activity in the connective tissue (Langevin et al. 2001). Acoustic and optical images of subcutaneous tissue with unidirectional needle rotation. **A** Fresh tissue sample imaged with ultrasound scanning acoustic microscopy; **B** the same tissue sample was formalin-fixed after ultrasound imaging, embedded in paraffin, sectioned, and stained for histology with hematoxylin/eosin. Scale bars: 1 mm. From Langevin et al. (2002) *FASEB J*, with permission

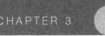

Table 3.2 Summary of proposed model of physiological effects seen in acupuncture that may serve to inform all forms of therapeutic bodywork

Traditional Chinese medicine concepts	Proposed anatomical/physiological equivalents
Acupuncture meridians	Connective tissue planes
Acupuncture points	Convergence of connective tissue planes
Qi	Sum of all body energetic phenomena (e.g. metabolism, movement, signaling, information exchange)
Meridian Qi	Connective tissue biochemical/bioelectrical signaling
Blockage of Qi	Altered connective tissue matrix composition leading to altered signal transduction
Needle grasp	Tissue winding and/or contraction of fibroblasts surrounding the needle
De qi sensation	Wave of connective tissue contraction and sensory mechanoreceptor stimulation along connective tissue planes
Restoration of flow of Qi	Cellular activation/gene expression leading to restored connective tissue matrix composition and signal transduction

Source: Langevin and Yandow (2002), with permission of John Wiley & Sons, Inc.

Identical to the the San Jiao's role in distribution of water, 'connective tissue plays a fundamental part in the body's water metabolism and the mechanism through which the body guides and distributes fluids' (Rolf 1977).

Gua sha physiology

Observation

What a provider observes when applying Gua sha is a gradual expression of small red petechiae (also sometimes brown, blue, very deep red or nearly black). The patient often feels exhilarated, invigorated, even excited. Acute pain is immediately affected, and sometimes completely resolved. Nausea and vomiting cease (So 1987), wheezing and shortness of breath lessen or completely resolve, and so on. Research on the biomechanism of Gua sha, as well as recent research and modeling of the role of fascia in acupuncture and other therapeutic techniques, suggest specific mechanical and processial aspects of Gua sha have physiological significance, namely: the closely timed repeated press-stroking, the unidirectionality, and the intentional extravasation of petechiae and their resolution over time (Nielsen 2012).

Gua sha and the connective tissue model

While the biomechanism of manual therapies is not completely understood (Corey et al. 2009), transduction of force and stretch are thought to cause connective tissue innervations and restoration (Corey et al 2009; Farasyn and Meeusen 2009; Standley and Meltzer 2008; Iatridis et al. 2003) but only to specific kinds of connective tissue. Moreover, physical interventions differ in terms of intention, observable feedback, pressure, term of application, repetition, dosage, and so on.

There are at least three characteristics that distinguish Gua sha from other manual therapies that involve pressure or fascial stretch. Gua sha is characterized by: (1) closely repeated unidirectional stroking that intentionally presses into the fascia; (2) application is predominantly along a muscle and specifically not oscillating or across muscle tissue; and (3) the intentional creation of transitory petechiae and ecchymosis. In fact, the production of petechiae and ecchymosis requires closely timed repeated press-stroking that is unidirectional.

Connective tissue may respond to directionality as it does to tensile loading with collagen strands aligning in parallel arrangement along the direction of the loads imposed (Langevin and Huijing 2009) as in dense 'regular' connective tissue. Mechanotransduction in the rotation of an inserted acupuncture needle is facilitated along cleavages or concentrations of fascia in zones that coincide with ancient TEAM channels and acupuncture points. Langevin et al. (2002) have confirmed that the most common acupuncture points exist at these cleavage concentrations of connective tissue within and along meridian/fascial layers, suggesting that activation at these sites, in fact, augments a connective tissue response. Insertion of a needle off-site of an acupuncture point might activate a response but perhaps to a lesser degree than a known connective-tissue-rich point. This is borne out by studies comparing acupuncture points to control points, where control points demonstrate some therapeutic effect[1] (Haake et al. 2007).

Directionality: unidirectional stroking force

The directionality of manual therapy has specific response. Acupuncture needle rotation that is unidirectional produces more torque in the connective tissue and necessitates greater withdrawal force than bidirectional needle rotation, which is also connective-tissue responsive but dose-dependent (Langevin et al. 2007). What effect repeated unidirectional mechanics has on connective tissue, or how the effect is transferred throughout the system, is hypothesized based on recent connective tissue research, and discussed as a model below (Nielsen 2012).

One potential mechanism is the formation of nitric oxide, discussed below in terms of its role in pain modulation: Endothelin-1 (ET-1) and endothelial constitutive nitric oxide synthase (ecNOS) mRNA expression has been shown to be time- and mechanical force dependent (Ziegler et al. 1998b). Specifically, the effect of unidirectional force or stress differs

---

[1] Connective tissue signaling, enhanced at connective tissue-rich sites that coincide with the main acupuncture points, might illuminate how acupuncture practice persisted for 2000 years: a provider did not have to be that good in terms of precise point location. Some affect was seen as the connective tissue is always penetrated. If adept in point location, main point concentrations of connective tissue are accessed and a better effect elicited.

from oscillating or alternating force or stress in vascular endo-thelium (Ziegler et al. 1998a). Gua sha is always applied with unidirectional stroking.

Moreover, blood circulation is predominantly unidirectional throughout the system while capillary beds have at least some bidirectional interaction with the surrounding tissue. Since unidirectional needle mechanics produces unique fibril activity in the connective tissue, it may be that for certain conditions the direction and kind of mechanical intervention is specific: that unidirectional press-stroking force may invigorate blood flow and fascial mechanics differently than oscillating press force. In fact, Standley and Meltzer (2008) show that anti-inflammatory cytokine secretion is activated by directionality of myofascial release: pressure and shear that create uni-axial fibroblast strain can account for improved range of motion (ROM), decreased edema, reduced analgesic requirements and 'long-term benefits despite short-term treatment'.

Gua sha increases surface perfusion

Research using laser Doppler scanning performed on 11 healthy subjects at the University of Duisburg-Essen in Germany (Nielsen et al. 2007) showed a 400% increase in surface micro-perfusion at the area treated for over 7 minutes immediately following treatment, and a significant increase for the full 25 minutes studied. There are no other reports using laser Doppler imaging that show a sustained microcirculation increase of this magnitude in the medical literature. For example, massage has been shown to increase microperfusion slightly while engaged, but is not sustained when massage is stopped (Mars et al. 2005). Acupuncture needling has demonstrated increase in microperfusion at a needle site by as much as 75% but is not maintained longer than 5 minutes after needle withdrawal (Sandberg et al. 2003). One study showed a slight short-lived increase in microperfusion at LI 11 with acupuncture at LI 4 (Kuo et al. 2004).

An increase in perfusion would be expected with Gua sha given that one can easily observe petechiae and ecchymosis. Tian et al. (2009) also demonstrated increased perfusion in rabbits from Gua sha. What is significant about the Gua sha perfusion study in humans (Nielsen et al. 2007) is that:

- Gua sha increases surface microperfusion in the area treated *but not* outside the area treated;
- Gua sha immediately reduces pain local to *and* distal to the treated area.

Hence there is a pain-relieving process with Gua sha that is communicated to tissue distal to the area treated. One theory is the circulation of nitric oxide (NO).

Gua sha, nitic-oxide mediation and pain relief

One theory of the effect of mechanotransduction in skeletal muscles involves NO release initiating smooth muscle relax-ation and vasodilation (Findley 2009; Hocking et al. 2008). NO is an important mediator in both health and disease. It is an endogenous mediator of vasodilation, also having effects on platelet function, inflammation, and pain perception (Macken-zie et al. 2008). In preclinical studies NO was shown to help maintain gastric mucosal integrity, to inhibit leukocyte adher-ence to the endothelium, and to repair non-steroidal anti-inflammatory drug (NSAID)-induced damage, thus having a protective effect on the gastrointestinal tract (Lanas 2008). NO-based intervention may produce substantial pain relief by increasing circulation, decreasing nerve irritation, and decreas-ing inflammation (Hancock and Riegger-Krugh 2008). Release of NO as part of the process of increased perfusion and vaso-dilation is one hypothesis for the immediate pain relief expe-rienced locally and distally with Gua sha.

Gua sha and cervical arterial circulation

As seen in the Chapter 2, Gua sha is reported to be effective for neck pain, cervical spondylosis, as well as vertigo related to cervical problems. Braun et al. (2011) supported these reports in their randomized controlled trial (RCT) on Gua sha for neck pain. Two studies using transcranial Doppler ultrasound dem-onstrated an advantage to using Gua sha to effect a change in arterial blood flow, affecting pain and vertigo related to cervical pathology (Wang 2009; Wang et al. 2010).

Gua sha and immunity: heme oxygenase-1 (HO-1)

Providers familiar with Gua sha know that it can reduce a fever and alter the course of an acute infectious illness as well as reduce inflammatory symptoms in chronic illness. Many of the articles on the history of Gua sha relate its effect in fever and cholera (see Chapter 2). Wang et al. (2009) found immune response stimulated in fevered rats treated with Gua sha, and Zeng (2003) found a benign increase in white blood cells (WBCs) in humans with fever treated with Gua sha. A Harvard study using bioluminescent imaging with a mouse showed that Gua sha upregulates gene expression for an enzyme that is an anti-oxidant and cytoprotectant, heme oxygenase-1 (HO-1), at multiple internal organ sites immediately after treatment and over a period of days following Gua sha treatment (the mouse studied was unharmed) (Kwong et al. 2009). HO-1 and its catalysates (biliverdin, bilirubin and carbon monoxide (CO)) exhibit not only anti-oxidative but also anti-inflammatory effects (Xia et al. 2008). For example, augmentation of HO-1 expression attenuates allergic inflammation: HO-1 plays a pro-tective role in allergic disease in part by inhibiting Th2 cell-specific chemokines (Xia et al. 2008). Kwong's group provide the first study to show an immediate and sustained immune response from a traditional East Asian modality that has direct relevance to the treatment of internal organ and inflammatory problems.

HO-1 regulates cell cycle and anti-smooth muscle hyperpla-sia providing protection in many disease models, such asthma, organ transplant rejection, inflammatory bowel disease and experimental autoimmune encephalomyelitis, even though the immune pathological mechanisms of these diseases are dis-similar (Xia et al. 2008). Upregulation of the enzyme HO-1

Table 3.3 Trials and studies specifying the biological mechanisms of Gua sha from the Chinese- and English-language database (references included below)

Intervention	Basis	Condition/subjects	Reference
Gua sha	Theoretical neurological physiology	Neurodermatitis in human subjects	Liao 2010
Gua sha	Laser Doppler scanning and frozen section histomorphology	Perfusion in rabbits	Tian et al. 2009
Gua sha	WBC, bilirubin, IL-1, IL-6, SOD	Effect on fever in rats	Wang et al. 2009
Gua sha on Jingluo + exercise vs. exercise vs. quiet group	RCT 24/12/6/6 Glucose reserve and serum enzyme	Effect on exercise endurance, glucose reserve and serum enzyme of rats	Liu et al. 2009
Gua sha along meridian	Benign increase in WBC	Fever in human subjects	Zeng 2003
Gua sha	Examination vascular morphology	Sha, human postmortem	Yu et al. 2008
Gua sha, acupuncture and traction vs. intravenous TMP	RCT 86/46/40 Transcranial Doppler ultrasound of cervical vertebral artery	Cervical spondylosis in human subjects	Wang 2009
Gua sha + pricking bloodletting vs. control	Transcranial Doppler ultrasound of cervical vertebral artery	Cervical spondylosis vertigo in human subjects	Wang et al. 2010
Gua sha (English)	Laser Doppler scanning	Surface perfusion in human subjects	Nielsen et al. 2007
Gua sha (English)	Bioluminescence imaging	HO-1 regulation in mouse	Kwong et al. 2009
Gua sha (English)	Active chronic hepatitis B; HO-1, anti-inflammation	$n = 1$ active chronic hepatitis B, human subject	Chan et al. 2011
Gua sha (English)	Inactive chronic hepatitis B and healthy subjects	4 inactive CHB 9 healthy subjects	Chan et al. 2012

CHB, Chronic hepatitis B; HO-1, heme oxygenase-1; IL-1, interleukin-1; IL-6, interleukin-6; SOD, superoxide dismutase; WBC, white blood cells.

has been reported to be effective in the control of hepatitis B virus (HBV) infection and offers hepatoprotection in animal models (Farombi and Surh 2006; Immenschuh et al. 2010; Protzer et al. 2007; Wunder and Potter 2003). Induction of HO-1 results in decreased hepatitis C virus (HCV) replication, as well as protection from oxidative damage, suggesting a potential role for HO-1 in antiviral therapy and therapeutic protection against hepatocellular injury in HCV infection (Zhu et al. 2008). In fact, as seen in Chapter 2, Gua sha is used to treat symptoms of acute and chronic hepatitis in China.

Chan et al. (2011) describe a case in a Western journal where a single Gua sha treatment in a patient with active chronic hepatitis reduced levels of liver enzymes alanine transaminase (ALT) and aspartate transaminase (AST), modulated T-helper (Th)1/Th2 balance and enhanced HO-1, which they suggest is responsible for the hepatoprotective effect (see Chapter 9). In this case, and in general, Gua sha may be effective in transiently reducing the inflammatory injury to the liver when chronic hepatitis B moves into the immune active phase indicated by liver function test. To provide a comparison, Chan's group (2012) looked at the effect of Gua sha on liver function in normal subjects and subjects with inactive chronic hepatitis B. They established that while Gua sha provides benefit to an inflamed liver (Chan 2011) it does not cause any significant change in liver function in healthy subjects whose immune response is working. They were also able to discount

the hepatoprotectant effect of Gua sha as placebo since subjects were unaware of their liver status and are not able to manipulate 'liver status' response via expectation. This evidence points to the need for a larger trial to establish to what degree and at what dosage Gua sha might maintain hepatoprotection in patients with active hepatitis.

Gua sha has also shown significant beneficial effects on exercise endurance, glucose reserve and serum enzyme in rats. This correlates with provider reports of Gua sha's benefit for athletic fatigue (Fang et al. 2008), chronic fatigue (Ruan 2008; Wang 2002) and stress (Liu 2009; Geng 2010). Table 3.3 lists studies and trials on the physiology of Gua sha, West and East.

Summary

A global physiological role for connective tissue functionally connecting all parts of the body with one another was suggested over 2000 years ago by the traditional East Asian channel system. Current models hypothesize that certain layers of connective tissue may be a functioning organ, one that may tie together all body functions. The ancients called this mediator of all influences the 'San Jiao'.

Identifiable cleavages of fascia associated with acupuncture channels may be the very tracks that facilitate transduction of signals within the body's contiguous network of connective tissue, expressing also to internal organs. Unidirectional acupuncture needle rotation propagates a unique response in the connective tissue. Nitric oxide synthase (ecNOS) mRNA expression has been shown to be time and mechanical force dependent (Ziegler et al. 1998a). Specifically, the effect of unidirectional force or stress differs from oscillating or alternating force or stress in vascular endothelium (Ziegler et al. 1998a). Anti-inflammatory cytokine secretion is activated by directionality of myofascial release: pressure and shear that create uni-axial fibroblast strain (Standley and Meltzer 2008) like that propagated by the unidirectional pressured stroking of Gua sha.

The transitory therapeutic petechiae exhibit Gua sha's extravasation of blood within the capillary bed that is measured as an increase in surface microperfusion (Nielsen et al. 2007).

The breakdown of hemoglobin upregulates HO-1, CO, biliverdin and bilirubin that are anti-inflammatory and cytoprotective (Xia et al. 2008). Studies show the anti-inflammatory effect of Gua sha has a therapeutic impact in inflammatory conditions, such as active chronic hepatitis, where liver inflammation indicates organ breakdown that over time can lead to premature death (Chan et al. 2011). The physiology of HO-1 may also explain Gua sha's anti-inflammatory effect in other responsive clinical conditions, such as fever, cough, asthma, bronchitis, emphysema, mastitis (Chiu et al. 2010), gastritis, musculoskeletal conditions such as neck pain (Braun et al. 2011), migraine (Schwickert et al. 2007), postherpetic neuralgia (Nielsen 2005), and so on. The implications are profound and predict an expanding role for Gua sha in treating inflammatory conditions.

References

Ahn, A.C., Colbert, A.P., Anderson, B.J., et al., 2008. Electrical properties of acupuncture points and meridians: a systematic review. Bioelectromagnetics 29 (4) (May), 245–256.

Ahn, A.C., Park, M., Shaw, J.R., et al., 2010. Electrical impedance of acupuncture meridians: the relevance of subcutaneous collagenous bands. PLoS One 5 (7), 11907.

Ahn, A.C., Wu, J., Badger, G.J., et al., 2005. Electrical impedance along connective tissue planes associated with acupuncture. BMC Complement Altern Med 5 (2), 10.

Braun, M., Schwickert, M., Nielsen, A., et al., 2011. Effectiveness of Traditional chinese 'Gua Sha' Therapy in patients with chronic neck pain; a randomized controlled trial. Pain Med January 28.

Chan, S., Yuen, J., Gohel, M., et al., 2011. Guasha-induced hepatoprotection in chronic active hepatitis B: A case study. Clin Chim Acta 412, 1686–1688.

Chan, S., Yuen, J., Gohel, M., et al., 2012. Does Gua sha offer hepatoprotective effect to chronic inactive hepatitis B carriers? A built-in design to control subject expectation. J Altern Complem Med in press.

Chiu, J.-Y., Gau, M.-L., Kuo, S.-Y., et al., 2010. Effects of Gua-Sha therapy on breast engorgement: a randomized controlled trial. J Nurs Res 18(1) (March), 1–10.

Corey, S.M., Stevens-Tuttle, D., Langevin, H., 2009. Sensory innervation and development of a model of connective tissue inflammation in the low back of the rat: implications for the future study of low back pain pathophysiology. Fascia Congress 2009 November 22, 2009.

Epler, D.C., 1980. Bloodletting in early Chinese medicine and its relation to the origin of acupuncture. Bulletin of the History of Medicine 54, 337–367.

1980. The Essentials of Chinese Acupuncture. Foreign Language Press, Beijing, China.

Fang, L., Fang, M., Liu, Y.-C., 2008. Research advances of traditional Chinese medicine therapy in treating sports fatigue. Journal of Chinese Integrative Medicine 12, 1305–1310.

Farasyn, A., Meeusen, R., 2009. Effect of deep cross-friction myotherapy on pressure pain thresholds on patients with non-specific low back pain. Fascia Congress 2009 November 22, 2009.

Farombi, E., Surh, Y., 2006. Heme oxygenase-1 as a potential therapeutic target for hepatoprotection. J Biochem Mol Biol 39, 479–491.

Findley, T., 2009. Fascia Research II: second international fascia research congress. IJTMB 2 (3) (Sept.), 4–9.

Gallaudet, B., 1931. Description of the Planes of Fascia of the Human Body. Columbia University Press, New York.

Geng, Y., 2010. Gua sha conditioning three kinds of sub-health symptoms: fatigue, insomnia and neck and shoulder pain. Zhonghua Yangsheng Baojian 1, 18.

Haake, M., Muller, H., Schade-Brittinger, C., et al., 2007. German Acupuncture Trials (GERAC) for Chronic Low Back Pain. Arch Intern Med 167 (17), 1892–1898.

Hancock, C.M., Riegger-Krugh, C., 2008. Modulation of pain in osteoarthritis: the role of nitric oxide. Clin J Pain 24 (4) (May), 353–365.

Hocking, D., Titus, P., Sumagin, R., et al., 2008. Extracellular matrix fibronectin mechanically couples skeletal muscle contraction. Circ Res 102 (3), 372–379.

Iatridis, J.C., Wu, J., Yandow, J.A., et al., 2003. Subcutaneous tissue mechanical behavior is linear and viscoelastic under uniaxial tension. Connect Tissue Res 44 (5), 208–217.

Immenschuh, S., Baumgart-Vogt, E., Mueller, S., 2010. Heme oxygenase-1 and iron in liver inflammation: a complex alliance. Curr Drug Targets 11, 1541–1550.

Jinkui Yaolue Fanglun, 1987. Synopsis of Prescriptions of the Golden Chamber. New World Press, Beijing.

Juhan, D., 1987. Job's Body, a Handbook for Bodywork. Station Hill Press, Barrytown, New York.

Julias, M., Edgar, L.T., Buettner, H.M., et al., 2008. An in vitro assay of collagen fiber alignment by acupuncture needle rotation. Biomed Eng Online 7, 19.

Kuo, T.-C., Lin, C.-W., Ho, F.-M., 2004. The soreness and numbness effect of acupuncture on skin blood flow. Am J Chin Med 32 (1), 117–129.

Kwong, K.K., Kloetzer, L., Wong, K.K., et al., 2009. Bioluminescence imaging of heme oxygenase-1 upregulation in the Gua Sha procedure. J Vis Exp 30 (August 28), 1385.

Lanas, A., 2008. Role of nitric oxide in the gastrointestinal tract. Arthritis Res Ther 10 (Suppl 2), 4.

Langevin, H., 2006. Connective tissue: a body-wide signaling network? Med Hypotheses 66 (6), 1074–1077.

Langevin, H.M., Bouffard, N.A., Churchill, D.L., et al., 2007. Connective tissue fibroblast response to acupuncture: dose-dependent effect of bidirectional effect of needle rotation. J Altern Complement Med 13 (3) (April), 355–360.

Langevin, H.M., Churchill, D.L., Cipolla, M.J., 2001a. Mechanical signaling through connective tissue: a mechanism for the therapeutic effect of acupuncture. FASEB J 15 (12) (October), 2275–2282.

Langevin, H.M., Churchill, D.L., Fox, J.R., et al., 2001b. Biomechanical response to acupuncture needling in humans. J Appl Physiol 91 (6), 2471–2478.

Langevin, H.M., Churchill, D.L., Wu, J., et al., 2002. Evidence of connective tissue involvement in acupuncture. FASEB J 16 (8) (April), 872–874.

Langevin, H.M., Huijing, P.A., 2009. Communicating about fascia: history, pitfalls, and recommendations. IJTMB 2 (4), 1–6.

Langevin, H.M., Yandow, J.A., 2002. Relationship of acupuncture points and meridians to connective tissue planes. Anat Rec 269 (6) (15), 257–265.

Liao, R., He, Y., Tang, D., 2010. Gua sha treatment mechanism of neurodermitis. J Tradit Chin Med 6, 1124–1125.

Liu, R., Ma, Y., Wang, B., et al., 2009. The study of Jingluo Guasha on exercise and the activity of glucose reserve and serum enzyme of rats. Journal of Nanjing Institute of Physical Education (Natural Science) 3, 33–35.

Lu, G.-D., Needham, J., 1980. Celestial Lancets. A History and Rationale of Acupuncture and Moxa. Cambridge University Press, Cambridge.

Maciocia, G., 1989. Foundations of Chinese Medicine. Churchill Livingstone, Edinburgh.

Mackenzie, I.S., Rutherford, D., MacDonald, T.M., 2008. Nitric oxide and cardiovascular effects: new insights in the role of nitric oxide for the management of osteoarthritis. Arthritis Res Ther 10 (Suppl 2), 3.

Mann, F., 1977. Scientific Aspects of Acupuncture. Heinemann Medical, London.

Mars, M., Maharaj, S., Tufts, M., 2005. The effect of compressed air massage on skin blood flow and temperature. CardiovascJ of S Afr 16 (4) (July/Aug), 215–219.

Nielsen, A., 2005. Postherpetic neuralgia in the left buttock after a case of shingles. Explore (NY) 1 (1) (January), 74.

Nielsen, A., Knoblauch, N., Dobos, G., et al., 2007. The effect of 'Gua sha' treatment on the microcirculation of surface tissue: a pilot study in healthy subjects. EXPLORE: The Journal of Science and Healing 3, 456–466.

Nielsen, A., 2012. Gua Sha. In: Schleip, R., Findley, T., Chaitow, L., et al (Eds.), Fascia, the Tensional Network of the Human Body. Elsevier, Edinburgh.

O'Connor, J., Bensky, D. (trans), 1981. Acupuncture: A Comprehensive Text. Shanghai College of Traditional Chinese Medicine, Shanghai.

Porket, M., 1974. The Theoretical Foundations of Chinese Medicine Systems of Correspondence. MIT Press, Cambridge, MA.

Protzer, U., Seyfried, S., Quasdorff, M., et al., 2007. Antiviral activity and hepatoprotection by heme oxygenase-1 in hepatitis B virus infection. Gastroenterology 133, 1156–1165.

Rolf, I., 1977. Rolfing: The Integration of Human Structures. Harper and Row, New York.

Ruan, J., 2008. Gua sha treatment of chronic fatigue. Family Doctor 15, 39.

Sandberg, M., Lundeberg, T., Lindberg, L.-G., et al., 2003. Effects of acupuncture on skin and muscle blood flow in healthy subjects. Eur J Appl Physiol 90 (1-2) (September), 114–119.

Schatz J., Larre C., Rochat de la Valle E., 1978. Structures de l' Acupuncture Traditionelle. Vol I. Notions D'energétique Fondamentale. Senart-Typo/Ecole Européene d'Acupuncture, Paris.

Schleip, R., Findley, T., Chaitow, L., et al (Eds.), 2012. Fascia, the Tensional Network of the Human Body. Elsevier, Edinburgh.

Schwickert, M.E., Saha, F.J., Braun, M., et al., 2007. [Gua Sha for migraine in inpatient withdrawal therapy of headache due to medication overuse.]. Forsch Komplementmed 14 (5) (October), 297–300.

So, J.T.Y., 1987. Treatment of Disease with Acupuncture. Paradigm Publications, Brookline, MA.

Standley, P.R., Meltzer, K., 2008. In vitro modeling of repetitive motion strain and manual medicine treatments: potential roles for pro- and anti-inflammatory cytokines. J Bodyw Mov Ther 12 (3) (July), 201–203.

Tian, Y., Wang, Y., Luo, M., et al., 2009. Comparative study on Gua sha influence on histomorphology and skin blood perfusion volume in rabbits. Journal of External Therapy of Traditional Chinese Medicine 6, 8–9.

Unschuld, P., 1985. Medicine in China, a History of Ideas. University of California Press, Berkeley, CA.

Unschuld, P., 1986. Nan Ching, The Classic of Difficult Questions. University of California Press, Berkeley, CA.

Wang, M., 2009. Gua sha acupuncture and traction cervical vertebral artery clinical observation. Journal of Huaihai Medicine 4, 342–343.

Wang, Y., Gao, M., Wang, Y., et al., 2010. Observations on the improving effect of gua sha (dermal scraping) and pricking bloodletting interventions on vertebroarterial blood supply during frequent occurrence of vertigo. Shanghai Journal of Acupuncture and Moxibustion 6, 375–376.

Wang, Z., 2002. Chronic fatigue nemesis: gua sha holographic scraping of foot. Medicine and Health Care 10 (5), 17.

Wang, Z.K., Jiang, Y., Zhang, Q.-J., et al., 2009. Changes of bilirubin, SOD, IL-1, IL-6 and WBC count before and after Gua sha treatment in rats. Journal of Beijing University of Traditional Chinese Medicine 9, 618–620.

Wunder, C., Potter, R.F., 2003. The heme oxygenase system: its role in liver inflammation. Curr Drug Targets Cardiovasc Haematol Disord 3, 199–208.

Xia, Z.W., Zhong, W.W., Meyrowitz, J.S., et al., 2008. The role of heme oxygenase-1 in T cell-mediated immunity: the all encompassing enzyme. Curr Pharm Des 14 (5), 454–464.

Yu, R.-T., Lou, X.-F., Tang, M.-L., et al., 2008. Anatomical study of vessels in the area of the back by using Gua sha (scraping therapy). J Wenzhou Medical College 2, 151–153.

Zeng, S., 2003. Analysis of leukocyte (WBC) change before and after Guasha along Meridian. Heilongjiang Journal of Traditional Chinese Medicine 1, 41–42, 54.

Zhu, Z., Wilson, A.T., Mathahs, M.M., et al., 2008. Heme oxygenase-1 suppresses hepatitis C virus replication and increases resistance of hepatocytes to oxidant injury. Hepatology 48 (5) (November), 1430–1439.

Ziegler, T., Bouzourene, K., Harrison, V.J., et al., 1998a. Influence of oscillatory and unidirectional flow environments on the expression of endothelin and nitric oxide synthase in cultured endothelial cells. Arterioscler Thromb Vasc Biol 18 (5) (May), 686–692.

Ziegler, T., Silacci, P., Harrison, V.J., et al., 1998b. Nitric oxide synthase expression in endothelial cells exposed to mechanical forces. Hypertension 32 (2) (August), 351–355.

Further reading

Finando, D., Finando, S., 1999. Informed Touch, a Clinician's Guide to the Evaluation and Treatment of Myofascial Disorders. Healing Arts Press, Rochester, VT.

Myers, T., 2009. Anatomy Trains: Myofascial Meridians for Manual and Movement Therapies. Churchill Livingstone Elsevier, Edinburgh.

Ni, Y., 1996. Navigating the Channels of Traditional Chinese Medicine. Oriental Medicine Center, San Diego, CA.

Schleip, R., Findley, T., Chaitow, L., et al (Eds.), 2012. Fascia, the Tensional Network of the Human Body. Elsevier, Edinburgh.

San Jiao

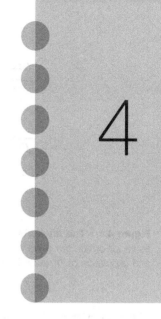

4

*It is no part
of prudence to cry down an art,
And what it may perform deny
because you understand not why*

(Hudibras)

The San Jiao has been a 'stone in the shoe' of every acupuncture student. Westerners have politely forgiven the concept of the San Jiao as prescientific. Although we understand that traditional East Asian Internal Organs are not equivalent to the Western internal organs, thankfully almost all of them bear the same names. The San Jiao did not have the same linguistic 'good fortune'. Translators, even modern Chinese, have at times apologized for the San Jiao as antiquated. It was this wincing that aroused my interest. The concept of the San Jiao informs counteractive medicine and techniques like acupuncture and Gua sha, even more so now through an understanding of the hypothesized role of connective tissue signaling. The concept of the San Jiao changed from prescientific to prescient. The channel system of traditional East Asian medicine suggested the proposed physiological model of connective tissue functionally connecting all parts of the body (Langevin 2006). What follows here is how this concept is discussed in the classical Chinese medical texts, some of the earliest medical texts known.

Etymology of the characters 'San Jiao'

'San' means three. According to Larre and Rochat de la Vallee (1992):

> Three is the number of all that is held between two poles, yin and yang, Heaven and Earth. Three is the number of man because man, being between heaven and earth, best represents the influx of heaven and earth in a perpetual exchange … All exchanges, all transformations of life, take place here at the level three.

The ancients regarded the San Jiao as 'the medium through which the process of transformation occurs within the human body'. The concept of fire exciting humors in the body coincides with the vapors that rise from cooking rice that is Qi and the Greek concept of wind arising from digestion of food (see Table 3.1 and Figure 4.1).

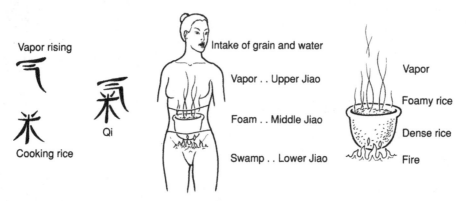

Figure 4.1 ● The ancients regarded the San Jiao as the medium through which transformation occurs in the body ● Qi is seen as vapor or humors rising from food rendered or spoiled by fire. The Upper, Middle and Lower Jiao each have a role in the transformation and circulation of Qi, coordinated and governed by the San Jiao.

Table 4.1 In Chinese, 'Jiao' is thought to depict a phoenix rising from flames, an image of transformation from death to rebirth. The San Jiao is seen as 'the medium through which the process of transformation occurs within the human body' (Weiger 1965)

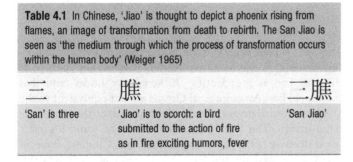

三	膲	三膲
'San' is three	'Jiao' is to scorch: a bird submitted to the action of fire as in fire exciting humors, fever	'San Jiao'

Principles observed in nature were attributed to the human body. The ancient Chinese, like the ancient Greeks, assumed the existence of some kind of heat source in the body (Unschuld 1985). In the Chinese model, the San Jiao administered this heat, regulating transformation and circulation of life humors in the three burning spaces, upper middle and lower body sections (see Figure 3.1 and Table 3.1, as well as Figure 4.1 and Table 4.1). Humors operated in the body as water did in the external setting.

The conveyance of water to where it was needed, as irrigation, and away from where it was unwanted was crucial to the survival of the community. This responsibility was administered by the state. The life-sustaining symbolism taken from waterworks is seen in this 3rd century BC quote from the Confucian work *Lu-shih ch'un-ch'iu* (Unschuld 1985):

> Flowing water and the pivot of a door do not rot because of their constant movement. The relationship between form and influences (Qi) is the same. If the form does not move, the essence (Jing) does not flow; if the essence does not flow, the influences will stagnate.

Thus, the concept and import of ceaseless flow was conferred to the body. Hence the human organism's form and function in Chinese classics is rendered in the language of the natural environment where the community appropriation of food and water is essential to the survival of the population (see Figure 4.2).

In classical texts the body is divided into three sections, three burners or heaters: the three Jiaos (see Figure 4.1). The San Jiao is said to regulate all water passageways; according to the analogy, it is the 'official' responsible for maintaining the 'ditches'. It also regulates Fire in the three burning centers or Jiaos. The Qi influences (i.e. Ying, Wei and Yuan Qi) are transformed from water and cereal and the San Jiao circulates these three Qi. The *Nei Ching* 'documents the development of the San Jiao from a designation of functions' symbolizing state appropriation of water and grain, whereas the *Ling Shu* suggests that it includes the designation of a tangible entity (Unschuld 1985). The San Jiao's expression is at the Li, which is understood as lining or pores, a pivot between outside and inside that is itself not outside or inside, therefore without form, but has form.

San Jiao and Li: lining, pores, pivot, no form, form

The 81 chapters of the *Nan Ching* text sought to clarify issues from the oldest text the, *Huang di Neijing*. The *Nan Ching* established, for example, the theory of the Path of Qi via the back Shu points and front Mu points, as well as the Yuan source points. The *Nan Ching* also contains discourse on the San Jiao. The 25th and 38th issues of the *Nan Ching* speak of the San Jiao as having name but no form. Ting Chin states in his commentary to the 25th Difficult Issue:

> If the Triple Burner has no form, how can passageways of water emerge from it? How can it be thick or thin? How can it be like mist or fog or foam or a ditch? How can it emit influences in order to supply warmth to the flesh? And if the enclosing network of the heart has no form, how can all the evil influences settle in this network enclosing the heart? They obviously did not know that the heart enclosing network is a small bag providing a network internally and an enclosure externally. Thus, the name already states that it is an 'enclosing network'.

Commentary by Kato Bankei to the 38th issue states:

> ... the Triple Burner is not a proper palace. However, without its influences all the other palaces could not fulfill their functions of

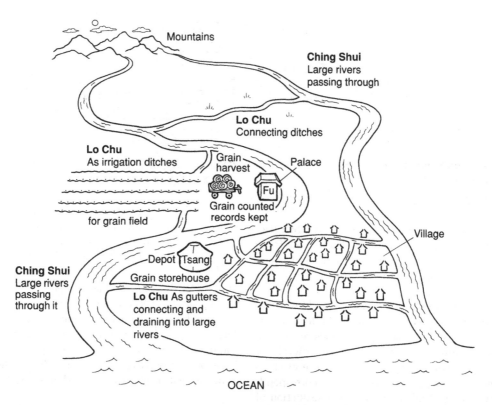

Figure 4.2 • The ancients imagined that Qi, Blood and Fluids sustained the human body as water and grain sustained the community • The Yang organs, Fu, were seen as palaces where grain was measured. The Yin organs, Zang, were seen as depots where grain was stored. The meridians corresponded to rivers and ditches, Ching Shui and Lo Chu (Jing and Lo). The San Jiao corresponded to the agency that administered the supply of food and water and organized the defense system.

emitting, intake, revolution, and transformation. It is not a proper palace; hence, it steams inside of the membrane; it moves in between the palaces and depots. It resembles an external wall. Hence it is called external Palace.

Ting Chin also states: 'The San Jiao is a large bag supporting the organism from the outside and holding it inside'.

A similar view was held in early Western medicine that to prevent stagnation of fluids, friction was considered to affect the cellular membrane surrounding the whole body under the skin (Kaim 1756):

> The cellular membrane, surrounding the whole body under the skin, and the muscles within it, and penetrating their fibers, is the most powerful seat of the watery humors which stagnate under the skin in anasarca [a condition in which body tissues contain excessive fluids], leukophlegmatia [white inflammation], and chlorosis [iron deficiency anemia] …

The *Ling Shu* and the *Su Wen* describe the San Jiao as completely enclosing each of the Internal Organs (Unschuld 1986). The membranous structure of the San Jiao is compared to the structure of the Xin Bao, Pericardium or Heart Protector, in the Chinese medical classics. The Xin Bao is a membrane or bag that encloses the heart, detaining evil influence, preventing penetration to the Heart. Likewise the San Jiao is a bag, a membrane that surrounds the entire body and each individual Organ. It forms a network of interconnecting bags. Like the Xin Bao, the San Jiao detains evil influence, preventing it from

ultimately penetrating to the Kidneys. As stated in Chapter 2 of the *Ling Shu*, the Kidneys own the Shao Yang (the San Jiao and Gall Bladder).

The early Western anatomists' cellular membrane (Kaim 1756) is clearly the subcutaneous fascia, called the Cou Li in traditional East Asian medicine.

Cou Li

The classic medical text *Jinkui Yaolue, Synopsis of Prescriptions of the Golden Chamber* (1987) warns against intrusion of pathogenic factors through the Cou Li. According to Epler (1980), Cou Li means 'pores' in much of the *Su Wen*. Open pores allow penetration of exogenous factors and allow their release through sweat. Closed pores are a barrier to exogenous factors or hold the exogenous factor in, once present. Epler notes that some commentators of the *Su Wen* translated Cou Li as 'between the skin and underlying musculature'. This coincides with the current definition in the *Chinese–English Medical Dictionary* (Ou Ming 1988):

> The Cou Li is striae, the natural lines of the skin and muscles and the spaces between the skin and muscles. It serves as an entrance and outlet for the flow of vital energy and blood and one of the routes for the excretion of body fluid, and as a barrier against the exogenous evils.

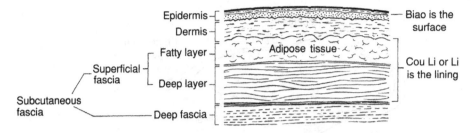

Figure 4.3 • Western and Eastern surface anatomy • Biao is the surface. The Cou Li, or lining, corresponds to the superficial fascia in Western anatomy. Arteries, veins, nerves, lymph vessels and nodes run through the deep layer of superficial fascia and Jing Lo vessels also run through this layer. Wei Qi moves through the fatty layer.

Here the Cou Li is the anatomical expression of the San Jiao. The *Ling Shu*, Chapter 47, confirms 'The Bladder and Triple Heater (San Jiao) have their correspondence and resonance in the most external structure of the body, the Cou Li' (see Figure 4.3).

The correspondence of the San Jiao to the Cou Li is essential to understanding the model for the curative effect of Gua Sha, acupuncture and, for that matter, any hands-on physiotherapy. When stimulating the body surface superficially or penetrating it, as with acupuncture or Gua sha, the effect is conducted internally by way of the Cou Li, that corresponds to fascial connective tissue and the potential transduction of chemical and mechanical signaling (as discussed in Chapter 3). As the outermost of the San Jiao's interconnecting network of bags, the Cou Li links the exterior of the body with the Internal Organs. Likewise, what is internal is conducted and reflected at the surface: 'the external envelope is where the inner motion is visible' (Larre and Rochat de la Vallee, 1992).

The workings of body Qi, Food and Fluid is isomorphic to the workings of a sustained community (see Figure 4.2). The Protective Wei Qi, like a guard, moves outside the vessels. The constructive Ying Qi moves inside the vessels. The original Source or Yuan Qi comes from heaven, but is sustained and replenished by the balanced function of the whole. In the community, the state is seen as the agency or 'fire' that regulates all transactions. In the body the San Jiao regulates all transactions in the three Jiaos by circulating the three Qi.

Wei Qi

The Wei is greasy and slippery and cannot enter the channels or vessels but resides in between the skin and the muscles, at the Cou Li. Functionally, Wei Qi warms the muscles, fills up the skin, opens and closes the pores to protect the body from penetration of Cold and Wind (*Ling Shu*, 100 BC). Wei assumes form as body fat, the adipose tissue of the superficial fascia. Wei Qi is an aspect of body resistance within the Cou Li and is controlled by the San Jiao. Hence, the San Jiao governs at the Cou Li and takes form at the Cou Li.

When an exogenous evil penetrates the Cou Li it progresses inward within the network of bags that connect the surface with the internal organs. The *Su Wen* states:

> This is the origin of all diseases. Evil always attacks first at the skin and hair and then comes into the area between the skin and the

flesh. It comes in and stays at the Lo vessels. If it does not leave, it transmits to and enters the meridians. If it does not leave, it transmits to and enters the Fu and gathers at the Intestines and Stomach.

At the Cou Li, the San Jiao protects from but also conducts pathogenic factors such as Wind, Cold, Damp, Heat and Dryness. Like the Pericardium membrane, the Xin Bao, which detains the 'evil', preventing entrance to the Heart, the San Jiao detains but also *conducts* exogenous evil or pathogenicity. The Cou Li provides a pathway that diverts the causative agent from the seat of life, the Ming Men at the Kidneys.

Ying Qi

Like connective tissue, it is said there is nothing the San Jiao does not envelope, including the vessels that hold the Blood and conduct the Ying Qi. Ying is the nourishing, constructive aspect. Ying flows in the blood vessels and channels, while Wei Qi flows outside the channels. Ying suffuses the entire body through the vascular system and the meridian system. According to Ross (1985) Ying and Blood are often synonymous. The Blood carries Ying, but Ying is not contained only in Blood. Ying Qi is the Qi activated when a needle is inserted in an acupuncture point (Maciocia 1989).

When the 'Ying and the Wei are out of balance' the patient is said to sweat without resolution. This sweat is loss of the Ying through the pores. The Wei is said to have gone inside and the Ying is said to have gone outside. Hence there is no protection and the constructive aspects are scattered. This is one scenario of chronic fatigue syndrome, where an illness is trapped at the Shao Yang. The patient is vulnerable to any outside influence due to the lack of protection. Her nourishing aspects are spent externally, rather than retained and incorporated within.

Yuan Qi

'Yuan' means 'original, primordial source'. It is our life force endowed by heaven, manifest through our parents, accumulated in the Kidneys and circulated by the San Jiao. The ideogram for Yuan, '原', represents three springs gushing out of a cliff. An image emerges of the San Jiao force of Fire 'gushing' Water in the three body zones, accessed at points CV 17, CV 12 and CV 6.

The San Jiao Fire is the Yuan Yang, original Yang of the Gate of Life (Ming Men). It is the original constituent of all Yang function. The Water is the Yuan Yin, the original constituent of all Yin, substance and fluid. When Fire meets Water in the body, a transformation into Qi takes place.

Larre and Rochat de la Vallee (1992) state: 'There is no vital Water without Fire to transform it and no Fire of life without Water to fix and express it'. The creative tension between 2, Fire and Water, the motive and the quiescent, becomes 3, *san*, continuous transformation. This is the formula for life as our ancestors expressed it. The Yuan not only suffuses the body with motive force but is a catalyst in the formation of Ying, Wei, Qi and Blood. Yuan is itself, in turn, 'persistently regenerated' by those very products. It accumulates or resides in the Kidneys at the Ming Men and, through the San Jiao, reaches the entire body. It can be directly accessed at the Yuan Source points at the extremities, or at CV 17, CV 12 or CV 6 at the front of the body.

The San Jiao regulates water passageways

Jin Ye

In the commentary to the 66th issue of the *Nan Ching*, Yang explains:

> The location between the two kidneys is called the great sea, *ta-hai*; another name is 'submerged in water', *ni shui*. Inside it is the spirit-turtle. It exhales and inhales the original influences. When the original influences (yuan) flow out of the tan tien (3 inches below the navel) they penetrate the four extremities as wind and rain; they reach everywhere.
>
> (Unschuld 1986)

The term 'hai' refers to 'the internal environment of the body as a 'sea within a sea' (Liu and Liu 1980). Body Fluid is a constituent of Blood when in the blood vessels. When it is outside of the blood vessels, it stays in the slit of the body organs (Academy of TCM 1979). All organs and tissues within the body are individually or collectively surrounded by and in direct contact with the Body Fluids, Jin Ye, as though afloat yet duly adhered to a base and properly anchored. The body itself virtually exists in an external envelope of fluids. (Liu and Liu 1980).

Chapter 36 of the *Ling Shu* states: 'The Qi of the Triple Burner goes to the muscles and skin and is transformed into fluids (Jin). Other body fluids do not move and are transformed into liquids (Ye).'

Jin Ye are Body Fluids. Jin fluids circulate with the Wei Qi at the body exterior as an agency of protection and nourishment to the skin and muscles. Jin leave the body as clear light fluids: sweat, tears, saliva and mucus. The Lungs and the Upper Jiao of the San Jiao control movement and expression of Jin.

Ye fluids are more dense and turbid. They circulate with the Ying Qi at the interior, lubricating the joints and orifices (eyes, ears, nose, mouth). Ye are controlled by the Spleen and Kidneys and the Lower Jiao of the San Jiao. Ye leave the body as

discharges that could be said to be heavier in the sense that they contain more waste.

Observing mist, foam and swamp

The form of fluid is specific to the Jiao. This can be directly observed. The fluid of the Upper Jiao is a mist associated with the vapor that rises to the Lungs from the Stomach, Spleen or Kidneys and is dispersed by the Lungs throughout the body. The vapor described is like the exhalation mist observed in winter.

The Middle Jiao fluid is described as thicker, as a foam or a muddy pool. It is associated with the contents of the stomach in the process of transformation. This can be observed when the stomach rebels and the foamy contents are vomited.

The Lower Jiao rules discharge. Its fluid is the dregs, i.e. stool and urine, described as a swamp. Swamps are a mixture of dark mud and water and they stink. The Lower Jiao, like a swamp, vaporizes some of its fluid, which rises like mist back up to the Lungs. The swampy discharge of the Lower Jiao can be observed in the stool.

The San Jiao controls Jin Ye fluids and one control valve is the Bladder. It can be observed that when a living body becomes suddenly cold the Cou Li and muscles at the surface contract, the pores close and the Bladder fills. The body excretes clear, light yellow fluid. Hence the association of the San Jiao, Bladder and urine in the *Su Wen* and *Ling Shu*.

The San Jiao regulates the entire cycle of Jin Ye circulation and the intercommunication of fluids throughout the Body. The *Su Wen* states that the Upper Jiao resembles fog, the Middle Jiao resembles foam and the Lower Jiao resembles a swamp. This is reminiscent of the character for Qi – the vapor rising from the foamy boiling of the denser rice (see Figure 4.1).

The Triple Burner is a palace acting as central ditch; the passageways of Water emerge from it. It is associated with the Bladder and it constitutes the palace of uniqueness.

When the pores (*tsouli, couli*) are sealed tightly and the skin is thick, the Triple Burner and the Bladder are thick too.

> The lower section of the Triple Burner is located exactly at the upper opening of the Bladder ... From there the clear portions enter the Bladder where they become influences and urine ... The lower section of the Triple Burner masters discharge but not intake; it serves as transmitter.
>
> (Unschuld 1986)

The *Ling Shu*, Chapter 47, states that the Kidneys connect with the San Jiao, and the Bladder and San Jiao have their resonance at the Cou Li (Larre and Rochat de la Vallee 1992).

Gao Huang, Huang Mo, Mo Yuan: internal network of bags

The Bladder is called Pang Guang or Gao Huang. Gao Huang also refers to the greasy membrane or Li, the lining between the Heart and diaphragm. It is also the name of acupoint BL 38 (TCM BL 43), 'gao huang shu'. One of the five main apucunture points, gao huang shu directly accesses this abdominal membrane or fascia. The *Su Wen* states: 'The Wei Qi goes between the skin and tissues and flesh. The Wei keeps the 'Huang Mo' warm. The Wei scatters to the chest and abdomen'. 'Mo' means membrane. Huang Mo, like Gao Huang, describes the greasy membrane between the Heart and diaphragm.

The membrane source, Mo Yuan, refers to the membrane found between the viscera and the wall of the trunk. Called the greater omentum, peritoneum or mesentery, it refers to the fascia of the abdominal cavity. According to the *Wen Re Jing Wei, the Warp and Woof of Warm Febrile Diseases*, 'The membrane source is connected to the muscles externally and is close to the stomach internally. It is the gateway to the Triple Burner and, in fact, is at the half-exterior, half-interior level of the body' (Bensky and Barolet 1990).

Gao Huang, Huang Mo and Mo Yuan, then, are the internal aspect of the San Jiao; the internal network of bags that connects with the external bag, the Cou Li.

The Shao Yang belongs to the Kidneys

Half-interior, half-exterior

The Shao Yang describes the sides of the body traversed by the San Jiao and Gall Bladder vessels. The Shao Yang is said to be half Biao, half Li. It represents not just the lateral aspect of the body but a distinct place within the entire body surface envelope, the half-inside, half-outside, the Cou Li and Mo Yuan. The Shao Yang is the pivot from 'outside to inside', the mediator (see Figure 4.4).

Shao Yang symptoms

The Shao Yang exhibits a mix of symptoms of the Exterior and Interior (see Table 4.2). A Shao Yang disorder is *between* the outside and inside. The place 'between' is specifically the Cou Li and Mo Yuan, the fascial network.

Table 4.2 Three Yang stages of acute illness. Symptoms of the Shao Yang are a mix of symptoms of the Tai Yang and Yang Ming stage

Tai Yang	Shao Yang	Yang Ming
Chills, aches Aversion to/fear of Cold/Wind	Chills, then fever, then chills	Aversion to/fear of heat
Cold/Wind	Not simultaneous	
No fever, pathogen has not penetrated to deep heat response	Aches No appetite, sweat does not resolve fever	Fever (with chills), fast pulse, thirst, sweat = Four Bigs
Frequent urination	Dysuria	Scant urine due to Heat

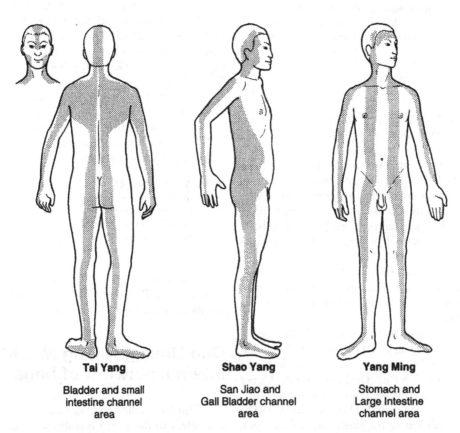

Tai Yang
Bladder and small intestine channel area

Shao Yang
San Jiao and Gall Bladder channel area

Yang Ming
Stomach and Large Intestine channel area

Figure 4.4 • Areas of the body associated with the Tai Yang, Shao Yang and Yang Ming • The acute symptomatology of disorders at these areas is described in Table 4.2. Some symptoms can linger or become chronic reflecting a persisting stasis.

Before thermometers were used to measure body temperature, fever was detected by touch or by report of the patient. The chills of a Shao Yang disorder alternate with fever, but the fever is not high. The patient may feel hot and be hot to the touch but a Shao Yang fever would not register high on a thermometer. This is because the fever is not coming from the inside, where true heat resides, but from half-in, half-out. An increase in fever indicates the pathogen has deepened and reached Yang Ming Fire.

Alternating fever as in malaria, or Babesiosis (a Lyme disease coinfection) express at the Shao Yang.

What are the possible outcomes of the Shao Yang stage? The pathogen (chill) can sink deeper into the body, creating hotter signs: Yang Ming. Or the pathogen can vacate the Tai Yang and Shao Yang regions, the Biao and Li, in resolution. A third possibility is for the illness to become chronic, with continued bouts of chills, slight fever, feeling achy and never quite well. This indicates that the pathogen is lodged in the Shao Yang or that the Shao Yang is retaining the pathogen. This is one scenario of chronic fatigue.

Treating illness with aspects at the Shao Yang

Any chronic illness may have a Shao Yang component. Just as the Shao Yang is the pivot between outside and inside, a chronic 'Shao Yang' patient is never quite sick, never quite well (see studies on using Gua sha for treating 'sub-health' in Chapter 2). Any bodywork that manipulates or penetrates the body surface, stimulating the Cou Li or fascia, affects the Shao Yang, the Mo Yuan and, hence, the Internal Organs. The global physiological role of the Li, which may wholly or in part correspond to connective tissue, structurally and functionally connecting all parts of the body, may leave no aspect unaffected by treatments such as Gua sha. Just as water quenches thirst, so too would the most thirsty aspects be noticeably quenched by directed stimulation.

Psychospiritual implications: inside–outside

> When influences are balanced and one's mind reaches into the distance, happiness and joy originate.
>
> (Unschuld 1986)

The Organs and Zang Fu patterns of Chinese medicine have their psychospiritual as well as their physical expressions. For example, Liver constraint, expresses as various Qi stagnation syndromes. There is frustration, anger, obstructed will and creativity. Liver Qi is never said to be Deficient because it is the nature of the Liver to stagnate rather than wane. Liver Blood, on the other hand, can become Deficient. Each organ is a unique expression of an aspect of body and spirit.

The San Jiao mediates all stimulation from the universe 'outside' the body: Heat, Cold, Wind, Damp, Dryness, barometric pressure, the spirit that passes between humans, and what passes between humans and the spirit world. Ancients regarded the human being as a microcosm of the universe, in sympathetic resonance with the forces of the universe. The San Jiao is the physiological organization of an individual's every response – yes, no or maybe – to all that is.

> This refers not only to the fact of swallowing and excreting, but to everything that allows me to receive and introduce something into my body that is other than myself, something that comes from outside. It is also that which gives the ability to eliminate all that cannot be integrated and assimilated into my being. Between these two activities are all the transformations that are under command of the Triple Heater. The Triple Heater gives the unity to all these operations between entry and exit. The details of them may be governed by one organ or another, but the whole thing is governed by the Triple Heater, so it gives a unity to all this functioning.
>
> (Larre and Rochat de la Vallee 1992)

In sympathetic resonance, the body is balanced, fluid and flexible with the environment. Imbalance fosters the opportunity for intrusion. The *Shang Han Lun*, clause 97, says: 'When the Blood is Deficient and the Vital Resistance weak, the Cou Li opens, so the pathogenic factor intrudes'.

Furthermore, from a psychosocial perspective, when the Blood is Deficient the self-esteem may be low. If the Wei is also weak, there may be sensitivity to stimulation, including the thoughts and actions of others. The results are comparable to when the physical body is engaged in illness, as the body battles with a penetrating factor. The patient suffers pain, is preoccupied, out of balance within themselves and out of a healthy resonance with the whole.

Summary

The concept of the San Jiao regulating the three Qi at the Cou Li, or lining, via the ancient channel system informs not only ancient counteractive medicine and techniques like acupuncture and Gua Sha, but also an understanding of the models for connective tissue signaling: the physiological role of connective tissue connecting all parts of the body with one another. The San Jiao has changed from a prescientific to a prescient concept of function.

References

Academy of Traditional Chinese Medicine and the Guangzhou College of Traditional Chinese Medicine, 1979. Concise Dictionary of Chinese Medicine (trial edition). People's Medical Publishing House, Beijing.

Bensky, D., Barolet, R., 1990. Chinese Herbal Medicine: Formulas and Strategies. Eastland Press, Seattle.

Epler, D.C., 1980. Bloodletting in early Chinese medicine and its relation to the origin of acupuncture. Bulletin of the History of Medicine 54, 337–367.

Kaim, S., 1756. Dissertatio Inauguralis Medica de Frictionibus. Chipok R 1994 (trans). Kaliwodian Press, University of Vienna.

Jinkui Yaolue Fanglun, 1987. Synopsis of Prescriptions of the Golden Chamber. New World Press, Beijing.

Langevin, H., 2006. Connective tissue: a body-wide signaling network? Med Hypotheses 66 (6), 1074–1077.

Larre, C., Rochat de la Vallee E., 1992. Chinese Medicine from the Classics: Heart Master, Triple Heater. Monkey Press / Ricci Institute, Cambridge.

Liu, F., Liu, Y.M., 1980. Chinese Medical Terminology. Commercial Press Ltd, Hong Kong.

Maciocia, G., 1989. Foundations of Chinese Medicine. Churchill Livingstone, Edinburgh.

Ming, O. (Ed.), 1988. Chinese – English Dictionary of Traditional Chinese Medicine. Guandong Science and Technology Publishing House, Hong Kong.

Ross, J., 1985. Zang Fu, The Organ System of Traditional Chinese Medicine. Churchill Livingstone, Edinburgh.

Shang Han Lun, 1986. Treatise on Febrile Diseases Caused by Cold. New World Press, Beijing.

Unschuld, P., 1985. Medicine in China, A History of Ideas. University of California Press, Berkeley.

Unschuld, P., 1986. Nan Ching, The Classic of Difficult Issues. University of California Press, Berkeley.

Weiger, L., 1965. Chinese Characters, Their Origin, Etymology, History, Classification and Signification: A Thorough Study from Chinese Documents. Dover, New York.

Sha syndrome and Gua sha, cao gio, coining, scraping

5

Gua sha, cao gio, kerik, khoud lam, ga sal, coining, scraping

Gua sha is a traditional East Asian medicine healing technique that applies instrument-assisted unidirectional 'press-stroking' of a lubricated area of body surface to intentionally create transitory therapeutic petechiae representing extravasation of blood in the subcutis.

Gua sha is also known as *cao gio* (Vietnam), *kerik* (Indonesia), *khoud lam* (Laos), *ga sal* (Cambodia), coining or scraping, and has been used for centuries in Asia, in Asian immigrant communities, and by acupuncturists and practitioners of traditional East Asian medicine worldwide (Nielsen 2009) (see Chapter 1).

Sha

Sha is a polysemous term describing the presence of surface blood stasis associated with pain or sickness and the petechiae that are raised from applying Gua sha. Sha may be symptomatic (sha syndrome), asymptomatic, or mildly symptomatic and potentially pathogenic. Sha is literally translated as 'sand', 'sharkskin', or 'red, raised, millet-size rash' (Ou Ming 1988).

In ancient medical literature sha '沙' refers to cholera (see Table 5.1), wherein sha petechiae resemble cholera's end-stage rash, linking Gua sha to its history as treatment for fever and cholera (Mathews 1931; Weiger 1965) similar to techniques used for cholera in early Western medicine (see Chapter 1). Sha syndrome is characterized by different kinds and stages of fever responsive to Gua sha (Yang et al. 2007b) (see below).

Dr So liked the translation of sha as 'sand' or 'sharkskin', since the texture of sha petechiae is bumpy like sand on the skin, similar to a sharkskin. The raised bumps are most often red but can be blue, purple or black (see Plate Section).

Table 5.1 Sha'沙'refers to cholera in ancient medical literature but it also refers to sand in common language. Sha as petechiae feel slightly rough on the skin surface, like sand or sharkskin. Rash-like petechiae are characteristic of end-stage choleric dehydration (see Chapter 1). The oldest medical literature that describes the sickness of 'sha' or 'sha syndrome' is the *Shi Yi De Xiao Fang*, written by physician Yi-lin Wei in Yuan Dynasty (AD 1337). In Ming Dynasty (AD 1368–1644), the medical literature used another sha '痧'to refer the sickness of '沙'.

Ideogram	痧	=	疒	+	沙
Pronunciation	Shā		Nè		Shā
Modern language	Cholera		Sickness		Sand
Ancient medical language	Cholera		Sickness		Cholera, sand

Gua

Sha is intentionally brought to the body's surface by four methods: Gua sha, Pak sha, Tsien (Nieh or Niu) sha or by Ba guan, cupping. 'Gua' literally means 'to scrape or scratch' but is more accurately described as unidirectional instrument-assisted press-stroking. Scraping is a rather misleading term since there is nothing taken from the skin surface; it remains intact. 'Pak' means 'to slap', 'Tsien' means 'to pinch'. Tsien sha is used, for example, at the point 'yin tang' between the eyebrows. Ba guan, i.e. cupping, raises sha by vacuum force created by suction or flame. The cup is then applied to the surface causing the flesh to 'tumify' into the cup, resulting in extravasation of blood (Cao et al. 2010; Chirali 1999; Manz 2009).

Gua sha and Ba guan have similar therapeutic intentions but different mechanisms. While both may be warming, fire cupping (or moxibustion) may be more suitable for warming a cold abdomen. Cupping is essential for bloodletting, called wet cupping, applicable in early stages of eczema, for example. Whether a practitioner uses Gua sha or Ba guan comes down to personal preference. In my experience Gua sha does more to stretch the tissue and underlying fascia and is easier to execute over a large area. Gua sha is easier in that cap instruments can be discarded, whereas cups are not intended as disposable instruments and require decontamination and/or sterilization before reuse (see Safety protocols, Chapter 6).

Sha syndrome

The oldest known medical literature that describes 'sha syndrome' or sickness of 'sha' was the *Shi Yi De Xiao Fang, Effective Formulas Tested by Physicians for Generations* (1337), written by physician Yi-lin Wei in the Yuan Dynasty. Dr Wei prescribes the treatment for 'sha' as '...scraping at the neck, elbows and knees using wet hemp until there was an increase of blood in skin which appeared as small red spots.' The description for cholera treatment or treatment of 'Sha syndrome' in the famous Korean text printed in 1613, the *Dongui Bogam, Mirror of Easter Medicine* by Dr Heo Jun is the same as that in the *Shi Ye De Xiao Fang*.

The *Chinese–English Medical Dictionary* (Ou Ming 1988) defines sha syndrome as:

A disease caused by the exposure of Wind, Cold, Summer-Heat or wetness evil in summer or autumn leading to blockage to meridians; manifested as chilliness, fever, distension and pain of the body, or vomiting and diarrhea, or rigidity and numbness of extremities.

There are three significant points to this definition. The first is the notion of disease caused by exposure to the Elements.

Disease caused by exposure to the Elements

The notion of atmospheric factors causing disease is found in every culture. Epler (1980) cites Chapter 62 of the *Su Wen* that dates from the 2nd century BC where *hsieh* describes a range of 'pathogenicity', including external disease, that is, disease attributed to exposure to external elements that in turn affect the exterior of the body with agency to progress internally. It is associated with atmospheric factors, especially wind and rain, or with food and drink.

Exposure can lead to illness or exacerbate symptoms of any existing condition. Wai feng, evil wind, enters from outside the body (Liu and Liu 1980). External factors in excessive of that manageable by the body's defense system, are heteropathic, and become harmful to the body's orthopathic Qi thus causing illness. The body's defensive barrier, Wei Qi, is a circulating shield of warmth and regulatory processes that protects from penetration of external excesses. Wei Qi can become weakened by improper diet, lack of sleep or by the effects of stress or illness. Externally the Wei Qi is challenged by repeated unprotected exposure to changes in external conditions like temperature, wind, dampness, and so on. The wisdom of Chinese medicine emphasizes prevention of illness by carefully clothing, resting and feeding ourselves. Those who do not eat or drink at the proper time impair the Internal Organs and deplete the Blood and Qi. That can in turn weaken the Wei Qi allowing entry of injurious influences.

We may think such considerations irrelevant to modern times. Housing and central heating shield us. We are at once protected from the Elements and less aware of them. However, changes in temperature from cozy central heating to the wet, cold wind or from summer's heat to air-conditioning challenge the body's regulatory mechanisms. We are spared extended exposure to a harsh climate, but the contrast between our indoor and outdoor environments can also be an immune stressor.

When an outside agent violates the body, penetration advances with recognizable signs. The Elements act within the body like they act outside. Methods of intervention are specified accordingly.

Elements act in the body like they act outside

If an Element is able to penetrate the body's resistance, it is the 'character' or 'nature' of the Element that invades the body. The inner Qi is disturbed in a manner characteristic of the Element.

Cold

Cold causes the body to contract. It slows things down just like a stream freezing over. 'Just as Cold causes the water in rivers to freeze so it is said to cause the Blood in the vessels to congeal' (Epler 1980). Cold inhibits circulation, causing things to 'collect' and get stuck. Pain from Cold is marked by symptoms of chill, contraction, cramps and spasms.

For decades conventional medicine has maintained that respiratory infections are caused by viruses and bacteria, purging the historical association of colds with exposure to 'chill' and humans from their place in nature (Douglas 1969). Recent study, however, supports the role of exposure as contributing to illness. Acute cooling of the body surface (Eccles 2002) and inhaling of cold air (Mourtzoukou and Falagas 2007) causes reflex vasoconstriction in the nose and upper airways, and this vasoconstrictor response inhibits respiratory defense and promotes the onset of common cold symptoms by converting an asymptomatic subclinical viral infection into a symptomatic clinical infection. Researchers also found cooling of the feet led to cold symptoms onset in some subjects (Johnson and Eccles 2005). Moreover, thermoregulatory responses are altered by repeated cold-water immersion (Young 1986). Hot drinks were found to be a beneficial treatment for relief of common cold and flu symptoms (Sanu and Eccles 2008). Cooling of the feet provokes symptomatic lower urinary tract infection in cystitis-prone women (Baerheim and Laerum 1992).

Thermographic imaging (see front cover) can show how cold penetrates the body when in a cool environment. It shows heat loss and penetration of cold by conduction. Body heat loss through convection, the normal rising of heat, happens continuously. A wind or draft expedites heat loss through convection by more quickly replacing the air that surrounds the body.

In other research, Vitamin D concentrations correlated with susceptibility to acute viral infections (Sabetta et al. 2010). Serum concentrations of 38 ng/ml or greater were associated with a two-fold reduction in risk of developing illness. Vitamin D is sourced through food and exposure to sunlight, and it is thought that Vitamin D deficiency contributes to seasonal flu epidemics, especially in climates where cold winters reduce exposure to sunlight. This research supports the importance of spending some time outside every day, and for some, to supplement with Vitamin D in fall and winter.

Dampness

Dampness acts inside like it acts outside. It causes things to be wet, sluggish, to collect as edema and to pour down as diarrhea or discharge. The pain of Dampness is a steady, heavy ache that stays in one place. While it is thought that even in early China cholera was known to come from drinking tainted water, cholera symptoms (chills, fever, vomiting and unremitting diarrhea and dehydration) were treated as manifested forms of exposure to cold and damp with Fire

Heat. As discussed in Chapter 1, sha is also translated as cholera and Gua sha is a treatment indicated for cholera and cholera-like disorders.

Dryness

Dryness deprives the body of moisture, injuring all functions dependent upon fluid. Fluids conduct all body nourishment and elimination, as well as facilitating movement itself. Fever, fluid loss or inability to drink create internal Dryness that can be life-threatening.

'Outside' Dryness injures the skin and the Lungs first, causing dry skin, dry cough and thirst. Research has shown that dry air promotes respiratory viruses to become trapped in mucosa and reproduce. Also, influenza viruses stay alive longer in dry air, favoring transmission (Lowen et al. 2007). As Dryness persists, its effects deepen in the body, causing dry stool, dark infrequent urine, fatigue and stiffness. Dryness can also lead to internal Wind that appears as dizziness or spasms.

Heat

Heat causes things to stir, to agitate. Heat raises body temperature overall or at one site and dries fluids, causing elements to concentrate. Pain from Heat feels hot and irritable, and dense. The Heat of fever causes excessive internal motion. Hippocrates understood fever to arise from excessive motion. He believed frictioning could augment the vital force and excite a warm fever in even the most 'frigid dropsical person', creating Heat as therapy (Kaim 1756).

Wind

Wind moves. It can penetrate the Cou Li, (lining, pores) carrying other Elements into the body. 'Outside' Wind affects the skin, head, throat and Lungs first. Wind is also responsible for advancing the illness inward to the body interior.

Wind acts inside like it acts outside. Wind pain can be of sudden onset, tending to move around or shoot, and it can cause rigidity like a tree straining against a steady gale.

The common effect of the penetrating nature of Cold, Dampness, Dryness, Wind and sometimes Heat is 'blockage to the channels'. This is the second significant point of the sha-syndrome definition: outside excesses obstruct the inner Qi.

Bu tong ze: tong; tong ze: bu tong
No free flow: pain; free flow: no pain

Like Hippocratic medicine, traditional East Asian medicine uses aphorisms. According to one traditional saying, pain is caused by obstruction in the flow of Qi or Blood. The ceaseless flow of Qi is a body concept analogous with the ceaseless flow of water in nature. Obstruction causes problems. Herein lies the curative principle of acupuncture. Acupuncture is the mechanical stimulation of points with needles, the effect of which is to move Qi. Moving Qi removes obstruction, reestablishing the normal free flow and, thus, resolving pain. If the

Blood is stuck, acupuncture alone will not resolve it and techniques like Gua sha are needed.

Distinguishing pain: Shi/excess or Xu/deficient

The pain of obstruction is considered an excess or Shi pain. Excessive Shi pain comes from invasion of external factors, stuckness of Qi, Blood, Dampness/Fluids and/or Food or from Organ dysfunction that allows excess of substances to concentrate. When things collect there is abundance, and that inappropriate surplus causes pain. The bottleneck in the flow of Qi, Blood, Food, Phlegm or Fluids creates a shortage somewhere else. Hence, obstruction can lead to Deficiency.

There is also pain of a Deficient or Xu nature. Deficient types of pain are duller in character than a Shi pain and are associated with 'not enough' Qi, Blood or Body Fluids. When there is a shortage of Qi, Blood or Body Fluids, the force in their flow is compromised allowing substances, Blood, Body Fluids, mucus or food to collect. So Deficiency can lead to obstruction. Because there is less force behind the obstruction, the pain is duller.

A practitioner is able to distinguish a Shi from a Xu condition by the quality of pain, the texture and color of sha and the patient's response to Gua sha. This will be detailed in Chapter 6.

Symptoms measure climatic penetration

The third significant aspect of the definition of the sha syndrome is the subjective symptoms. We recognize 'chilliness, fever, distension and pain of the body, or vomiting and diarrhea, or rigidity and numbness of extremities' as early stage symptoms of an acute flu. The traditional East Asian perspective interprets: 'Wind Cold produces chilliness. The presence of Wind, Cold and Dampness at the level of the muscles produces generalized soreness and pain' (Bensky and Barolet 1990).

The body's resistance to Wind Cold is evidenced by fever. Advancement to the Middle Jiao is marked by vomiting and diarrhea. Rigidity and numbness of the extremities is evidence of severe obstruction by Wind.

In traditional East Asian medical diagnosis particular attention would be paid to the signs that dominate. Chills predominating rather than fever indicates penetration has not reached past the surface or Tai Yang region. Fever and sweating with thirst indicate the external influence has reached the body's deep heat response. Sweating may resolve the fever or may not. Both fever and sweating can eventually deplete Body Fluids. Thirst is a sign that the fluids are depleted or not circulating.

What is the location and nature of the pain? Dr So and the classical elders taught that the area of greatest pain is the original site of penetration. Changes in stool and urine and even characteristics of vomit all help to place the patient on a continuum of diagnostic and prognostic perception, from which is fashioned a treatment, applying the principles of traditional East Asian medicine. The proper response to the above signs is to first treat the Exterior.

Xian biao hou li: first treat the Exterior, then the Interior

Another important aphorism that guides treatment deals with prioritizing: *xian biao hou li*. To treat an Interior condition when there is also an Exterior pathogenic factor may drive the Exterior factor into the Interior, making the patient worse. For this reason, treatment of chronic conditions is postponed until the acute condition is gone. For example, purgative herbs are not given in an acute external illness. A purgative would cause the stool to move down and out, drawing the external factor in at the surface.

Therefore, the principle of releasing the Exterior is applied first. When the external factor is resolved, Interior chronic patterns can be treated, often in subsequent sessions.

Clause 1.15 of the *Synopsis of Prescriptions of the Golden Chamber* (Jinkui Yaulue Sanglun 1987) states:

> When a patient with a chronic disease is affected by a new disease, the new disease should be given priority in treatment, after which the chronic disease can be treated. Chronic disease cannot be cured within a short time, while a new disease can be treated easily as it has not penetrated deep into the Interior. Generally speaking, patients with chronic diseases lack body resistance, permitting pathogenic factors to invade the Interior in a short period of time. If timely treatment is not directed at the new disease, it will aggravate and complicate the chronic disease.

In an acute illness it is thought that the body is trying to push out the penetrating external factor, as in fever culminating in a sweat. The proper therapeutic response is to help the body push. The method is called 'releasing the Exterior'.

Gua sha terms of action

Gua sha dredges the channels

Chinese-language articles consistently refer to Gua sha as dredging the channels, an action that is stronger in terms of clearing stasis than acupuncture's stimulation of Qi. These ancient channels or meridians are consistent with planes or cleavages of connective tissue (Langevin and Yandow 2002), the same connective tissue that is intimately associated with all other tissues including organ systems, now recognized in models as a 'body-wide mechanosensitive signaling network' (Langevin 2006). Dredging the channels relieves local stasis, as Gua sha stretches the tissue along the planar boundary that is responsive to both depth and direction of manual stimulation, propagating mechanical and chemical signaling within the connective tissue matrix, which may potentiate tissue morphogenesis associated with healing (Langevin et al. 2001).

Gua sha vents Heat

Heat stress reduces cerebral blood velocity and markedly impairs orthostatic tolerance in humans, leading to Heat syncope (Wilson et al. 2006). Physiological studies show that increased skin blood flow effectively conducts away heat caused by increased metabolic activity (Schubert et al. 1994). Increased surface microperfusion from Gua sha vents Heat in heat-stressed humans, linking Gua sha to its well known effect in reversing heatstroke and increasing orthostatic tolerance (Wilson et al. 2002).

As demonstrated in Chapter 7, Gua sha's ability to vent Heat shows as an immediate reduction in Tongue redness that is sustained after treatment.

Gua sha releases the Exterior

Dr So taught that there are two ways to resolve sha. One is diaphoresis from a true fever (or from diaphoretic medicines) termed 'releasing the Exterior' in traditional East Asian medicine (TEAM); the other is to Gua sha. The natural mechanism for ridding the body of heat is evaporation through sweating (Thornton 1799–1800). Gua sha mimics sweating and releases the Exterior by venting Heat, moving Qi, Blood and Jin fluid, stabilizing the 'pores', the Li lining, and halting penetration of Wind, Cold, Damp or Heat. Any pathogenic factor is said to be weakened, while the body's Wei antipathogenic Qi is fortified.

Gua sha is applied to prevent onset of illness and to expedite resolution of acute illness. If already sick, the patient may get sicker for a day and then recover rather quickly. If the onset is at the earliest stage, however, penetration is often resolved without illness. The *Shang Han Lun* talks in great detail about herbal decoctions to release the Exterior through diaphoresis or therapeutic sweating. In protracted illness, weakened patients or repeated but weak diaphoresis, sha stasis may not be completely resolved. Therefore, checking for and applying Gua sha is important even when a patient reports they had fever with sweating.

Fever may also express Heat in the form of a rash or petechiae, as in measles, chicken pox, shingles or cholera. Gua sha is essential to reduce this Heat and may be applied sequentially to completely resolve Heat toxin (see Chapter 9).

Gua sha's release of the Exterior promotes a speedy resolution and rebound to health and prevents progression of illness to chronic unresolved syndromes like chronic cough, sinusitis, diarrhea or fatigue. The wisdom of 'first treat the Exterior, then the Interior' extends to all patients presenting with any Exterior signs: pain or constriction or evidence of sha upon palpation. Gua sha treatment prevents potential acute illness. It also resolves external pain and constriction shifting any chronic internal disturbance associated with it.

Gua sha resolves Blood stagnation

Cold and Wind obstruct not only the Qi but the Blood as well. The *Su Wen* states:

> A Cold Qi may lodge within the Blood of the Lo [vessels]. The Blood becomes congealed and is not able to flow into the large Jing [vessels]. The Blood and Qi are retained, unable to course through …

(Epler 1980)

> When a person is exposed to the wind, either lying down to rest or walking about, his Blood will be affected. The Blood then coagulates within the flesh and the result is numbness in the hands and the feet. When it coagulates within the pulse the Blood ceases to circulate beneficially; when the Blood coagulates within the feet, it causes pains and chills.

(Veith 1966)

Gua sha 'lets blood' within the tissue. This blood is not let from the skin, but appears as small petechiae or ecchymotic patches confirming stuck Blood at the surface. If there were no stagnation of Blood, Gua sha or any other surface frictioning would only be rubefacient, bringing blood to the surface in a pink blush. When surface frictioning reveals sha, stuck Qi and Blood have been moved.

Internal Blood stasis pain is an excess Shi pain, more intense than the pain of stuck Qi. It is described as boring, stabbing or torturous. Stuck Blood pain can be experienced on a scale of persistently bothersome to intolerable. In addition to pain, Blood stasis also impedes the new production of Blood and obstructs the dissemination of fluids throughout the body (Bensky and Barolet 1990).

Gua sha moves Blood externally and internally, promotes Blood production and improves dissemination of fluids. Proper dissemination of fluids is imperative to the all body function. Given its ability to move stuck Qi and Blood, release the Exterior, vent Heat, disseminate fluids and stimulate creation of new Blood, Gua sha becomes a relevant tool of treatment for almost any presenting disorder.

Gua sha as scraping, coining, spooning

A literal and oft heard translation of Gua sha is as scraping, and it is sometimes also known as coining or spooning. I avoid using the term 'scraping' because it misleads. Gua sha is more accurately described as instrument-assisted 'press-stroking' of a lubricated surface. Scraping implies something is removed, or scraped off, which is not the case. Scraping also implies injury, which is not the case with Gua sha. 'Coining' comes from the use of family or community coins to apply Gua sha (cao gio; Van Nguyen and Pivar 2004), 'spooning' from the use of Chinese soup spoons. These last two point to contingency: using available smooth-edged instruments to perform Gua sha in the home and the kitchen, not only in the clinic.

Introducing Gua sha to your patient: terms

A practitioner's introduction of Gua sha can influence a patient's comfort and receptivity; calm and adept technique that includes presentation will instill confidence in a patient. If a patient is familiar with traditional East Asian medical concepts then explaining that Gua sha dredges the channels, releases the Exterior, resolves Blood stagnation, vents Heat, disseminates Fluids, tonifies Blood, warms what is cold and cools what is hot, is appropriate. If a patient is more familiar with Western terminology then Gua sha can be explained as creating transitory therapeutic petechiae associated with increased surface microperfusion, increased upregulation of the genetic expression of heme oxygenase-1 (HO-1), stimulation of the immune system and evidence of pain reduction and anti-inflammatory effect that is sustained over time. Or a provider can use concepts from both models. Or, in simple terms, 'when substances become stuck function is slowed and there is often pain: Gua sha moves what is stuck and resolves pain'.

What is important to communicate is that the mechanism of Gua sha is unique and necessary in certain presentations; that Gua sha relieves pain, and that science is now able to explain some of the biology of the benefits of Gua sha. Chapter 6 details how to apply Gua sha and how to present Gua sha to a patient. A Gua sha handout can be found in Appendix A. It is recommended to give a handout explaining Gua sha every time it is performed.

References

Baerheim, A., Laerum, E., 1992. Symptomatic lower urinary tract infection induced by cooling of the feet. A controlled experimental trial. Scand J Prim Health Care 10 (2) (June), 157–160.

Bensky, D., Barolet, R., 1990. Chinese Herbal Medicine: Formulas and Strategies. Eastland Press, Seattle.

Cao, H., Han, M., Li, X., et al., 2010. Clinical research evidence of cupping therapy in china: a systematic literature. BMC Complement Altern Med 10 (1) (November 16), 70.

Chirali, I.Z., 1999. Traditional Chinese Medicine: Cupping Therapy. Churchill Livingstone, Edinburgh.

Douglas, R.G., 1969. Exposure to cold environment and rhinovirus common cold: Failure to demonstrate effect. NEJMq 279, 743.

Eccles, R., 2002. Acute cooling of the body surface and the common cold. Rhinology 40 (3) (September), 109–114.

Epler, D.C., 1980. Bloodletting in early Chinese medicine and its relation to the origin of acupuncture. Bulletin of the History of Medicine 54, 337–367.

Jinkui Yaulue Sanglun, 1987. Synopsis of Prescriptions of the Golden Chamber. New World Press, Beijing.

Johnson, C., Eccles, R., 2005. Acute cooling of the feet and the onset of common cold symptoms. Fam Pract 22 (6), 608–613.

Jun, H., 1613. Dongui Bogam: Mirror of Eastern Medicine. Korea: Medical Center for the Royal Family of the 1392–1910, Joseon Kingdom.

Kaim, S., 1756. Dissertatio inauguralis medica de frictionibus. Chipok R 1994 (trans). Kaliwodian Press, University of Vienna.

Langevin, H., 2006. Connective tissue: a body-wide signaling network? Med Hypotheses 66 (6), 1074–1077.

Langevin, H.M., Churchill, D.L., Cipolla, M.J., 2001. Mechanical signaling through connective tissue: a mechanism for the therapeutic effect of acupuncture. FASEB J 15 (12) (October), 2275–2282.

Langevin, H.M., Yandow, J.A., 2002. Relationship of acupuncture points and meridians to connective tissue planes. Anat Rec 269 (6) (15), 257–265.

Liu, F., Liu, Y.M., 1980. Chinese Medical Terminology. Commercial Press Ltd, Hong Kong.

Lowen, A.C., Mubareka, S., Steel, J., et al., 2007. Influenza virus transmission is dependent on relative humidity and temperature. PLoS pathogens 3, 1470–1476.

Manz, H., 2009. The Art of Cupping. Thieme Medical Publishers, New York and Stuttgart.

Mathews, R.H., 1931. Mathews' Chinese–English Dictionary. Harvard University Press, Cambridge, MA.

Mourtzoukou, E.G., Falagas, M.E., 2007. Exposure to cold and respiratory tract infections. Int J Tuberc Lung Dis 11 (9) (September), 938–943.

Nielsen, A., 2009. Gua sha research and the language of integrative medicine. J Bodyw Mov Ther 13 (1) (January), 63–72.

Ou, Ming., (ed.), 1988. Chinese–English Dictionary of Traditional Chinese Medicine. Guandong Science and Technology Publishing House, Hong Kong.

Sabetta, J.R., DePetrillo, P., Cipriani, R.J., et al., 2010. Serum 25-hydroxyvitamin D and the incidence of acute viral respiratory tract infections in healthy adults. PLoS One 5 (6), 11088.

Sanu, A., Eccles, R., 2008. The effects of a hot drink on nasal airflow and symptoms of common cold and flu. Rhinology 46 (4), 271–275.

Schubert, V., Perbeck, L., Schubert, P-Å., 1994. Skin microcirculatory and thermal changes in elderly subjects with early stage of pressure sores. Clin. Physiol 14 (1), 1–13.

Shang Han Lun (Treatise on Febrile Diseases Caused by Cold), 1986. New World Press, Beijing.

Thornton, R.J., 1799–1800. How Nature Increases or Rids Herself of the Animal Heat. In: The Philosophy of Medicine: Or, Medical Extracts on the Nature of Health and Disese, Including the Laws of the Animal Oeconomy, and the Doctrines of Pneumatic Medicine. Vol 2 of 5. http:galenet.galegroup.com/servlet/ECCO: Eighteenth Century Collections Online, Gale Group; 630.

Van Nguyen, Q., Pivar, M., 2004. Fourth Uncle in the Mountain. A Memoir of a Barefoot Doctor in Vietnam. St. Martin's Press, New York.

Veith, I., 1966. Huang Ti Nei Ching Su Wen (The Yellow Emperor's Classic of Internal Medicine). University of California Press, Berkeley.

Wei, Y-L., Shi Yi De Xiao Fang: Effective Formulas Tested by Physicians for Generations; 1337.

Weiger, L., 1965. Chinese Characters. Their Origin, Etymology, History, Classification and Signification. A Thorough Study from Chinese Documents. Dover Publications, New York.

Wilson, T.E., Cui, J., Zhang, R., et al., 2002. Skin cooling maintains cerebral blood flow velocity and orthostatic tolerance. J Appl Physiol 93 (1) (July), 85–91.

Wilson, T.E., Cui, J., Zhang, R., et al., 2006. Heat stress reduces cerebral blood velocity and markedly impairs orthostatic tolerance in humans. Am J Physiol Regul Integr Comp Physiol 291 (5) (November), 1443–1448.

Yang, J-s., Zhao, M-l., Wang, Y-y., et al., 2007. [Studies on treatment based on differentiation of syndromes of SHA syndrome in Sha Zhang Yu Heng. Zhonghua Yi Shi Za Zhi 37 (2) (April), 76–79.

Young, A.J., 1986. Human thermoregulatory responses to cold air are altered by repeated cold water immersion. J Appl Physiol 60, 1542–1548.

Application of Gua sha

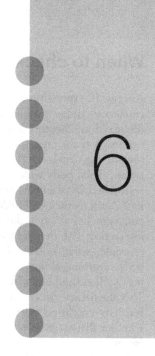

6

When to check for sha

Always. In every situation: check for sha. The body's surface connective tissue is a membrane, the Cou Li in ancient terms discussed in Chapters 3 and 4 as one of the largest and most extensive body organs, where electrical, cellular and tissue remodeling signals are thought to be responsive to mechanical forces. This 'body-wide mechanosensitive signaling network' researched by scientists today was understood by traditional East Asian medicine (TEAM) for over 2000 years in a medical paradigm based on ordinary human sensory awareness and interaction with the body, environment, health and illness. For example, when outside Cold conditions are greater than a body's warming ability, cold penetrates the membrane, stagnating Qi, Blood and Fluid (see thermogram image on book cover). This stagnation can communicate a deeper stagnation. Therefore any condition warrants checking for surface stagnation, whether that stagnation is considered a causative or coexisting factor.

Suspect sha when there is pain anywhere. Gua sha may fully or partially resolve a presenting problem; it will almost always help. In addition, the response to Gua sha adds important diagnostic and prognostic information.

How to check for sha: pressing palpation

Dr So discovered a way to palpate for the presence of sha surface stagnation. When examining a patient and palpating for Ah Shi or trigger points, make an impression in the flesh with several fingers of the hand (see Figure 6.1, Plate 1). Then quickly pull your hand away. If you can see the places where your fingers pressed and those areas are slow to fade to normal flesh color there is sha (Figure 6.2, Plate 2). The pressure from your fingers blanches the flesh, that is, displaces Blood. If there is a smooth flow of Qi and Blood in the flesh, blanching will disappear right away. If the blanching disappears gradually, it means the Blood is slow to return. This indicates the Blood is obstructed or congealed, which is evidence of sha. Simply put, pressing palpation causing blanching that is slow to fade confirms the presence of sha.

If a patient presents with pain that is helped by massage but the pain returns immediately after, it is a good indication of sha. If a patient has a sudden stiff neck, wakes with a body kink or reports pain that comes and goes, think sha. Chronic pain problems almost always involve sha.

Where to check for sha

This is as simple as it is important. If the presenting disorder resides in or affects the upper body or upper extremities, check for sha at the upper back, neck and shoulders. If the problem is in the Internal Organs, check the back for areas of tension, Ah Shi points and sha. Treat the upper back for the Upper Jiao problems, the middle back for Middle Jiao problems, and the lower back for lower abdomen problems. It is

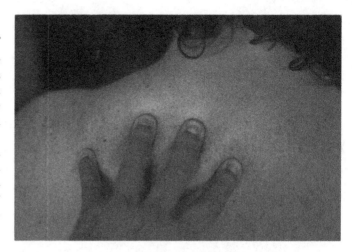

Figure 6.1 • Pressing palpation • Checking for sha, the practitioner presses her fingers onto the flesh and immediately withdraws them (see also Plate 1). See Figure 6.2.

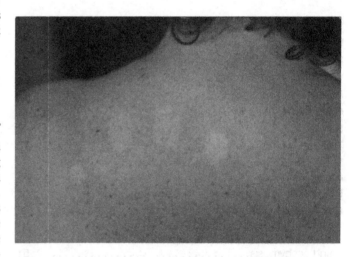

Figure 6.2 • Blanching that is slow to fade • Pressing palpation (Figure 6.1) that results in blanching that is slow to fade indicates sluggish surface perfusion, or sha 'Blood stasis' in surface tissue (see Plates 1, 2 and 3).

by way of the Path of Qi that a Jiao's Internal Organs are affected by treatment of the back (see Figure 3.1).

For problems of the lower extremities, hips and pelvis, check for trigger points and sha at the lower back, sacrum and buttocks (see Figures 6.3 and 6.4).

For problems along the back itself, check the entire back for sha, as above can affect below, and below can affect above. For example, if the presenting pain is at the upper back, treat the site but also check the mid-back and the low back, even the back of the legs. If the problem is in the mid-back, treat the site but also check the upper and lower back. If the problem is at the lower back, needle and Gua sha at the low back but first check and treat accordingly the mid-back, upper back and even legs for trigger points and sha.

For musculoskeletal problems a general rule of thumb, or palpating finger, is to check along the channel or meridian that

Figure 6.3 • Horizontal Path of Qi • The Upper, Middle, and Lower Jiao with the Back Shu points and their associated organs.

Upper Jiao
Disorders affecting the head, neck, chest, Heart, Lungs and upper extremities.

Middle Jiao
Disorders affecting the Stomach, Spleen, Liver, Gall Bladder and trunk.

Lower Jiao
Disorders affecting the Kidneys, Bladder, Intestines, genitals, reproductive system, pelvic region and lower extremities.

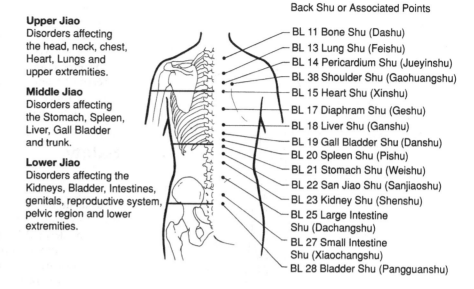

Back Shu or Associated Points

- BL 11 Bone Shu (Dashu)
- BL 13 Lung Shu (Feishu)
- BL 14 Pericardium Shu (Jueyinshu)
- BL 38 Shoulder Shu (Gaohuangshu)
- BL 15 Heart Shu (Xinshu)
- BL 17 Diaphram Shu (Geshu)
- BL 18 Liver Shu (Ganshu)
- BL 19 Gall Bladder Shu (Danshu)
- BL 20 Spleen Shu (Pishu)
- BL 21 Stomach Shu (Weishu)
- BL 22 San Jiao Shu (Sanjiaoshu)
- BL 23 Kidney Shu (Shenshu)
- BL 25 Large Intestine Shu (Dachangshu)
- BL 27 Small Intestine Shu (Xiaochangshu)
- BL 28 Bladder Shu (Pangguanshu)

Figure 6.4 • Horizontal Path of Qi • The Upper, Middle and Lower Jiao with the Front Mu points and their associated organs. The Yuan Qi can be accessed at CV 17 at the Upper Jiao, CV 12 at the Middle Jiao and CV 6 or CV 4 at the Lower Jiao.

Upper Jiao
Disorders affecting the head, neck, chest, Heart, Lungs and upper extremities.

Middle Jiao
Disorders affecting the Stomach, Spleen, Liver, Gall Bladder and trunk

Lower Jiao
Disorders affecting the Kidneys, Bladder, Intestines, genitals, reproductive system, pelvic region and lower extremities.

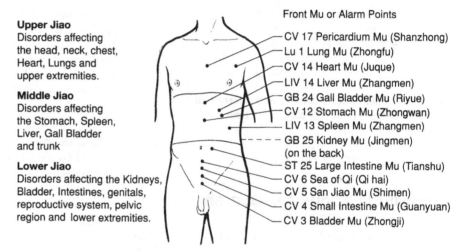

Front Mu or Alarm Points

- CV 17 Pericardium Mu (Shanzhong)
- Lu 1 Lung Mu (Zhongfu)
- CV 14 Heart Mu (Juque)
- LIV 14 Liver Mu (Zhangmen)
- GB 24 Gall Bladder Mu (Riyue)
- CV 12 Stomach Mu (Zhongwan)
- LIV 13 Spleen Mu (Zhangmen)
- GB 25 Kidney Mu (Jingmen) (on the back)
- ST 25 Large Intestine Mu (Tianshu)
- CV 6 Sea of Qi (Qi hai)
- CV 5 San Jiao Mu (Shimen)
- CV 4 Small Intestine Mu (Guanyuan)
- CV 3 Bladder Mu (Zhongji)

passes through an area of pain or stagnation, as well as directly at or near the site itself. Figures 6.5 and 6.6 illustrate this.

Consider areas where there is known referred pain or a known effect from Organ disharmony. For example, with eye problems one would check the upper back and neck because constriction of Qi or Blood in the upper back and neck can affect the head and eyes. It might also be wise to check the area of Liver and Kidney Shu points at the back, since the eyes open to the Liver and sight is influenced by the Kidneys. For ear problems check the Kidney area of the back as well as the Gall Bladder and Triple Burner (San Jiao) meridian paths for Ah Shi points and sha. For nose problems, treat the upper back and neck, the entire Lung area at the back (the nostrils open to the Lungs) as well as the BL 20 area of the back (the Spleen owns the nose). And so on.

Keep in mind that the connective tissue is concentrated at the body channels/meridians. Local treatment for a problem is propagated internally via the Path of Qi; distal treatment is propagated as well by the channels associated with concentrations of connective tissue planes.

Risk in ignoring sha

Unresolved sha leaves a patient vulnerable to tightness, tissue strain, pain, and illness, and/or their recovery from illness is protracted and incomplete. Blood and Fluids stagnating at the surface membrane mitigate circulation of warmth and Wei Qi. Hence the Exterior is porous to penetration by Cold or Wind. There is potential for chronic weakness or fatigue. Pain resulting from stagnation will persist until the stagnation is resolved. Chronic pain leads to decreased activity and compromised range of motion. Moreover, other forms of manual intervention may feel good in the moment but result in more pain and deter a patient from seeking further care.

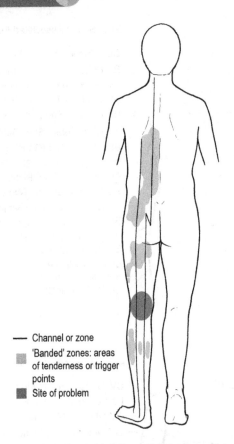

— Channel or zone

■ 'Banded' zones: areas of tenderness or trigger points

■ Site of problem

Figure 6.5 • Palpate for tightness and referred pain on the channels that pass through an area of pain • Back, low back and hip areas shown are often reactive in knee problems, for example. Gua sha can be applied to the back and buttocks for relief of knee pain (see also Plate 12).

Contraindications for Gua sha

It is inappropriate to apply Gua sha directly to an area that has just been injured, where there is bruising or abrasion. As an injury heals, if pain remains then look for sha.

Do not apply Gua sha when there is sunburn, rash or a break in the skin. If a bleeding technique is required at a rash site, such as in the case of eczema, cupping may be used. Gua sha should not be done over pimples or moles (see Figures 6.7 and 6.8). A mole or pimple can be covered by a finger of the practitioner's other hand and the area around the site can be Gua sha-ed. Figure 6.7 shows a practitioner doing Gua sha while protecting a mole with the other hand.

Gua sha should not be applied to the abdomen of a pregnant woman. Gua sha should be applied with care to extremely Deficient patients or not at all. However, Gua sha is indicated in most cases of Deficiency.

It is not necessary to apply Gua sha if it has just been done on a patient. The petechiae should have completely disappeared before considering Gua sha at a site.

Gua sha is not contraindicated in diabetes, or in patients taking anticoagulant medication who have a stable INR (international normalized ratio) or who have blood thinning disorders like Von Willebrand's disease (Nielsen 2002). If a provider is concerned, application may be applied over a small area to observe the petechiae and ecchymosis appearance. With Gua sha, as with all bodywork, transmission of bloodborne pathogens is prevented by following safety recommendations.

Safety

The most prevalent complication reported in the Western medical literature for Gua sha is the misattribution of the transitory therapeutic petechiae and ecchymosis as a burn, bruise or dermatitis caused by abuse, pseudo-abuse, battery, pseudo-battery or torture (discussed in Chapter 2). To prevent misinterpretation of sha petechiae, it is recommended to provide a patient with a handout that explains Gua sha (see Appendix A). It is also the case that some actual complications may not be widely recognized or may not have been reported yet in the literature. Gua sha instruments are commonly used on different patients. In certain cases, after repeated press-stroking, the lubricant on the instrument can take on a pinkish tone suggesting extravasated blood cells may cross the skin surface with potential risk of bloodborne pathogen exposure. Preventing risk of exposure to bloodborne pathogens with Gua sha can be accomplished by (Nielsen et al. 2012):

* gloving both hands for Gua sha procedure
* using disposable press-stroking devices, i.e. a single-use smooth-edged metal cap (see Figure 6.9 below); note that used Gua sha instruments must be cleaned and disinfected even if intended for disposal
* cleaning immediately after use with soap and water, then sterilizing or disinfecting metal or stainless steel instruments designed for re-use with a high-level, registered hospital-grade disinfectant[1]
* decanting lubricant into disposable treatment-sized containers to prevent cross-contamination, or using lotion from a pump dispenser as lubricant
* following safe sequencing of palpation, gloving, needling, use of lubricant, application of procedure and clean-up.

Press-stroking devices that are made of materials such as horn or bone are not suitable for heat or chemical sterilization and are therefore no longer appropriate for clinical use.

Treating infants and children

Gua sha is very effective in children, particularly because kids tend toward Excess and Gua sha is so effective at venting heat and resolving Excess. Children are most often treated for acute illness, fever, respiratory problems, cough, bronchitis or wheeze

---

[1]Professional Disposables International (http://www.pdipdi.com) makes alcohol-based germicidal disposable wipes (Super Sani-Cloth, purple top) that are bactericidal, tuberculocidal, and virudical, tested to be effective against 26 microorganisms including TB, Influenza A (H1N1) and MRSA. Wiping the outside and inside of the instrument is required, and drying for at least 2 minutes. If patient exposure to the presence of dried chemical disinfectant is a concern, then flushing the instrument with clean water after disinfection and air drying is recommended.

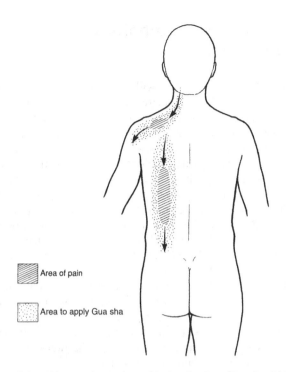

Area of pain

Area to apply Gua sha

Figure 6.6 • 'Above, through and below' rule • Sha should be raised 'above and end below' the trigger point or area of pain while keeping each stroke line from 4–6 inches in length, completely raising sha at a stroke line before moving to begin the next stroke line.

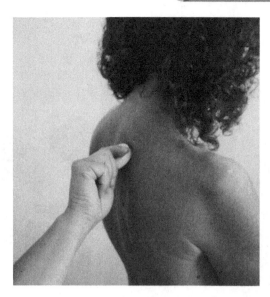

Figure 6.8 • Improper procedure • The practitioner is failing to cover and protect a mole that could be disturbed by Gua sha. Also the angle of the Gua sha tool is not ideal: the hand holding the tool should be touching the skin as well as the tool.

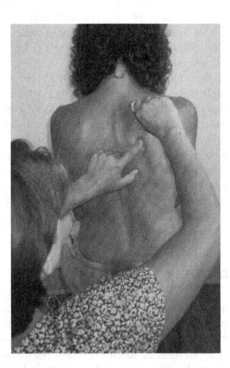

Figure 6.7 • The practitioner covers the mole with her finger while applying Gua sha above and below it. This prevents damage to the mole. Any pimple or eruption should be protected in the same way.

associated with asthma or reactive airways, and also for digestive problems.

Always treat a child in the presence of a parent or responsible guardian. Have the parent watch while you are applying Gua sha and explain while applying. Always provide a handout. Check in with the child frequently as to pressure and comfort. Watch their expressions and body language.

If treating an infant or toddler, have the parent lay on the table face up and the child lay chest down on the parent. Have the parent remove the child's shirt. Nursing infants can nurse if they like. Apply rather bland lubricant with a slow light massage. Apply Gua sha lightly, smoothly but still with closely repeated press-stroking. Be sure to bury the instrument within hand contact as detailed below.

Gua sha just until the sha breaks the surface. This is enough to resolve stagnation in a young child and will interrupt an asthma attack and alter the course of bronchitis, croup, even whooping cough. If the child is older, continue for a few strokes past the first appearance of petechiae. Typically it will be at this point that the child will start to move away, scrunch up their shoulders or wince. Take that as a cue to move to the next stroke line. Proceeding in this way, the child will allow the treatment.

Tools for Gua sha: round, smooth-edged instrument and lubricant

Historically any smooth-edged instrument was suitable. In Asia common soup spoons and coins were used, or Gua sha instruments were fashioned from jade, or cow or

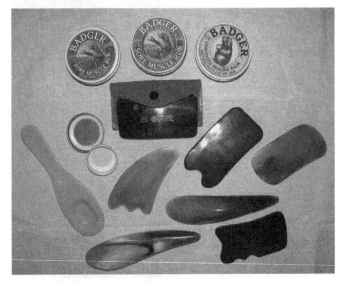

Figure 6.9 • Tools • Gua sha is applied with a smooth round-edged instrument. In China this may be a soup spoon or slice of water buffalo horn specifically made for this purpose but cannot be repeatedly heat or chemically disinfected/sterilized (see Safety guidelines above). Some tools are fashioned with curves to move over joints . A simple metal lid with a rounded lip is the most comfortable tool I have found (center left) and can be disposed of after one use. The warming, cooling and neutral lubricants shown are vegetable-based and made by Badger Balm. (www.badgerbalm.com)

water-buffalo horn. Dr So taught us to use the metal lid from a Vicks VapoRub jar, which are now plastic and not appropriate. Any metal lid that has a rounded lip can be used, though a thinner gauge is more suitable. The smoothness allows the object to press into the flesh and fascia without breaking the surface skin (see Figure 6.9). Moreover, it is easier to use a simple lid because it can be easily discarded. Baby food jar lids are not recommended because they do not have a true lip and are too blunt. While some practitioners like the notion of a jade or water buffalo instrument, they are also blunt and the blunter an instrument is the more discomfort to the patient.

It is necessary to use something to lubricate the skin. The lubricant is applied to the surface, not to the instrument. Peanut oil was commonly used; some doctors in China have fashioned oil concentrates using blood-moving herbs.

Dr So used Vick's VapoRub because he liked the viscosity and the damp-resolving penetration of camphor. More importantly, he thought that most people in the United States had good associations with Vicks and that familiarity would relax the patient. However, Vicks VapoRub is made from Vaseline, which is a petroleum product. It is fine in a pinch, as is simple peanut or olive oil. The company Badger Balm makes preparations of oils, beeswax and organic essential oils in various combinations: warming, pungent, cooling, and mild. These preparations serve as more environmentally friendly lubricants and are available in many health food stores, sports and camp shops, and even some pharmacies.

Preparation: morphology and palpation

While a discursive interview will establish a cognitive rapport, palpation establishes a somatic rapport that also tunes the patient in and connects the patient and provider. While taking a proper history and clarifying presenting symptoms, including pain and sensation, palpate areas directly or indirectly related to the presenting problem and inquire if there is pain while feeling for tightness. Experienced practitioners will know how to look at problem's morphology: the location, quality and mutability of its nature. Inexperienced practitioners can discover just as much by searching and asking. Repalpation after treatment will help to clarify change and improvement, so this first step is crucial to focus treatment within and beyond each session.

Gua sha can be used without acupuncture needling. It can be done by anyone, anywhere and does not require acupuncture treatment. For acupuncturists it is better to apply needles before Gua sha to make the treatment most effective. However, there is widespread use of Gua sha in the domestic sector without attendant acupuncture needling.

An acupuncturist will want to needle main points in an area and nearby or related trigger points. Trigger points alone should not be needled absent the appropriate main points that are the primary conduits of channel propagation. Dispersive technique is often used: needling to obtain 'de qi' several or more times. De qi involves a particular sensation at a point, sometimes fasciculation, sometimes a needle grasp, a trajecting of sensation, and a sense of release. A patient new to acupuncture will benefit from fewer points and milder stimulation at first.

While needling is thought to move Qi, when Blood is stuck, as in the presence of sha, moving Qi can congest an area more, as in the case of increased pain after acupuncture or massage alone. Needle stimulation congesting the Qi facilitates the expression of sha from Gua sha.

I do not show a patient a picture of Gua sha before applying for one simple reason: most people have no relationship to appearance of petechiae except in relation to injuries like road rash, illnesses that include surface rashes, or a hickey or love bite when young. None are great associations. I explain Gua sha as I am doing it, I make sure the patient is comfortable at every step, I repalpate to discover change or areas that need more work and when I am done I ask the patient to move and let me know how they feel. Then I show them their own sha. Patients do not care how the sha looks because the change in symptoms is so dramatic.

How to apply Gua sha

Gua sha is repeated, closely timed, unidirectional press-stroking with a smooth-edged instrument over a lubricated area of the body. After palpation, identification of an area to be treated and application of lubricant, place the smooth-edged instrument just above the area to be Gua sha-ed. The instrument edge should be at a low angle to the skin (see Figure 6.10). Then move down the area with a moderate amount of

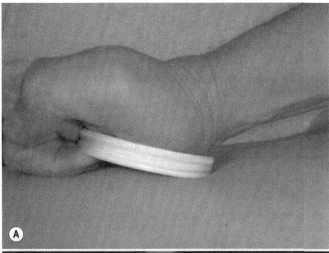

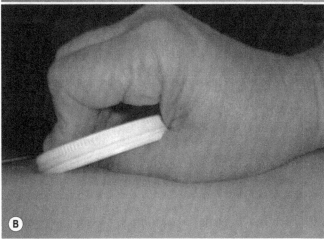

Figure 6.10 • Proper angle and correct use of instrument
The instrument moves over the surface of the skin as it is pressed into the flesh: **A** Press-stroking right to left using pressure from the heel of the hand; **B** Press-stroking left to right using the fingers to press). Closely timed, repeated unidirectional press stroking produces transitory therapeutic petechiae and ecchymosis. Note contact in addition to the instrument, hand to flesh. This hand contact while stroking 'blurs' the sensation of the instrument (Nielsen 2009).

pressure, pressing the smooth edge into the flesh. If the stroke is moving away from the provider, the fingers lead touching the flesh, and the heel of the hand applies the pressure to the back of the instrument. If the stroke is toward the provider, the extended thumb makes contact with the flesh, and the fingers apply pressure to the front of the instrument (see Figure 6.10). Note in either direction, there are two areas of contact with the patient: an aspect of the hand and the edge of the instrument. The sensation of the instrument pressing into the fascia is blurred by the touch of the provider's hand.

Typically it takes anywhere from six to 15 strokes to raise sha. It can take as little as four strokes or more than 15 depending on the depth of the sha and the pressure used. One can do Gua sha with very light pressure; this might require more strokes than if done with more pressure but the sha will come up. Or Gua sha can be applied with more pressure and fewer

strokes may be needed. It should not cause pain to the patient, though it may be slightly uncomfortable as the sha is near complete expression.

A stroke should only be 4–6 inches long. Strokes are repeated at a stroke line raising all of the sha before moving to adjacent tissue.

'Above, through and below' rule

Always start the stroke above the area to be treated. When Gua sha is complete, sha should extend to below the area of interest (see Figure 6.6). This is the 'above, through and below' rule. Note that an area of treatment might be quite large and the rule does not mean the stroke itself should extend beyond 4–6 inches. A stroke that is too long discourages expression of sha petechiae. 'Above, through and below' means that collectively the sets of stroke lines will include above, through and below the area of interest.

Appearance of transitory therapeutic petechiae and ecchymosis

Gua sha intentionally creates transitory therapeutic petechiae and ecchymosis. All the petechiae will gradually blend into areas of ecchymosis. There is little discomfort for most patients if done correctly using pressure agreeable to the patient.

Students new to Gua sha typically do not apply enough pressure and do not thoroughly raise sha. Even after petechiae begin to appear one must continue in the stroke line until all the sha is up. You will know that all the sha is up when continued strokes no longer increase the number of petechiae or change the color of them.

Then there are other students who over stroke, applying too much pressure or too many strokes, resulting in excess ecchymosis (Plate 24). As with any technique, practice and with different kinds of subjects will help develop an adeptness in and confidence with Gua sha. One does not expect to see lines of sha that would match meridian lines, and producing stripes is just incomplete technique. The end picture should be as if an area were completely painted.

The transitory therapeutic petechiae and ecchymosis of Gua sha do not signify bruising. Bruising represents damage to an area of tissue from a blow or shear force. With Gua sha blood cells are extravasated from the capillary bed of surface tissue without damage to the capillaries themselves (Nielsen et al. 2007). The sha that emerges as petechiae then immediately changes to ecchymosis and then begins to fade. These changes represent function within the circulatory bed, the movement and removal of the extravasated blood and resulting anti inflammatory and immune stimulation (see Chapter 3). For most patients the sha completely fades in one to three days, whereas the damage to tissue related to bruising takes longer to resolve.

Sequence of stroke lines

As in the sequencing of pulse taking, it is recommended that a consistent sequence be followed whenever performing Gua sha. With the pulse a practitioner proceeds by feeling first for the entire quality of the pulse, then maybe the rate, then perhaps the individual Organ qualities starting with the inch pulse. When applying Gua sha establish a method, a sequence order, and stick to it.

The recommended order is to start at the Du mo, complete Gua sha at the midline of the back, and then proceed to the Hua tuo jiaji area lateral to the spine, then to the first Bladder channel, and then to the more lateral Bladder channel (see Figure 6.11). Keep the strokes even. Do not dig at a spot. Follow the contour of the body down and laterally. Strokes at the occiput go up into the hairline. Follow the rule of 'above, through and below' discussed above. Avoid making stripes: complete Gua sha evenly over an area.

For problems with extremities, Gua sha is applied to the appropriate area of the torso, back or front, and then into the extremity. The same holds for the head, which is an extremity. First Gua sha the upper body, then, for example, at the scalp for migraine or cluster headaches (Plates 24 and 25).

What to tell the patient before, during and after gua sha

Below is a quick reference of points to include when using Gua sha in practice while discussing with the patient.

GUA SHA IN PRACTICE: POINTS TO INCLUDE WHILE TREATING AND TALKING WITH YOUR PATIENT

INTRODUCING GUA SHA: PAIN AND TEMPERATURE SENSATION

Pain: does the patient have pain, where and when? 'Does it hurt when I palpate here...or here?'

'Does the area feel cold or hot to the touch?' Does the patient report cold or hot at an area?

'Does heat comfort the pain?' This means the pain is related to cold.

'Does cooling comfort the pain?' This means the pain involves heat or inflammation.

'Pressing palpation shows me where there is sha.'

'Gua sha is a technique used to release the effects of Elements like, Cold, Heat, and Wind in the surface of the body. Cold acts in the body like it acts outside: it slows things down and causes things to collect and congest. When things congest there is pain. Gua sha is a treatment for pain and congestion'

COMMUNICATE WHILE APPLYING GUA SHA

Explain by saying: 'This technique is called Gua sha. Now I am going over the surface with a smooth edge. Where the blood is stuck in the subcutaneous fascia, it comes up little red dots that look like a hickey. That fades in 2–4 days.'

Check in with the patient in terms of amount of pressure when applying Gua sha. Just as the sha is near complete expression there may be discomfort. Let the patient know they can say: 'stop, lighter, or more pressure is OK'.

How does the treated area feel?

Does the patient have pain now: 'How does it feel when I palpate this area'?

'Is there tenderness, warmth, cold?'
This information helps direct treatment.

INTRODUCE PATIENT TO THE CHARACTERISTICS OF THEIR SHA

Show the patient their sha in a mirror and provide them with a handout explaining Gua sha (see Appendix A). Explain that the sha often appears more concentrated at the site of pain. If the sha is dark it indicates a longer-standing problem. If it is light, it may be fairly recent. The brightness of the sha begins to fade as the practitioner lightly massages the area. How fast the sha fades over days points to the strength of the patient's circulation.

RECOMMENDATIONS TO THE PATIENT AT THE END OF THE SESSION

'Avoid exposure to the sun and wind until the sha is gone. Keep the area covered.'

If activity has been limited, 'increase it slowly so that capacity may be rebuilt.'

The pain may be gone but the area may still be weak and unstable.

'Avoid excessive cold, sour or salty food or fluid. Cold causes contraction, which makes pain worse. Sour is the flavor of the Liver, which owns the nerves. Sour flavors increase pain and nervousness. Salty foods tend to increase swelling and worsen pain.'

FOLLOW-UP

Ask the patient to keep track of how they feel in subsequent days to fill you in at the next appointment. This is the most important information whether seemingly positive or negative, listen with equanimity.

'Did the pain resolve, return? Is it as intense as before? If the pain is episodic, are the episodes as frequent?' Is the patient able to do more before tiring? Is the patient doing too much too soon? Answers to these questions are important guides to completely resolve a problem.

Stop clause

Patients have varying levels of tolerance. Some can sleep through Gua sha; others find it uncomfortable, a few impossible. I have found that a patient will be on the verge of saying 'stop' just as the surfacing sha is almost complete. The more fearful a patient is of the technique or in life generally, the more uncomfortable any therapeutic 'push' will be.

Communicate clearly about the 'stop clause'. This means that the patient can moan, groan, swear or express any other cathartic vocal release. But if they want you to take a break, then you expect to hear 'stop'.

Sometimes patients who can't say 'no' in their lives will needlessly endure discomfort during treatment and find it difficult to ask for an adjustment in pressure. Just the practice of saying 'stop' and taking breaks during Gua sha can be a useful reframe response to pain. And for the practitioner, 'stop' means stop. Do not proceed without the patient's consent.

Completing treatment

When Gua sha is complete, wipe the oils off the skin with paper towels. Lightly massage and repalpate the area of hand numbness, who could once again feel his hands directly after Gua sha: 'Now that's what I'm talkin' about'. Or the 40-year-old patient who had severe back pain after a blow from a bat during a Brooklyn mugging in his teenage years, immediately resolved from Gua sha: 'How come no one ever told me about this?' There are immediate reactions to Gua sha. Gua sha provides immediate relief, comfort and warmth and patients will say they don't care how it looks. However, I still show the patient their sha with a mirror while discussing recommendations and fielding questions. Gua sha can frighten patients and their loved ones at home, even if the patient feels better. A practitioner is a teacher as well as a provider and must teach about the technique when performing it, and provide a handout with explanation (see Appendix A). It should be mentioned that patients can have an emotional even angry reaction to the lifting of long standing pain. It is important to maintain a compassionate presence for emotional reactions but neither solicit nor rebuff any expression of emotion. Allow things to transpire.

The color of sha, how quickly it surfaces or fades is diagnostic and prognostic, and is discussed below.

Leaking

Another aphorism from traditional medicine to 'stop leaking' is obvious when a patient is losing blood, or fluid, but less so when the leaking is of the Qi, Jing or Shen. For these too, before attempting restoration 'first stop the leaks'. This applies to excessive menstrual bleeding, sweating, urine, exercise, sex, work, illness, stress, drugs like pot, cocaine, amphetamines, any lack of sleep, and ongoing stress from work or relationships. A patient's situation may necessitate referral to psychotherapy.

For the overworked or depleted patient, excessive coffee drinking is like having a little hole in the bottom of their boat. There is a constant tiny leak. As a diuretic taken daily, excessive coffee depletes the body of water-soluble nutrients including B vitamins and vitamin C, as well as minerals such as calcium and magnesium. This will exacerbate any painful condition as well as fatigue the patient, increasing the desire for more coffee. Because caffeine occupies adenosine receptor sites, and adenosine relaxes muscles so they may return to and maintain their resting length, consistent caffeine intake can lead to muscle strain, tears and contractions, causing and retarding healing of injuries. Caffeine also contributes to hot flush disorder in menopausal women. The diuretic activity severely depletes the Yin, which is already in decline at this age. Depletion of Yin unroots the Yang, which flashes chaotically up and out to the surface. Soon the unchanneled Yang also becomes depleted and the patient becomes cold between hot flushes.

Increased urination frequency abuses the Kidneys and weakens Yang areas associated with the Kidneys, such as the back and knees. It is strongly recommended that caffeine be removed from the diet altogether in these conditions. Chronic painful conditions are more likely to resolve with treatment when provider and patient have stopped the leaks. After recovery, coffee can be resumed in moderation.

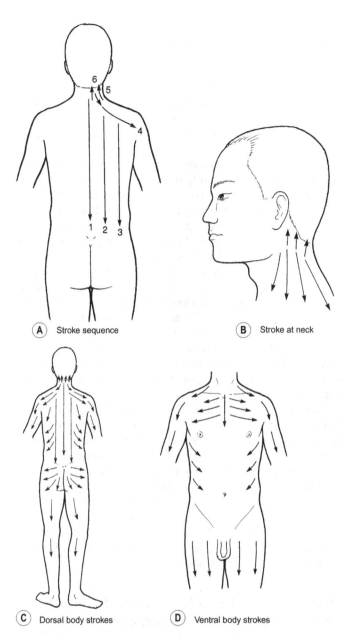

Figure 6.11 • Gua sha stroke-line sequence • A Back: proceed from midline outward. **B** Neck: strokes go down except for upper neck where strokes go into hairline. **C** Dorsal body strokes go down. At the lateral back the strokes follow the body contour. **D** Ventral body strokes follow the body contour. The lines indicated in these images are to suggest direction of stroking for Gua sha, and not meant to suggest that Gua sha results in 'stripes'.

interest; ask the patient to move around with attention to the presenting problem. Discuss the points under Recommendations to the patient, above. A point of clarification to providers: I am often asked if the direction of stroking is specific to disorders, or supposed direction of Qi within a channel. Gua sha should be applied along the muscles regardless of channel direction, that is, in whatever way is easiest to raise the sha. After Gua sha, light massage and repalpation can address the channel direction if desired.

Part of completing the treatment is assessing the impact on the patient. To quote a well-known jazz pianist I treated for

Color, appearance and resolution of sha

The color of sha, how quickly it surfaces and how fast it fades gives the practitioner information. If the sha surfaces quickly, it is more recent; if hard to raise, it is thought to be deeper and more long-standing.

Sha is blood extravasation and so is always red. Yet there are variations in the color of sha and these are of interest. The color of sha is used to corroborate other signs and symptoms, and not as a single determinant outside the context of other signs and symptoms. Images of the color of sha are shown in the Plate Section:

- Bright red sha may indicate Wind Heat, more recent penetration (Plate 21).
- Pale red sha can corroborate Blood deficiency (Plate 6).
- Dark red sha reflects more intense heat stasis (Plate 9).
- Purple or black sha reflects very old stagnation (Plate 9).
- Blue sha relates to cold, Liver Qi constraint or Heart problems (Plate 7).
- Brown sha, similar to dry brown menstrual blood, is associated with Yin deficiency and is sometimes seen in diabetes (Plate 10).
- Yellow pigmentation is normal to sha fading, and is indicative of bilirubin and biliverdin (see 2-day-old sha, Plate 5)
- Sha for person of color also appears as petechiae that redden the skin (Plate 4).

Fading

If the sha fades quickly, the circulation is good. If more slowly, then that area is perhaps not so well served by the Blood. This may be due to insufficient Qi, Blood or Yang. As sha fades, it becomes lighter, perhaps a bit brown, and finally the surface may appear yellowish before sha hyperpigmentation disappears. This discoloration is the effect of bilirubin and biliverdin reflecting the breakdown of hemoglobin that in part produces the anti inflammatory and immune protective action (see Chapter 3) (Plate 5).

Relief

Assessing Gua sha in acute disorders: what to expect from treatment

If an acute disorder is of recent onset, Gua sha can extricate the surface stasis and pathogen with comfortable easing of symptoms. If the onset is less recent with more severe stasis, Gua sha may create a crisis: that is, a temporary worsening of symptoms as pathogenic stasis occupying different levels resolves (Nielsen, 1996). Changing Tongue signs will correspond with the trajectory of healing, indicating the depth and direction of an acute disorder (see Chapter 7).

For example, applying Gua sha at the very beginning of a cold or flu, may prevent any further respiratory symptoms. If the intervention occurs somewhere in the middle of the illness, fever or pain may actually intensify, and then decline over the next 24–48 hours. If the intervention is given at the recovery stage of an acute illness when there is no longer fever, but palpation (press and blanche technique) and Tongue examination (red with or without red points) reveal residual pathogenic heat and sha, then Gua sha essentially clears what is left and is comforting, lifting the fatigue associated with fever sequelae. There would be no worsening of symptoms.

Acute pain is most often associated with a Shi Excess condition that responds differently from a Deficient one: Excess is associated with more sha. The sha is deep in color: red, purple or black. The darker the sha, the longer the Blood has been stuck. Gua sha resolves the pain immediately and any associated internal pain is likewise affected. Relief is pronounced and range of motion immediately expanded.

Sha always represents stasis which is an Excess; sha related to Deficiency can be red and even replete, but is less so than in Excess. In Deficiency the sha can appear throughout an area but not be abundant. It can be dark or light but is thin-looking. At root may be Deficient Blood or that Qi and Blood do not move well and stagnate. Pain associated with Deficiency is dull, achy and lingering. Deficiency pain also responds to Gua sha immediately due to the resolution of stasis, but gradually some pain, which may be slight, may return.

Dull lingering pain that recurs points to Deficiency. It shows that even with a resolution of stasis, the new Blood-return to the area does not supply enough warmth or nutrients. The muscles hurt once again and are, in a sense, starving. Gua sha can be applied sequentially, but further evaluation and treatment is required to tonify (Bu) and supplement Qi and Blood through food, adjustment of activity, acupuncture and herbs. A provider might ask what and when does this patient eat? What hours do they keep? How much do they work and doing what? Does behavior represent a kind of 'leaking'? Or is there a hypofunctional problem at root?

Assessing Gua sha in chronic disorders; what to expect from treatment

Patients have relationships with their chronic disorders and the common expectation is that chronic disorders are slow to change, with regard to the patient's presenting complaints as well as indicators such as Tongue. Most chronic disorders have features of stasis, and features of Deficiency with hypo- or hyperfunction. In what way the stasis yields to Gua sha, and how deeply that movement reaches into the Interior enlightens prognosis. How much a condition has the potential to change can often be sensed in the first treatment. Gua sha is an essential tool to shift not only the stasis symptoms but to create the possibility of change. This can be experienced firsthand within the session, and can serve to break the stalemate often seen in chronicity.

Treating a chronic disorder over time requires continually checking for sha stasis, and reapplying Gua sha as needed at least every two weeks. But if, for example, a patient presents a week after Gua sha treatment with symptoms of sha, questions must be asked regarding their behavior and in relation to

Wei Qi function. Does the patient sleep with some clothing or are they exposed to night chill; do they drink wine or other alcohol daily? Is the patient exposed to air conditioning? To what extent is their Wei Qi functioning, and in what way might it be challenged.

If a patient with a chronic problem has Gua sha, say, weekly or biweekly the provider will notice that the sha lightens, that is, typically early applications of Gua sha result in dark or very red sha. Over time as the stasis resolves and the heat is vented the sha that does appear is lighter in color, a fresher red. The features of stasis, including pain, resolve as well.

In chronic or acute disorders there can be responses that are between an extreme Deficiency and Excess. The Excess aspect is most responsive to Gua sha in the short term. The patient feels great, the provider feels adept. But this should not deter the use of Gua sha in Deficiency, where Gua sha can not only relieve stagnation but support creation of new Blood. Gua sha is absolutely indicated in Deficient conditions, in weak patients or patients who are menstruating. This is a common question in Gua sha seminars, but not so much from the perspective of TEAM. The timing, term, amount and quality of Blood at menstruation is informative for TEAM. Menstruation should not be considered by nature a state or stage of debilitation. For an interesting discussion on sources of taboos related to menstruation see *The Woman in the Body* (Martin 1987).

What follows are details as to the proper position and technique for application of Gua sha for conditions specific to areas of the body. *Gua sha: Step-by-Step*, a teaching video/DVD in English or German, is recommended as a visual aid to proper application of Gua sha (Nielsen 2002).

Treating the upper back, neck, shoulders and head

Position

The rule for Gua sha positioning is that the area to be treated should be exposed but relaxed. If a pain is experienced only in a certain position or movement, attempt to situate the patient close to the position that elicits the pain while keeping the area relaxed. Seat the patient with their arms relaxed in their lap. If the arms are raised to brace against a table or back of a chair, the muscles of upper back and neck bundle together, greatly reducing their availability to proper palpation and to Gua sha (see Figure 6.12 for correct and incorrect positioning). Patients will often automatically raise their arms for the support of something to lean on. This can indicate stress, fatigue in the back and or a Deficiency of the Central Qi that is engaged when holding the body erect.

I have the patient sit facing the treatment table. I double over a pillow, placing it between them and the table. Their hands remain in their lap and the pillow gives them some cushioning as they lean forward against the table. I place a

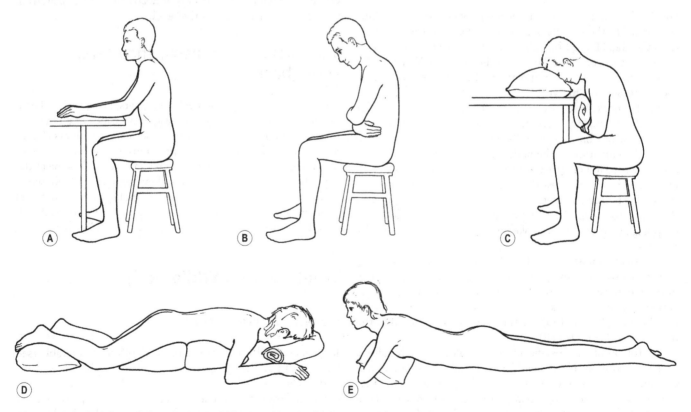

Figure 6.12 • For Gua sha to neck, shoulders and upper back • A Incorrectly seated: arms are raised onto table. **B** Correctly seated: hands are resting in lap, head tilted forward. **C** Correctly seated: leaning forward against table with hands resting in lap; head and torso are supported by pillows. **D** Correctly prone: back is supported, neck is relaxed. Good for treatment of entire dorsal body. **E** Incorrectly prone: because the back is arched, neck is tightened.

smaller, firmer support under the forehead. In this position, unlike any other, the areas of the neck and upper back are exposed but relaxed. The patient is not having to hold themselves up; they are supported.

Body Support Systems (www.bodysupport.com) makes a Body Cushion that patients can lie on in a prone position. With this device, the upper back and neck can be accessed at the same time as mid back, lower back, hip and legs. (see Figure 6.12D).

Technique: Gua sha to upper back

First treat the spine or Governing Vessel Du mo (see Figure 6.11). The skin over the spine should be relaxed, not taut. Flatten the instrument considerably and stroke lightly. Complete this line before moving laterally right or left. Follow the sequence in Figure 6.11A: the Hua tuo line, then the first Bladder channel (1–1½ inches lateral to the back midline). Avoid making stripes. This part of the Bladder channel contains the Shu points associated with the Internal Organs. Figure 6.3 shows the Shu points and lists their associated Organs.

When the sequence is complete on one side of the spine, repeat the procedure, if desired, on the other side (Plate 8). Gua sha should be applied in 4–6 inch length strokes resulting in sha 'above, through and below' the area that needs treatment.

Technique: Gua sha to shoulders

For shoulder, upper back or trapezius problems be sure to Gua sha medial to the scapula. Figure 6.3 shows that this area contains the Gao Huang Shu point, one of the five most important points on the body, also known as the shoulder Yu point, BL 43 (Bl 38). This is a main point for the entire shoulder area and diaphragm or 'mo yuan'.

At the neck base stroke along the top of the shoulder outward and slightly down toward the top of the scapula. Keep the stroke line length at 4–6 inches. Allow the strokes to follow the curvature of the body. Soon you will gain a feel for exactly what kind of stroke suits the musculature. Again, complete the sha in one area before moving on. Moving off one stroke line before completing is referred to as 'going shopping'. Returning to complete it will sting the patient. So don't 'go shopping'; complete each stroke line before moving over to the next one.

Gua sha is almost always done North to South, that is, using downward strokes especially when the patient is sitting. The more lateral aspects of the body as well as the shoulders are better treated with strokes that follow the angle of the muscle (see Figure 6.11C and D). At the occiput, stroke up into the hairline (see Figure 6.11B).

Painful problems specific to the shoulders can require a change in position. If the shoulder hurts only in a certain position, then it can be important to have the patient assume that position. Often only a particular position or motion will expose the site that can be needled, released and then Gua sha-ed. Positioning of the arm is critical in treating frozen shoulder. Positioning is just as relevant when you are applying Gua sha without needling.

If you need to Gua sha the latissimus dorsi proximal to the arm, it is necessary to have the arm extended and supported to expose the muscle (see Figure 6.13C). For treatment of the upper arm see below.

Technique: Gua sha to neck

The neck can best be treated in a seated position shown in Figure 6.12B and C. If the head is dropped too far forward the muscles of the neck become too tight to effectively Gua sha. If pain and restriction are coming from the lateral neck, feel free to apply Gua sha to the sides of the neck. One can also follow the sternocleidomastoid muscle downward. One should remember the neck is more sensitive than the back so proceed tenderly. Some patients get the shivers or feel ticklish at the neck.

Technique: Gua sha to scalp

In cases of fixed focal pain at the head or in the scalp as in migraine or cluster headache, Gua sha is typically applied to the upper back, neck and shoulders (Plate 24) and then finally to the scalp. A lubricant is not usually necessary for scalp treatment. Pull the hair up and Gua sha stroke across the section of scalp that is exposed. (See Plate 25). Gua sha until petechiae appear. Then expose the scalp just above or below so that the entire foci of pain is addressed. This specific treatment is very effective for migraine, cluster headache or focal pain from lasting injury or trauma to the head.

Indications: head, neck, shoulders, upper back

Any pain or disease of the neck, eyes, ears, nose, throat, head, shoulders, upper back, chest, breast, arms, hands or elbows can reflect stagnation in the upper back, neck and shoulders (Plates 8, 10 and 11). This includes any problems of the upper extremities. Lung problems are especially responsive to Gua sha at the upper back, including cough caused by bronchitis, emphysema, asthma and pneumonia and also psychological or emotional problems including depression, anxiety, panic disorders, ADD, ADHD, nightmares, insomnia and so on (see Chapter 9).

Treating the middle body

Position: middle body

To treat the mid-back region a prone position is preferable (see Figures 6.13 and 6.14). If you do not have a table with a face cradle, you can use a pillow to support the body mid-section so that the back is not arched. A regular sized bed pillow placed under the patient lengthwise supports from the shoulders to the pubic bone. This prevents back strain. The head is turned to one side but the position can be changed every few minutes to prevent neck strain. A table or Body Cushion with a face

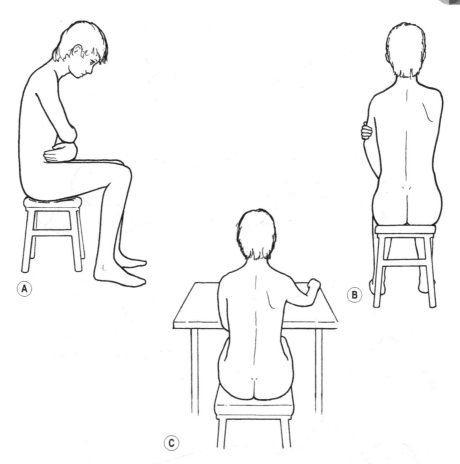

Figure 6.13 • Seated positions for treatment of the neck, shoulders and upper back including the area between scapula •
A Hands resting in lap, head tilted forward. **B** Right hand clasping left upper arm. **C** Right arm is stretched out onto table.

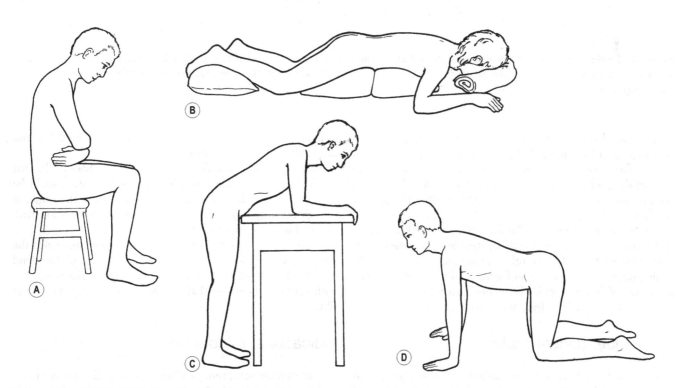

Figure 6.14 • A–D Positions for Gua sha to mid- and low back • C and **D** can be used to treat the low back, iliac crest and waist.
D Exposes the ischium and hamstring area.

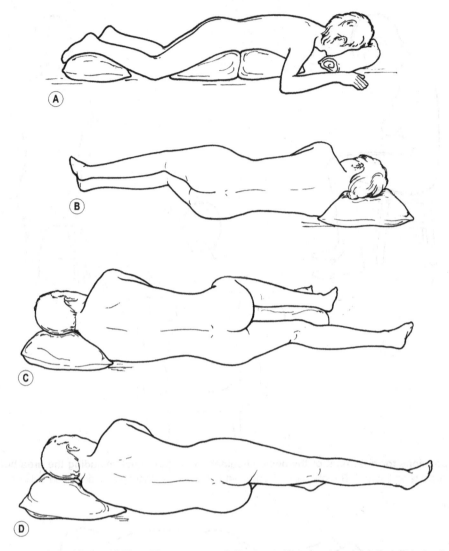

Figure 6.15 • For treatment of the hips and Shao Yang areas • A Prone position: for dorsal sciatica. **B** Lateral recumbent position: for lateral sciatica. **C** Lateral recumbent position: top leg drawn up, bottom leg straight. **D** Lateral recumbent position: top leg extended, bottom leg drawn up.

cradle is ideal and can even accommodate a pregnant patient (see Figures 6.14B and 6.15A). Feet can be supported or if using a flat table, can extend over the edge of the table to prevent the back arching. Arms rest along the sides of the body, not up over the head unless on a Body Cushion. The patient is relaxed.

Some patients cannot lie flat on a table at all. Have them sit leaning forward against the table, arms in lap, forehead supported by a firm pillow or rolled towel (see Figure 6.12C). Sitting upright in a chair, as in Figure 6.14A, is also fine. The advantage of being completely prone is access to other areas of the back, back of the legs, arms and neck.

Technique: middle body

Palpate Ah Shi points or trigger points in the area as well as along related channels locally and distally. Treat these as well as related main points with needles, if using acupuncture. Gua

sha as before, GV line first, then just lateral to the spine, and after that just lateral to that line.

When complete, one does not expect to see lines of sha that would match meridian lines. No stripes. The sha should be brought up over the entire muscle area lateral to the spine, as though coloring in an entire area. When one side is finished, proceed to the opposite side.

If you want to extend the Gua sha over the lateral ribs the strokes should follow the contour of the ribs angled down and outward (see Figure 6.11C and 6.11D). Move the flesh over with your other hand so that you do not leave stripes over the ribs.

Indications: middle body

Any presenting symptom or disorder of the abdomen, upper, middle or lower, will be touched by sha resolution of the mid-back. For example, any abdominal pain, feeling of fullness, congestion or stuckness, from a simple stomach ache, nausea or vomiting to stomach ulcers, gastritis to colitis, gallstones or gallbladder inflammation, diarrhea to constipation, hepatomegaly to splenomegaly, constrained Liver Qi to congealed Blood tumors. Sha resolution releases the Blood that is stuck at the surface and affords more complete Blood and lymph flow to the tissues and Organs in the body cavity. The effect persists for days and is both anti inflammatory and immune stimulating (see Chapter 3). In traditional medical terms, the effect is to move Blood, vent heat, cool areas that are hot and warm areas that are cool (Plate 8).

One must keep in mind that in traditional terms health reflects the proper flow of Qi, and movement of Phlegm, Food, Blood and Fluid. The destructive consequences of accumulation are the 'meat and potatoes' (or 'tofu and rice') of Chinese medicine. What might appear as a subclinical condition to a Western doctor and warrant the response 'There is nothing wrong with you' will usually fall into the category of accumulation and or dysfunction for a doctor of traditional East Asian medicine, because almost every disease or disorder begins as stuck Qi, and then exhibits signs of accumulation of Food, Fluid, Phlegm or Blood. Prevention of illness, with resulting increase in longevity and quality of life, is directly dependent on the ability to perceive and correct early signs.

Treating the lower back

Low back pain is a common presenting complaint. Whether the pain is muscular in origin or involves discs, tendons or ligaments, application of Gua sha will facilitate healing.

Position: lower back

This area can be treated in prone, sitting, standing and leaning positions, sometimes on all fours (cat/dog position) (see Figure 6.14D). The area to be treated should be exposed with the muscles relaxed and supple, always ensuring that the patient is comfortable.

Technique: lower back

Palpate the most tender points in the area of the lower back. Mark them, but before treating (with needles or Gua sha) palpate the mid-back, upper back and along the back of the leg for Ah Shi trigger points or areas where the muscles and fascia are constricted. Tender points in these areas can be distal trigger points for the lower back. Apply Gua sha first to the middle back, then to the lower back area of pain, finally to related areas of the hip and thigh, following the 'above, through and below' rule.

Sequencing of treatment of the lower back is the same as for the upper and mid-back. Start with the GV line and follow the sequence in Figures 6.11A and C. Complete one line before beginning the next, taking care to not create stripes therefore missing areas of sha.

The quadratus lumborum muscle attaches the bottom of the ribs to the iliac crest. Injury to this muscle is common with back strain. To thoroughly Gua sha this area, stroke along the bottom of the ribs outward. In addition, stroke just along the top of the iliac crest, from the center outward. The best position for this is leaning over a table.

Sometimes a sitting, leaning or cat position better exposes the iliac crest and gluteus medius area (see Figure 6.14C and D). With the torso lengthened and exposed it is important that the Gua sha strokes penetrate into the area. The effects are remarkable, with the patient often rising and moving immediately, relieved of pain.

Indications: lower back

Gua sha of the lower back is imperative in the treatment of any lower back strain or pain, including disc problems. In addition, any abdominal or lower abdominal problem with or without referred pain to the back should be treated with Gua sha to the back and lower back. These include, but are not limited to, intestinal, anorectal or genitourinary problems, pelvic floor dysfunction and pain, and history of abdominal surgery or trauma. The lower back is always treated in any lower extremity problem, including fractures, sprains, strains, difficulty walking for any reason, arthritis of knee, lower leg or foot, tarsal tunnel syndrome, Morton's neuroma, plantar fasciitis, heel spurs, and so on (Plate 17).

Treating the hips

Position: hips

The hips can be treated in the prone or lateral recumbent position (see Figure 6.15).

Technique: Gua sha to hips, prone position

In the prone position, palpate and needle the sacral and lateral sacral areas as well as channels distally that course through the hip and sacral area. There are trigger points here for the knee and leg. Gua sha strokes should follow anatomical lines, from sacral edge outward and slightly downward. When these areas are treated the Qi and Blood can flow properly to the extremity. Treating the extremity without clearing the corresponding trigger points on the body can result in a worsening of the extremity condition. Dredging the channels reestablishes a circuit that both feeds and drains the distal problem area with Qi and Blood.

Indications: Gua sha to hips, prone position

Treatment of the hip area is appropriate for local pain or to release back-to-front any problem of the pelvic region. This includes any menstrual, uterine, ovarian, prostate, Bladder, Small Intestine or Large Intestine, rectal, prostate or genital problems. Local pain in the hips, the gluteus muscle group, the piriformis including sciatic pain can all be treated by this method, in the prone position.

Sciatica that trajects down the back of the leg (Bladder channel) most often emanates from just lateral to the sacrum (Plate 17). The prone position gives best access.

Technique: Gua sha to hips, lateral recumbent position

For sciatica that trajects down the side of the leg (Gall Bladder channel) to the lateral foot, the lateral recumbent position is best. The affected hip should face up. With bottom leg extended, the top leg should be bent forward and resting on a supporting pillow (see Figure 6.15C). This position opens the hip joint, exposing the involved channels. If there is hip pain in the lateral hip joint, ask the patient to bend their bottom leg while extending the top leg. This opens the joint for Gua sha to the area (see Figure 6.15D).

Palpation follows a course from above the site of pain to below, along the indicated zone or channel. Often the central trigger point is GB 30, the main sciatica point. Gua sha strokes follow the downward depression along the hip that this position creates. Stroke outward if treating the gluteus medius area. Gua sha may be uncomfortable if this area is especially fatty so be gentle with stroking. More repetitions of lighter strokes will gain the same results as harder strokes with fewer repetitions. Gua sha can also be done along the side of the thigh if the sciatic pain extends into the leg (see Plate 18, and sciatica case, Chapter 9). See section below for special consideration of fatty areas of the upper arm, hips and legs.

Indications: Gua sha to hips, lateral recumbent position

In addition to sciatica, Gua sha to the hip in the lateral recumbent position treats any leg problem: spasm, pain, numbness or leg paralysis, difficulty in walking for any reason, uneven leg syndrome (treat the long leg, see Long leg treatment, Chapter 9), any one-sided pelvic disorder, hip pain, any problem of the GB meridian, including temporal migraine, and hearing or ear problems, especially those associated with fullness of the Gall Bladder and Liver channel.

Treating the ischium

Position: ischium

The ischium is the sitting bone, the bottom of the body. Sha can be retained there from sitting on cold surfaces (see book cover) or from extended periods of sitting, a modern-day work-related condition. Applying Gua sha to the ischium directly may be necessary.

For ischium problems or any pelvic or pelvic floor dysfunction first apply Gua sha to the hip areas and possibly even the low back. Then the best way to access the ischium is to have the patient assume the cat/dog position (see Figure 6.14D), with underwear pulled up from the leg, so the ischium and back of the leg are exposed.

Technique: ischium

Gua sha downward starting above the affected area and going beyond. Be sure to check the back of the leg for involvement (see Chapter 9).

Indications: ischium

Indications include pain at the ischium, pain along the hamstring muscles and/or down the BL meridian in the leg. Hemorrhoids, rectal pain or prolapse, anal fistula and lymph drainage of the pelvic floor or pelvic floor dysfunction are treated by Gua sha at the ischium. Pelvic floor pain, epididimytis, vulvadynia, neurogenic bladder or pain from injury to the ischium are also indications for this area.

Treating the coccyx

Position: coccyx

Treatment of the coccyx region is best achieved in the prone or cat/dog position. The leaning position is suitable for patients who cannot assume the other positions (see Figure 6.14C).

Technique: coccyx

Lightly palpate and massage the area with oil, noting any tenderness and any knotty spasm above or below on the sacrum, back or legs. Be careful if using preparations with volatile oils, such as camphor in Vicks or eucalyptus or ginger in Badger Balm, since this area is so close to the sensitive skin of the anus. The volatility of the oil, should it somehow touch this area, can be uncomfortably stimulating though not harmful.

Gua sha strokes can descend from above, from the sacrum down over the coccyx. The strokes should be light. It is just as important to include the area lateral to the coccyx and lower sacrum.

Indications: coccyx

Apply Gua sha at the coccyx for coccyx pain, which can happen in the months following childbirth or from a fall or contusion that has developed into chronic sensitivity. It is also useful for any problem of the anus and rectum such as hemorrhoids, anal fistula, prolapse, rectal or anal pain or bleeding, or pelvic floor pain. Apply Gua sha around the coccyx but not directly at the coccyx if the patient has just been injured.

Treating special sites: ribs, chest, scapula and lateral body

Gua sha is most often applied to the areas considered above. However, it can also be applied to other sites, such as the ribs, chest, scapula and lateral body regions.

Position for chest

The chest can be treated in a seated or supine position (see Figure 6.16).

Position for ribs and lateral body

The ribs and lateral body can be treated in any position that exposes them comfortably, seated, prone, lateral recumbent or supine (see Figures 6.13, and 6.16A and B). You may need to ask the patient to shift positions, raise or extend the arms to expose the area of pain.

Position for scapula

The scapula can be treated with the patient sitting, arm resting in their lap if that exposes the scapular pain. They can also grab their elbows with each hand, allowing the arms to rest against the front of the body (see Figure 6.13A) or they can grasp the upper arm with the opposite hand (see Figure 6.13B). This position comfortably exposes the area between the two scapulae. If the pain is at the medial border of the scapula, ask the patient to extend their arm forward out on the table (see Figure 6.13C).

Sometimes pain will occur only with certain movements. Ask the patient to repeat the movement. The patient must assume the position that exposes the areas of pain in a relaxed posture.

Technique: Gua sha to ribs, scapula and lateral body

The strokes of Gua sha are unique at these sites. After completing Gua sha at the back, Du mo and Bladder channels, moving laterally it is best to follow the line of the ribs, stroking from the medial aspect of the back outward and slightly downward along the curvature. Pull the flesh over with your opposite hand so that you are not raising sha at the ribs alone and missing areas between the ribs. Completely raise the sha before moving, if necessary, around to the lateral ribs. Follow the rib lines under the arm, which can be raised but in a relaxed position to treat the axilla (Plate 12).

If the pain is around the scapula be sure to palpate for sha in all the possible positions, at the upper and middle back as well as the back of the upper arm. At the medial border of the scapula, Gua sha strokes can go down or from the center outward, though they should be short strokes.

Technique: Gua sha to chest

The chest sites are the sternum and ventral ribs. The sternum should be stroked from the top down to the xyphoid process. Remember it is a bony area so proceed gently, as you would on the spine, with more repetitions of less pressure, if needed. Flatten the instrument.

The ribs in the chest area are Gua sha-ed like the ribs of the back. Strokes proceed from the center of the chest outward following the curve of the rib.

You can Gua sha above and below the breast tissue, (see Plate 13) but take care not to wander too far onto the breasts of women or men. The breast area is distinctive, not because of the fatty tissue but because of the glands within the tissue. Gua sha can be applied to the breast area but only by an experienced practitioner and only when necessary, as in cases of mastitis or breast distension (Chiu et al. 2010).

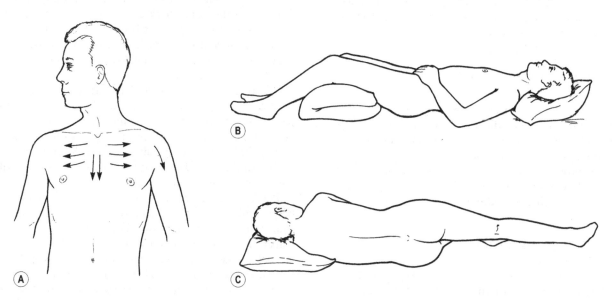

Figure 6.16 • Positions for treatment of chest and ribs • A Seated – exposure of chest. **B** Supine position. **C** Lateral recumbent position.

Indications: Gua sha to chest and ribs

These areas are essential to treat in cases of shingles where there is pain and to prevent postherpetic neuralgia (Nielsen 2005; see Chapters 2 and 9). In addition to Gua sha at the upper back, these areas are useful in the release of any Lung problem, chronic cough, asthma, emphysema or weakness in the Lungs. The back ribs and lateral body area on the right or left can be used in cases of hepatomegaly and splenomegaly. Gua sha may be applied to the chest and upper back in cases of bronchial cough or bronchial asthma, angina or esophageal reflux disorder.

It is important to Gua sha the area of the back between the scapulae, especially with the scapula moved forward, not only if there is pain at the site but for any problem of the Lung, Stomach, Spleen or Liver.

Treating the extremities

Position: extremities

The rule for treating extremity problems is to first treat the corresponding area of the torso, usually the back. Then go to the extremity. Have the area of the limb relaxed since sha cannot be completely released from an area of contracted muscles. This may be in a seated, prone or supine position.

For the top of the thigh or the foreleg, a sitting position or reclining with support under the knee is fine. For the back of the thigh, a prone position is the best, rather than standing. For the calf, a prone position is best.

The arm can be positioned with the patient either sitting or reclining. Be careful to use the position that best exposes and relaxes the painful area. To treat the upper arm in a reclining position, the arm should be at the patient's side, with the elbow bent and forearm resting on the body (see Figure 6.13B and C). To treat below the elbow, the arm can rest with the elbow bent or straight but not overextended or 'locked'. The wrist and hand should be relaxed.

Technique: extremities

The strokes of Gua sha on the extremities can go North or South. Sometimes you will want to do both to raise the sha completely. The strokes go along the channel of trajecting pain, along the muscle, not across it.

For a problem with a joint, you can apply Gua sha to muscles above, below and over the joint. Do not apply Gua sha over a joint that is 'hot', i.e. red, hot or swollen.

Indications: extremities

Gua sha is indicated for pain that extends through a limb. This can be as a result of injury that has not fully healed or from a condition that involves pain on the body trunk that extends into an extremity.

Sciatica often involves back and hip pain that passes down the leg. Arm pain, numbness or tingling can extend from the neck and back. In these situations it is appropriate to treat and Gua sha the extremity as well as the body proper (Plates 14, 15 and 18).

Painful joints can be treated by Gua sha to muscles above and below the joint and then at the joint itself (Plate 15). Gua sha can be used for any pain in a limb except directly at the site of recent fracture, contusion, abrasion or rash.

Other application considerations

Fatty areas of the upper arm, hip and leg

The upper arm, areas of the hip and upper leg tend to be more fatty in some patients, with more cellulite and or water retention. These areas are more sensitive to Gua sha. Care should be taken to not apply the same pressure and to not expect the same kind of sha to appear as would be in an adjacent area that is leaner.

Apply Gua sha with light strokes and when petechiae begin to appear, repalpate to check if the original pain is gone. If not, proceed carefully, checking in with the patient. More strokes with lighter pressure is recommended rather than heavy pressure. Acupuncture needling with de qi response before Gua sha, or within the Gua sha treatment, can help to raise the sha with fewer strokes.

Treating painful problems in particular fatty areas may take more than one session. It is also the case that raising any sha in a fatty area begins to thaw the area and the patient will experience relief.

Some disorders can require Gua sha at more than one site. If you are uncertain, check Chapters 8 and 9. Disorders that occupy a particular part of the body are addressed by Gua sha to that area. That is, whether a patient has a cough, chronic obstructive pulmonary disease (COPD), asthma or bronchitis Gua sha to the upper back and even chest area is indicated. Even if a particular diagnosis is not covered in this book, consider what area of the body it occupies or affects. Gua sha is applied by a problem's morphology: the location, quality and mutability of its nature.

Whether at the main body, extremity or odd body site once Gua sha is complete lightly massage the area treated. Ask the patient to sit up and move around and to move their head, neck, arms, etc. If the patient presented with any pain in the muscles ask if there is any pain still there. Most often 95–100% of the pain is gone. The areas you first massaged and palpated will be softer, less tight or ropey.

Repalpating an area that may have made the patient wince before will now feel very comfortable. If there is still a spot of pain or restriction, or if the most painful spot has moved, palpate and find the center of the pain, clean that area with alcohol and needle using strong stimulation. Ask if the patient has gotten the 'de qi' as you feel for needle response and grasp. Then lubricate and Gua sha that spot again. Start above, end below. Though the sha here may have seemed complete, now it will come up more and often darker in color.

Dr So used to speak of pain like numbers in a circle. The most painful Ah Shi points would be given the higher numbers and the less painful points the lower numbers. But as you clear the most painful spots, the ones previously less painful and less noticeable now become apparent, no longer in the shadow of the more painful spots. This can be confusing to both the patient and practitioner unless explained. The ancients called treating the pain pattern as 'Chasing the Dragon', or 'Chasing the Dragon's Tail', that is, tracking and treating the pain until the entire complex of pain is resolved. Sometimes the pain goes and when the patient returns in a few days, the pain is in a different area. This is the same phenomenon.

Review of rules

- Follow safety guidelines to prevent exposure or transfer of bloodborne pathogens.
- Explain and discuss Gua sha as you are treating your patient.
- Treat children with their parent or guardian in the room.
- Adjust stroke pressure to the comfort of the patient.
- Treat the body torso for any internal organ problem.

- Treat the body first for extremity problems; then treat the extremity.
- Do not treat the extremity without releasing sha on the body.
- Any area to be treated should be exposed but relaxed.
- Follow sequencing, starting at the middle part of the body and working outward in stroke lines.
- Gua sha along muscles not across them: dredge the channels.
- The provider's instrument-holding hand also makes contact with the flesh. Hand contact while stroking 'dims' the sensation of the instrument.
- Keep strokes to 4–6 inches in length.
- Don't make stripes.
- Don't 'go shopping': finish a stroke line before starting the adjacent stroke line.
- Complete Gua sha so that sha is raised 'above, through and below' the area of interest.
- Always show the patient their sha so it is not a shock to them later.
- Always give the Gua sha handout (Appendix A), even if you have treated this patient and given the handout before.
- Remember to be grateful for the gift that has been given to us by the ancestors of our medicine. Pass it on with gentleness, grace and compassion.

References

Chiu, J.-Y., Gau, M.-L., Kuo, S.-Y., et al. 2010. Effects of Gua-Sha therapy on breast engorgement: a randomized controlled trial. J Nurs Res 18 (March), 1–10.

Martin, E., 1987. The Woman in the Body. Beacon Press, Boston, MA, pp. 92–112.

Nielsen, A., 1996. Gua Sha as Counteraction: The Crisis is the Cure. J Chinese Med 50 (January), 5–12.

Nielsen, A., 2005. Postherpetic neuralgia in the left buttock after a case of shingles. Explore (NY) 1 (1), 74.

Nielsen, A., Author, 2002. Gua Sha: Step-by-Step. A Visual Guide to a Traditional Technique for Modern Practice. Kötzting, Germany: Verlag für Ganzheitliche Medizin;. 55 minutes.

Nielsen, A., Knoblauch, N.T.M., Dobos, G.J., et al., 2007. The effect of 'Gua sha'

treatment on the microcirculation of surface tissue: a pilot study in healthy subjects. Explore (NY) 3, 456–466.

Nielsen, A., 2009. Gua sha research and the language of integrative medicine. J Bodyw Mov Ther 13 (1), 63–72.

Nielsen, A., Kligler, B., Koll, B.S., 2012. Safety Protocols for Gua sha (Press-Stroking) and Baguan (Cupping). Complement Ther in Med in press.

Immediate and significant Tongue changes as a direct result of Gua sha*

7

Discovery in an ancient practice

Teachers say that they learn by teaching. The process of reviewing basic principles over and over highlights their essentiality. And then there are those moments when something is revealed that comes not from the teacher or from the student but rather from the interaction.

This occurred in 1996, in a Gua sha seminar I was teaching in Amsterdam. One of the acupuncturist participants asked me about a distended and very deep purple area on the lateral fore aspect of her Tongue that corresponded to a right shoulder injury. The class was learning to apply Gua sha to the upper back, neck and shoulders and proceeded to practice on one another. Within moments of having Gua sha applied to her back, her Tongue changed: the distension and the purple color were less. I instructed her seminar partner to extend the area of Gua sha laterally to the right scapula, corresponding to the Small Intestine channel, specifically the area of SI 11, 10 and 9 and to the LU 1 on the front of the body at the corresponding side (note: in Vietnamese medicine, these areas are included when applying Gua sha/cao gio for any Lung problem). The sha was pronounced and dark; a reexamination of the Tongue revealed the purple area was now completely gone (and did not recur). Her shoulder pain shifted significantly with increased range of motion and strength. But that was expected. The elimination of the distended purple area on the Tongue was a shock. After this event, we began to pay attention to Tongue changes before and immediately after Gua sha.

This is a departure from Tongue 'looking', in the modern traditional Chinese medicine (TCM) setting, which is typically done only once or twice at the beginning of the session because, so say the texts, the Tongue is not expected to change within

*Some of the content on immediate and significant Tongue changes as a direct result of Gua sha was first presented at the Anglo–Dutch Institute of Oriental Medicine International Acupuncture Conference in Amsterdam, November 1999, and first appeared in print in the German translation of the first edition of the Gua sha book as *Gua Sha, Eine traditionelle Technik für die moderne Medizin*, Verlag fur Ganzheitliche Medizi, ISBN 3-927344-51-6 (Nielsen 2000).

the session (Chen and Chen 1989; Kirschbaum 2000). To quote a respected text on Tongue diagnosis: 'Tongue body and coating colors are relatively unaffected by short term events or recent changes' (Maciocia 1995). Indeed, Tongue changes are expected to happen over time: days, weeks, even months, reflecting the gradual healing that takes place deep in the body as errant, excess or deficient substances and or systems reconcile.

From the perspective of classical Chinese medicine, as Dr So often said, 'the Pulse can lie but the Tongue never lies', meaning the Pulse could be influenced in the short term by stress, anger and even movement, but the Tongue is not altered by minor things. Most practitioners adept in Tongue observation would agree that the flesh color, the shape of the Tongue, as well as the presence of petechiae or points, are substantial indicators. Tongue moisture and coat shift more easily, reflecting the deepening or resolving of various states of acute pathology as in, say, a pathogenic Wind that obstructs Qi of the surface channels and, in turn, obstructs Fluids, making the Tongue appear to be wetter than normal. The Tongue coat is typically thicker before the first meal of the day and thins just from eating.

Yet, as a direct result of Gua sha I have documented Tongue changes that are not expected in the short term; changes that then shift 'how to think about a problem', and intervention in the short and long term.

It is worth mentioning that areas of the Tongue are not so strictly reduced to Organ associations in the classical perspective of Dr So's lineage. The Tongue is viewed according to Jiao, Upper, Middle and Lower; syndromes are differentiated according to 'involved' Jiao called 'San Jiao bian zheng' (see Figure 7.1). While it may be said that the Heart and Lungs reside in the Upper Jiao, Heat as redness at the fore aspect of the Tongue may well relate to focal inflammation in the sinuses and not relate to the anatomical heart or lungs at all while still the province of the traditional East Asian medicine (TEAM) Heart and Lungs. In this sense 'how to think about a problem'

may not always be limited to a primary *zang fu* focus, and certainly is not from the classical perspective that is responsive to specific morphology of a problem, its channel, and then related organs.

Immediate and significant Tongue changes as a direct result of Gua sha that have been observed with patients and in teaching seminars are presented here. What is important for the provider to assess is whether the Tongue has changed and how the change in Tongue flesh, color, shape, moisture and coat corresponds with immediate changes in other signs and symptoms. A conclusion need not be drawn; rather a noticing of the fluctuations that have occurred in an already fluctuating process is germane. Significant Tongue changes as a direct result of Gua sha adds to information that supports or detracts from 'how to think about the problem'.

Signs of stasis on the Tongue and body surface

Stases of body substances as well as system dysfunction appear on the Tongue as variations in color, shape, coat, fur and moisture (Kirschbaum, 2000; Maciocia 1995; Song, 1981). The very definition of pain in traditional East Asian medicine relates to some form of stasis. Sha stasis can relate to a spectrum of symptom severity, from the more superficial stiffness or myalgia, to bothersome pain, to severe fixed recurring pain, and further to actual 'hsieh' syndrome illness (see Chapter 5), where the 'pathogenic agent' has progressed from the surface Lo vessels, to the Jing vessels and the deeper tissues and organs. While channel communication can become disrupted or blocked, the channels '... may equally serve as a pathway for causative agents' (Epler 1980). Gua sha, then, not only relieves surface sha stasis but can also disrupt the process of pathogenic factors deepening into the body.

Qi stasis may or may not alter the Tongue presentation. Ongoing Qi stasis may produce stasis of other body substances. Blood stasis can appear as a darkening of the Tongue or as areas of the Tongue appearing blue or purple, or in some cases of Deficiency it will appear peachy in color. Heat stasis can appear as areas of increased redness; intensified Blood and Heat stasis as red or white points. When Fluids are not moving, all or part of the Tongue may be swollen or misshapen or may appear excessively wet, or even dry. Phlegm or Food stasis may appear as a thickened Tongue coat, and so on.

It is as important to examine the color and quality of the patients face, lips and body surface; it may be unremarkable at first look or may have discolored areas appearing blue or red, or the skin may redden from touch. The temperature of the surface may be warm or cool, but also may vary significantly even in areas proximal to one another. The presence of sha is confirmed by surface blanching that is slow to fade from pressing palpation (see Chapter 6, Figures 6.1 and 6.2; Plates 1, 2, and 3). A careful evaluation of history combined with palpation will reveal whether there are correlative symptoms of stasis or dysfunction deeper in the body. Removing this Blood stasis at the surface with Gua sha can, in turn, impact the deeper problem.

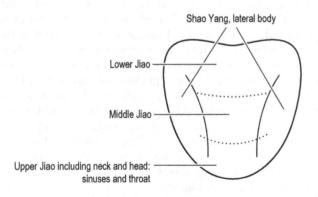

Shao Yang, lateral body

Lower Jiao —

Middle Jiao —

Upper Jiao including neck and head: — sinuses and throat

Figure 7.1 • The Tongue according to Jiaos • The classical East Asian medicine perspective in the lineage of Dr So starts with viewing the Tongue according to Upper, Middle and Lower Jiao, i.e. three-Jiao differentiation 'San Jiao bian zheng', before internal-organ differentiation 'zang fu bian zheng' where sections of the Tongue relate to organs. Note the fore aspect of the Tongue includes the head, neck, sinuses and throat as well as the organs of the chest.

Tongue looking

Consistency in the technique for viewing the Tongue is worth mentioning. The patient must extend their Tongue in a relaxed manner without opening the mouth too far. The Tongue should be extended for up to 5 seconds. Overextending the Tongue can cause the muscles to fatigue and may temporarily dry or redden the Tongue. Instruct the patient to retract, clear the mouth, swallow, and extend the Tongue again for a second look, and then possibly a third. Providers may want to draw an image of the Tongue making note of distinctive features to include in the patient's chart.

Observe the Tongue again directly after Gua sha, and again at the end of the session. Sequential looks at the Tongue will give the provider a sense of the depth and direction of a disorder and help to identify which features have or have not changed from Gua sha.

Changes in the color of the face, lips and body flesh are also important to note, as well as the relationship of these to Tongue color, and the relationship of sha color to Tongue color.

The Tongue before and after Gua sha

Tongue changes from Gua sha reflect the depth of transformation as a result of removing Blood stasis at the surface. Not all patients experience this and not all Tongues change immediately. However, even the smallest shift can clarify the depth, direction or range of a pathology or pattern. The sets of before and after photographs below and in the Plate Section show examples of significant Tongue changes commonly associated with Gua sha.

In general, the most profound Tongue changes occur after applying Gua sha to the upper back, neck, and shoulders, confirming the Tongue's direct correspondence with the Upper Jiao and indirect correspondence with the Middle and Lower Jiao. Documentation of immediate and significant changes in Tongue flesh color, shape and coat as a direct result of Gua sha are discussed below.

Gua sha and Tongue flesh color

Tongue becomes less red: Gua sha vents Heat

In cases of Heat, whether acute onset Wind Heat or more chronic Internal Heat, it is important to note the way in which the pathology is trending. Is the Heat increasing or decreasing, and in what way does the trend correspond to other signs and symptoms? Venting Heat is an intervention that not only relieves, regulates and cools, but can also 'tonify'.

In the years prior to protease inhibitors, many herbalists were prescribing tonifying herbs for human immunodeficiency virus (HIV) patients to address their extreme fatigue, only to find that their fatigue became worse or did not respond at all. A more adept herbalist recognized that theirs was pathogenic Heat-related fatigue, and developed formulae to clear that

Heat. The same therapeutic approach is used for post-fever fatigue, whether from an acute respiratory infection or from other infectious agents, as in dengue fever, Lyme disease, or even sequelae to heat stroke where residual pathogenic Heat dries fluids and suppresses Qi. Venting Heat is an essential therapeutic strategy that must be considered within the treatment session itself.

See Plates 19, 20 and 21: For subject 1 the red Tongue is associated with Wind Heat and early respiratory symptoms, as well as fatigued state, deficiency related to recent childbirth, nursing and student life (Plate 19). Her sha color (Plate 21) is a similar red color to that of the 'before' Tongue (Plate 19). Plate 20 is of her Tongue after Gua sha: the change in redness shows that Gua sha was able to vent Heat. There is slight coat observed and an underlying paleness that the 'before' Heat obscured. Childbirth, nursing and overwork can result in Blood deficiency. With the 'before' picture, an herbal formula might include blood nourishing herbs second to Wind Heat herbs, while the 'after' picture might reverse the order of emphasis in terms of dosage.

See Plates 22, 23, 24, and 25: Subject 2 had chronic cluster headaches with recurrent fixed pain at the side of the head. Her Tongue was very red, shiny and scalloped before Gua sha (Plate 22). After Gua sha to the back and neck (Plate 24), the focal area of cluster headache pain was treated at the scalp shown in Plate 25. After Gua sha subject 2's Tongue, lips and face are less red (Plate 23). Tongue scallops remain, but there is a slight increase in coat. Gua sha has vented Heat. Note that even with the dense ecchymosis from the student participant's over stroking, the sha is very similar in color to the 'before' Tongue (Plates 24 and 22).

Purple Tongue resolves: Gua sha moves Blood

See Plates 26 and 27: Subject 3 exhibits a deep purple and red Tongue with concentrated redness at front end and sides; the coat is concentrated on back right portion (Plate 26). After Gua sha the Tongue is less purple, less red, with a thicker coat overall (Plate 27). The coat at the back right portion is thicker, pasty and less rooted. Note the face and lips and nasi anni are also less red after Gua sha. Here Gua sha has vented Heat and moved Blood. The increase in coat points to a need for fluids.

Blue Tongue resolves: Gua sha harmonizes Blood and Gan Qi

See Plates 30, 31 and 32: Subject 3 exhibits a blue Tongue with a redder front rim (Plate 30). Immediately after Gua sha the blue aspect of the Tongue has almost completely resolved (Plate 31). The front end of Tongue is less red, less fluted. Plate 32 shows the same person two weeks later. The Tongue is fluted with a red scalloped front rim, showing an increase in Heat and Fluid stasis at the Upper Jiao related to new symptoms. The progression demonstrates that Tongue blueness can resolve from Gua sha, and remain resolved.

Peachy Tongue reddens: Heat concentrates

See Plates 28 and 29: Subject 4 exhibits a pale peachy Tongue (Plate 28). The peachier color at the front and sides represents Heat (a kind of redness) within Blood deficiency associated with the peachy color. After Gua sha (Plate 29) the peachy areas are darker, almost red, with appearance of points that are often associated with concentration of Heat; the coat is slightly increased, especially on the right. The face is a bit 'redder' as well. Heat appears to increase here further clarifying deficiency of Blood.

Changes in Tongue shape: Gua sha moves Qi, Blood and Fluids

See Figure 7.2 below. Subject 5 exhibits a Tongue that is asymmetrical, with one side larger than the other. Here the left side is swollen, distended and visibly larger than the right side (see Figure 7.2A), a sign that can be associated with injury and obstruction of the channels on the affected side. Though shown in black and white here, the Tongue color is rather normal: pink, pale and slightly blue.

Immediately after Gua sha the Tongue's left-sided swelling has changed. The Tongue has reddened slightly, particularly at the pockets of the side scallops, which appear darker (see Figure 7.2B). Figure 7.2C shows the Tongue two weeks later: the left-sided swelling remains resolved. The Tongue color is particularly fresh, and the Shen is bright.

Changes in Tongue coat

See Plates 33 and 34: Subject 6 exhibits a red fluted Tongue with a white coat a bit thicker at the right top (Plate 33). Immediately after Gua sha the Tongue is less fluted, slightly less red with remaining red sides but with an increase in coat (Plate 34). Notice the Stomach crack is somewhat 'healed' after Gua sha, i.e. the fur is filling in the area, indicating movement of fluids that moistens the flesh. However, the Tongue coat is thicker, which can point to a lack of fluids or dehydration. This subject had been up most of the night and his sleep deprivation and overwork was depriving the Yin. Increase in the Tongue coat after Gua sha should trigger an inquiry into the status of fluids and Yin. Gua sha moves Fluids and when there is not enough fluid, the Tongue coat will thicken. Gua sha also vented Heat for Subjects 1, 2 and 3 (above, and see Plates 19 through 27) but an increased coat in Subjects 3 and 6 points to need for fluids.

Summary of Tongue changes and their significance

The body is always changing. We are interested in understanding a problem in the context of what changes and what appears to stay the same. What is presenting right now? What can be said about its location, quality and mutability? How is the situation trending? Which aspects are more recent or superficial; which are more tenacious, deep, or stuck.

The Tongue is not a magnetic resonance imaging (MRI) scan of the internal organs. It should not be consulted like an MRI, but more like a rising or setting sun, indicating a building or declining of conditions, a very direct indicator of conditions at the surface and the Upper Jiao, reminding us that the Tongue is the bud of the Heart. Changes on the Tongue as a result of Gua sha give essential information about the depth, direction and potential of a problem to respond, resolve or worsen. Tables 7.1, 7.2 and 7.3 detail the most common immediate changes of Tongue flesh color, shape, and moisture/coat as a direct result of Gua sha. The color and texture of sha, as well as how fast it surfaces and how fast it fades, gives more information, and is discussed in Chapter 6.

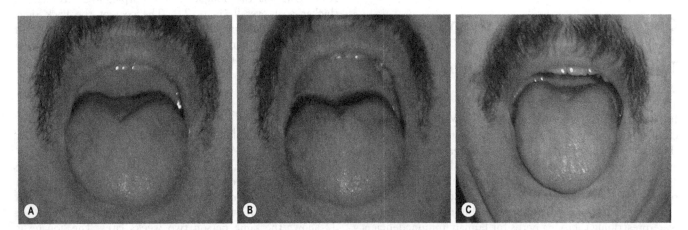

Figure 7.2 • Subject 5 presents with an asymmetrical Tongue • A The left side is distinctly larger and distended, associated with blockage of the channels on the left side of the body possibly from an old injury. **B** Directly after Gua sha the Tongue's left-sided distension is 'resolving'. The scallops are a bit redder (darker). **C** Two weeks later, the left-sided distension remains resolved. The Tongue color is fresh, the Shen on the Tongue is bright, the scallops have resolved.

Table 7.1 Significance of Changes in Tongue Flesh Color from Gua sha*

Tongue appearance	Immediately after Gua sha	Significance
Red	Less red	Heat is vented Areas remaining red indicate residual Heat
Pale	Reddens to 'normal'	Qi moved Qi and Blood quickened, warming
Pale, or pale with red areas	Reddens	Possible Yin deficiency, or not enough fluid Movement of Qi and Blood warms
Peachy	Becomes pink	Deficient Blood is quickened and nourished
Blue	Pinks to normal	Blood stasis is resolved Cold condition is warmed
Areas of purple	Turn normal pink	Blood stasis is resolved
Red points	Pale, flatten or disappear	Heat and Blood stasis resolving
White points/ thorns	Flatten tending to normal fur and pink or disappear	Heat and Blood stasis resolving

*As with all signs and symptoms, Tongue changes are considered in the context of the entire presenting picture: the location, quality and mutability of a problem or problems.

Table 7.3 Significance of changes in Tongue moisture and coat from Gua sha*

Tongue appearance	Immediately after Gua sha	Significance
Dry	Moistens	Fluids circulated
Drippy, wet	Resumes normal moisture Drier	Fluids astringed Harmonized
Normal	Dries	Fluids not enough, not moving
Thick coat	Becomes thin	Accumulated Dampness resolving
No coat	Becomes thin coat	Stomach Qi and Yin strengthened
Coat not rooted	Begins to root	Stomach Qi and Yin strengthened
Thin coat	Thickens or becomes drier	Damp collecting Possible lack of fluids, dehydration or unresolved pathogenic factor
Coat at specific area	Changes	Factors are either resolving or deepening at the corresponding Jiao, Channel or Organ
Tongue fur is cracked	Cracks 'heal', fur becomes 'grassy'	Blood is harmonizing, Yin is supported

*As with all signs and symptoms, Tongue changes are considered in the context of the entire presenting picture: the location, quality and mutability of a problem or problems.

Table 7.2 Significance of changes in Tongue shape from Gua sha*

Tongue appearance	Immediately after Gua sha	Significance
Swollen or thick	Reduces in size and shape	Fluids are astringed Tones Qi and Yang
Scalloped edges	Reduce in size or disappear	Fluids are astringed Tones Qi and Yang
Thin	Thickens or becomes scalloped (rare)	Fluids are collecting Consider internal Deficiency
One-sided swelling	Reduces: Tongue becomes symmetrical	One-sided channel stasis has resolved Qi and Blood moved
Swollen and pulls to one side	Reduces and corrects extension	Channel stasis and Wind resolved Channels nourished

*As with all signs and symptoms, Tongue changes are considered in the context of the entire presenting picture: the location, quality and mutability of a problem or problems.

Tongue changes and indications for herbal medicine

It is not unusual in practice in the Northeast United States to see some form of residual pathogenic Heat (Maciocia, 1995) in a patient's lingering symptoms. Often in winter a person is exposed to cold but also to an overheated indoor environment that is also quite dry. People will become overheated and dry and their Tongues will become red and dry. Research has shown that dry air promotes respiratory viruses to become trapped in mucosa and reproduce. Also influenza viruses stay alive longer in dry air, favoring transmission (Lowen et al. 2007). When such a person contracts a Wind Cold, there is rarely a recognizable Wind Cold stage; the problem immediately transforms to Wind Heat.

Correspondingly the Tongue will have reddening (with or without red raised points) at the front fore aspect. Heat-clearing herbs come immediately to mind, as an internal medicine response seems indicated. But after applying Gua sha, the redness may decline substantially, and the red points flatten, pale or even disappear. Now the Tongue can actually look pale, calling for reconsideration of medicines. Gua sha is able to vent and clear Heat, making visible the underlying terrain.

Alternatively, the reverse may happen, where Gua sha pinks the Tongue when the Tongue began as pale. This is an excellent sign, as the Qi and Blood have been quickened. But if the Tongue began as red, and becomes redder, then it is possible that a greater internal Heat or a deficiency Heat is now visible. In this situation, consider offering fluids to hydrate the patient and recommend more consistent hydration. Continue treatment and check the Tongue again at the end of the session. If the Tongue still remains red, then Heat-clearing herbs and Heat-reducing foods and behaviors are justified.

A myth in the Western acupuncture community holds that only herbs can address deeper dysfunction, particularly that associated with Blood stasis. The evidence presented here of immediate Tongue changes has demonstrated that Gua sha alone can not only vent Heat but move Blood, making significant changes that ramify deep into the body. This can, in turn, inform herbal prescribing if herbs are needed at all.

It is, therefore, recommended that providers palpate for and consider Gua sha in any stasis or pain presentation, whatever the stasis pattern, before prescribing herbs. Applying Gua sha and viewing the Tongue before and after Gua sha can inform the practitioner with regard to the depth and direction of a pattern and the ease of communication within the tissues. Furthermore, given the import of immediate changes from Gua sha, seeing no change in the Tongue is as significant as seeing an immediate change.

References

Chen, Z., Chen, M., 1989. The Essence and Scientific Background of Tongue Diagnosis. Oriental Healing Arts, Long Beach, CA.

Epler, D.C., Jr., 1980. Bloodletting in early Chinese medicine and its relation to the origin of acupuncture. Bull. Hist. Med 54 (3) (Fall), 337–367.

Kirschbaum, B., 2000. Atlas of Chinese Tongue Diagnosis. Eastland Press, Seattle, WA.

Lowen, A.C., Mubareka, S., Steel, J., et al., 2007. Influenza virus transmission is dependent on relative humidity and temperature. PLoS pathogens 3: 1470–1476.

Maciocia, G., 1995. Tongue Diagnosis in Chinese Medicine. Eastland Press; 1987, Seattle, WA.

Nielsen, A., 2000. Gua sha, Eine traditionelle Technik für die moderne Medizin. trans

Marcus Schmid and Suzanne Volcker. Verlag fur Ganzheitliche Medizin, Koetzting, Germany.

Song, T.B., 1981. Atlas of Tongues and Lingual Coatings in Chinese Medicine. Peoples Medical Publishing House, Beijing.

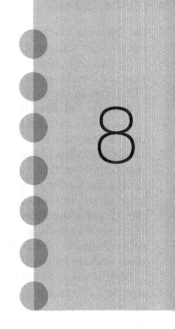

Classical treatment of specific disorders: location, quality, mutability and association

8

Classical 'diagnosis': location, quality, mutability and association

Gua sha is used alone or in combination with other therapies as is evident from the studies and articles published in Chinese and English. Gua sha is taught in acupuncture schools and is increasingly being taught in medical programs for physicians, nurses, massage and physical therapists. Depending on the scope of practice of these varied providers, Gua sha may be applied for a range of problems from acute or chronic illness to acute or chronic musculoskeletal problems.

How and when to use Gua sha within an acupuncture session is detailed in the tables below. If applying Gua sha alone, the middle column indicates where to treat for the condition named in the first column. These tables are adapted from an engaged classical perspective in the tradition of Dr James Tin Yau So: what is a problem's location, quality, mutability and association? If applying Gua sha it is assumed an aspect of a condition's quality is blood stasis, whether related to Excess or Deficiency, or related to Hot, Cold, Damp or Dry, etc. A condition's inherent mutability is of interest for interpreting a patient's response to any treatment. Gua sha always creates change; What effect does Gua sha have? What is the significance of a shift and what does it indicate in terms of the depth, direction, longevity and responsivity of a problem.

How to use these treatment tables

The following tables list specific disorders that respond to the application of Gua sha as might be seen in a general acupuncture practice. The points suggested in the first column are needled first to raise Qi in the area. One, two or three de qi responses are indicated at each point to both disperse and congest the Qi in the area. The technique of multiple strong de qi is considered dispersing; however, when there is sha, even a dispersing needling technique congests the area because of the sha stasis. Congesting the area promotes a more complete release from Gua sha.

The second column indicates where to apply Gua sha. If Gua sha is to be applied alone, these are the indicated areas. The points in the third column are needled after application of Gua sha, allowing the patient to relax. These tables and points should be considered as the core aspect of treatment; the provider may choose from these and then also individualize a treatment with additional points to respond to the patient's specific presentation.

Gua sha is relevant for the disorders listed with or without acupuncture. In addition to treating specific problems such as those listed in the tables, Gua sha should always be considered whenever there is pain, discomfort, compromised function or range of motion, alteration of senses, or any indication of sha stasis whether by palpation or Tongue indication.

Most of the acupuncture points suggested are empirical prescriptions of classical Chinese medicine, except for the TW gummy point popularized by Kiiko Matsumoto. Main acupuncture points are essential to tap the conduit system and additional trigger points and or Ah Shi points are expected to be applied according to the individual need of the patient, and so are not listed here. It is not recommended to acupuncture trigger points alone without accessing the channel system; nor is it recommended to acupuncture alone if there are indications of sha.

The disorders are organized by Jiao (see Chapter 4), beginning with the Upper Jiao, which includes disorders of head, neck, eyes, ears, nose, throat, chest, upper back and extremities. The Organs of the Upper Jiao are the Heart and Lungs. The Middle Jiao includes disorders of the trunk, back and middle ribs. The Organs involved are the Stomach, Spleen, Liver and Gall Bladder. The Lower Jiao includes disorders of the lower body, pelvis and lower extremities. The Organs involved are the Kidneys, Bladder, Intestines, reproductive and sexual organs. Aspects of Liver function belong to the Lower Jiao. Of course the Organ San Jiao, Triple Warmer, is accessed at its channel but also at any area of the body where the fascia is stretched, probed, pressured, poked or Gua sha-ed.

According to the functional system of traditional East Asian medicine, certain areas of the body relate to or associate with function even when seemingly distal from a presumed anatomical site. So, for example, for problems with the head, the upper back would be treated but also possibly the middle back or lower back, since the Liver and Kidneys relate to aspects of eyesight, hearing, and head pain. Or Gua sha might be applied to an extremity along a channel that accesses internal organ function, like the Heart channel for insomnia for example. Gua sha would still be applied to the upper back to address stasis of the Heart or upper body.

Upper Jiao disorders (Table 8.1)

For problems of the upper extremities, Gua sha would always be applied to the upper back and or chest area on the affected side, never to the extremity alone. As well, Gua sha can be extended from the upper body down the affected aspect of the arm, above, below and to a joint directly. The acupuncture points are not intended as a delimiting prescription but are suggested as options for core treatments to be adapted to a patient's specific presentation by the practitioner.

Table 8.1 Treatment of Upper Jiao disorders

Disorder	Needle	Gua sha	Needle
Influenza: Wind-Cold, Damp	GV 14, BL 12 BL 13, GB 20 BL 38	Gua sha to upper back, neck, shoulders, chest	LI 4, LU 7 LI 11
Acute head cold	GV 14, BL 12 BL 13, GB 20	Gua sha to upper back, neck, shoulders, chest	LI 4, LU 7 LI 11, LI 20
Sinusitis: touch the neck and forehead to assess for 'fever'; palpate occipital region for pain	GV 14, BL 12 BL 13, GB 20 GB 21 (needle GB 21 across the muscle)	Gua sha to upper back, neck, shoulders, chest	LI 4, LU 7 LI 11, LI 20, BL 7, ST2 LIV 2
Rhinitis	Same	Gua sha to upper back, neck, shoulders, chest	LI 4, LU 7 LI 11, LI 20, BL 7, ST 2 LIV 2, TW 5 BL 20, BL 23
Bronchitis	GV 14, BL 13 BL 38, GB 20, GB 21	Gua sha to upper back, neck, shoulders, chest	LI 4, LU 7 LI 11, CV 17 CV 22 LU 5, PC 6, SP 4 BL 20

Table 8.1 Treatment of Upper Jiao disorders—cont'd

Disorder	Needle	Gua sha	Needle
Asthma	GV 14, Ding Chuan, BL 13 BL 38 GB 21, GB 20 BL 15, ear Shen men	Gua sha to upper back, neck, shoulders, chest	LI 4, LU 7, or LU 9 PC 6, SP 4 CV 17, CV 21 CV 22, ST 36 or ST 40 BL 20, BL 23
Emphysema/COPD (Note: patients with a long-term breathing disorder are more vulnerable to pneumothorax because the lungs are closer to the surface. Only shallow needling is recommended)	Same BL 15, ear Shen men	Gua sha to upper back, neck, shoulders, chest	LI 4, LU 7, or LU 9 KI 6 or KI 7 PC 6, SP 4, Yin tang ST 36 CV 17, CV 21 CV 22 BL 18 or BL 20, BL 23
Cough	GV 14, BL 13 BL 38, GB 20 GB 21, BL20	Gua sha to upper back, neck, shoulders, chest	LI 4, LU 7, LU 9, LU 5, ST 36 PC 6, SP 4 CV 17, CV 21 CV 22
Deficient Yin, cough (Note: patients with COPD or any other long-term breathing disorder are more vulnerable to pneumothorax because the lungs are closer to the surface. Only shallow needling is recommended)	GV 14, BL 13 BL 38, GB 20 GB 21, Bl 23	Gua sha to upper back, neck, shoulders, chest	LI 4, LU 7, KI 6, LU 5, PC 6, SP 4 CV 17, CV 21 and/or CV 22 ST 36, Yin tang
Neck pain	GV 14, TW 15 TW 13, BL 10 GB 20, 21, Pak Loh, Ah Shi Neck + upper back; Bl 60 Bl 57 area per palpation	Gua sha to upper back, neck, shoulders; Gua sha into occiput, SCM lateral neck, LU 1 area chest	LI 4, LU 7 TW 3 or TW 4 TW 5, GB 41 SI 3, GB 39, TW gummy Check SCM, pectoralis and scalene areas for constriction
Thyroid problems, hypothyroid	GV 14, GB 20 BL 10, 11, 12 + 13, TW 13 Needle between cervical vertebra: 4–5, 5–6, and one eye division lateral to these points	Gua sha to upper back, occiput, back of neck, sides and SCM muscle Check TW channel on arms	LI 4, LU 7 LU 5, CV 22 ST 10, CV 17 BL 18, BL19, BL 20, BL 23 BL 31 to BL 32
Goiter, hyperthyroid	As above	Gua sha to upper back, occiput, back of neck, sides and SCM muscle Check TW channel on arms	Consider points above and KI 3 KI 6, KI 7 LI 11, ST 36 ST 40 TW4, GB 38 CV 22, points lateral to thyroid
Headache	GV 14, GV 15 GV 16, TW 15 or TW 16, GB 20 GB 21, BL 10 BL 12 or BL13, BL 38 (43)	Gua sha to upper back, neck, shoulders, sides of neck* Focal to site of scalp if pain is fixed (see Plate 25)	LI 4, LU 7 LI 11, ST 8 GV 20, GB 40 LIV 3 Extra points: Yin Tang, Tai Yang
Migraine, cluster headache, Fire of Stomach, Gall Bladder or Liver	As above GB 12, TW16	Gua sha to upper back, shoulders, neck, including sides* Focal to site of scalp if pain is fixed	As above, plus consider TW 5, GB 41 if one-sided; GB 38, LIV 2
Stagnant Blood, headache	As above but emphasize use of GV 20, GB 20 BL 10, BL 13 BL 17, BL 38 (43)	Gua sha to upper back, neck*, shoulders Focal to site of scalp if pain is fixed	Similar to above, but consider: SP 6, CV 6, SP 10, GB 40

Continued

Table 8.1 Treatment of Upper Jiao disorders—cont'd

Disorder	Needle	Gua sha	Needle
Back of head Tai Yang headache	General headache points above and GV 19, GV 16, GV 20, GB 20 BL 10, BL 12 BL 13, BL 38 (43)	Gua sha to upper back, both BL channels, shoulders, neck	Consider SI 3, BL 60, BL 62; if pain is occipital see treatment for sinusitis
Sinus headache, front Yang Ming, orbital	Headache points above with GB 20, BL 10 GV 16, BL 12, BL 13, BL 38 (43)	Gua sha to upper back, neck*, shoulders	LI 4, LU 7 LI 20 Yin Tang ST 8, GV 23 GB 14 ST 44, consider ST2, BL7
Side Shao Yang headache	Headache points above with GB 20, BL 10, GV 16, BL 12, BL 13, BL 38 (43)	Gua sha to upper back, neck*, shoulders, esp. TW channel	TW 5, GB 41, ST 8 Tai Yang extra pt, GB 40, GB 8 Check SCM, pectoralis and scalene areas for constriction
Top of the head Tsiue headache	Headache points above plus consider GV 20, BL 7	Gua sha to upper + mid-back, neck*, shoulders Focal to site of scalp if pain is fixed	LI 4, LIV 2, LIV 3, GB 38, check for sinusitis
Yin headache	Headache points above and: GB 20 BL 15, BL 17 BL 18	As above	LI 4, LU 7, LI 11, Yin tang, KI 3, BL 23
Deficiency Xu headache Xu headaches are dull and persistent. Survey diet in terms of what and also when a patient eats meals and check that meals are nutrient dense, including sources of protein	Headache points above emphasizing GV 20, GB 20, GV 14, BL 13	Gua sha to upper back, neck, shoulders Focal to site of scalp if pain is fixed	SP 6, ST 36 KI 3, LIV 3 BL 23, BL 20
Toothache	Headache points and include GV 20, GB 20, BL 13, TW 16	Gua sha to upper back, neck, shoulders	LI 4, ST 44 CV 24, ST 6 (lower teeth) GV 26, ST 7 (upper teeth)
Trigeminal neuralgia Advise patient to avoid wind, whether outdoors or indoors from fan, air conditioning or from any draft	GV 14, BL 13 GB 20, GB 21 BL 13 TW 15, TW 16 GB12	Gua sha to upper back, neck, shoulders Focal to site of scalp if pain is fixed	LI 4, LU 7, LI 11 Tai Yang extra pt, LIV 2, GB 37, 38, or 39 Levels: (Upper) ST 8, BL 2 GB 2, TW 21, TW 23 (Middle) GB 2, LI 20, ST 7 SI 19, ST 4 (Lower) ST 4, ST 6, ST 7, GB 2, SI 19, CV 24
Bell's palsy, facial paralysis (treat both sides of the face according to presentation)	GV 14, GB 20, GB 21, TW 15, BL 13	Gua sha to upper back, neck, shoulders	Bilaterally. Research shows there can be nerve damage on both sides of spine. LI 4, LU 7, GB 14, ST 4 ST 2, ST 7, ST 8, Tai Yang, extra pt, GB 2, SI 19, TW 21, ST 44

Table 8.1 Treatment of Upper Jiao disorders—cont'd

Disorder	Needle	Gua sha	Needle
Eye problems	GV14, BL 13, GB 20, TW 15, TW 16 BL 18, BL 19 BL 23	Gua sha to upper back, neck, shoulders	LI 4, LI 11 ST 8 BL 1, GB 1 GB 15 GB 37, SI 1 Extra pt Tai Yang
Ear problems	GB 20, GV 14 TW 16, TW 15 GB 12	Upper back, neck, sides of neck, shoulders	TW 3, TW 5, SI 3, SI 19 GB 2, TW 17, TW 21 BL 23, BL 18 GB 40
Temporomandibular joint disorder	GV 14, GB 20 TW 15, TW 16	Gua sha to upper back, neck, sides of neck, shoulders	GB 2, ST 7 ST 6, LI 4 ST 44 Check SCM and Scalenes for constriction
Herpes zoster, shingles head, neck or upper body (Treat shingles with acupuncture at initial signs of prodromal pain or outbreak even if patient is on medication. Add Gua sha as soon as lesions have healed. Treatment will prevent postherpetic neuralgia (PHN). If patient has PHN within 6 months to a year of an outbreak, emphasize repeated Gua sha treatment at the back and along the dermatome)	GV 14, BL 13 BL38, BL 15 BL 17, GV 20 Huato and BL channel points at the level of the affected dermatome	Gua sha is applied after lesions have healed. Upper back and neck for upper body shingles. Follow dermatome to axilla and front of the body (note: while tx is focused on affected side, palpate opposite side at dermatome level and treat if indicated)	LI 4, LIV 3, LI 11, SP 10 Yin tang 'Surround the Dragon' treatment: shallow needle insertion every inch along but outside of lesion scars. Point needles toward lesion. Set for 20–25 min. If shingles at level of eye see eye treatment above
Upper back pain, injury, fibromyalgia	GV 14, B 13, GB 20, GB 21, TW 13 TW 15, SI 14, BL 38 (43)	Gua sha to upper back, neck, shoulders to mid-back	LI 4, SI 3 TW 5, TW Gummy LI 11, LU 7
Chest pain, palpitation, angina, fibrillation, tachycardia	GV 14, GB 20 BL 10, BL 15 BL 17, GV 11	Gua sha to upper + mid-back, neck, shoulders, sternum	PC 5 PC 6, SP 4 HT 5, HT 7 Check chest muscles and ribs for constriction
Breast pain, distension, premenstrual syndrome, mastitis, fibrocystic breast condition	GV 14, GB 21 BL 13, BL 38 TW 15, GB 21 SI 11, BL 18	Gua sha to upper + mid-back, medial scapula border, neck, shoulders, sternum	LI 4, PC 6 SI 1, LU1 CV 17, ST 16 ST 18, ST 34 LIV 14 SP 10 ST 30 LIV 3, GB 34
Upper extremity problems	GV 14, GB 20 SI 14, TW 15 BL 13, BL 38 Ah Shi or trigger points by palpation	Gua sha to upper back, shoulders, neck, mid-back	LI 4, SI 3 TW 5, LI 11 palpate for constriction

Continued

Table 8.1 Treatment of Upper Jiao disorders—cont'd

Disorder	Needle	Gua sha	Needle
Shoulder pain, rotator cuff tear, bursitis, frozen shoulder (Alternate points when treating a chronic problem over time: point selection should be based on location of pain and where there is restriction in range of motion, i.e. follow the 'Dragons Tail')	GV 14, GB 20 GB 21, BL 38 TW 15, TW 14 SI 14, SI 11 SI 10, SI 9 LI 16, LI 15 LI 14, LU 1 LU 3	Gua sha to upper back, shoulder, neck, arm back, front + side	LI 4, LU 7 SI 3, SI 6 LI 11, TW 4 TW 5, LU 1 ST 39 Jianeiling
Upper arm injury/strain	GV 14, SI 14 SI 9, SI 10 SI 11, GB 21 LI 16, TW 15 TW 14, TW 13	Gua sha to upper back, shoulders, neck, arm back, front + side	LI 4, LI 11 LI 13, LI 14, LI 15 TW 5, TW 13, TW 14, TW 15, TW gummy SI 3, SI 6
Tennis elbow	GV 14, GB 20 GB 21, TW 15 BL 38, SI 14 SI 11, TW 14 SI 10, SI 9	Gua sha to neck, shoulder, upper back, arm above and below elbow on channel	LI 4, LI 10 LI 11, LI 12, TW 10, HT 3 TW 2, TW 3 TW 5, LI 5
Forearm injury/strain	GV 14, TW 15 LI 16, GB 20 GB 21	Gua sha to neck, shoulder, upper back, upper arm	LI 4, LI 10 LI 11 TW 5, Ah Shi
Carpal tunnel syndrome, wrist problems	GV 14, GB 20, GB 21, TW 15 BL 38, LI 16 LI 15, TW 14	Gua sha to neck, shoulder, upper back, arm above and below elbow on channel	LI 4, LI 5 LI 11, TW gummy LU 9, LU 11, PC 5 PC 6, PC 7 TW 4, TW 5 TW 6, SI 3
Joints of hand related to trauma or Bi syndrome arthralgia	GV 14, BL 13 TW 15, BL 38 LI 16, GB 20 GB 21, LI 15 TW 14	Gua sha to neck, shoulder, upper back, arm above and below elbow on channel	LI 4, LI 11 LI 10 PC 6, TW 5 Local pts on or between knuckles proximal or distal (Direct moxa on painful aspect of the joint)
Frostbite, fingertip snake boils (eruptions at fingertips from exposure)	GV 14, BL 12 BL 13, GB 20 TW 15	Gua sha to neck, shoulder, upper back, arm above and below elbow on channel	LI 4, LI 11 LI 10 PC 6, TW 5 Bleed Jing Well point

*Sternocleidomastoid muscle (SCM) can be treated on the side of headache pain

Middle Jiao disorders (Table 8.2)

For problems located in the Middle Jiao, Gua sha is applied to the back and may also be applied to the front and sides of the body. Treatment must also be considered above and below any area of the middle back. These considerations point to a need to not only treat a specific area of pain but also those areas that feed, drain or otherwise associate with a primary area or problem. The acupuncture points are not intended as a delimiting prescription but are suggested as options for core treatments to be adapted to a patient's specific presentation by the practitioner. Modern research has confirmed that most main acupuncture points are located at concentrations of connective tissue planes where propagation of mechanical and chemical signals from needling is enhanced. Therefore, main acupuncture points indicated for a problem are the essential core of treatment that can then be nuanced for the individual.

Table 8.2 Treatment of Middle Jiao disorders

Disorder	Needle	Gua sha	Needle
Abdominal or epigastric pain	BL 13, BL 18 BL 20, BL 21 BL 22	Gua sha to mid-back BL 12 to BL 22 Consider neck and GB 21 area	PC 6, SP 4, ST 36 CV 12, Yin tang
Lower abdominal pain	BL 17, BL 18, BL 20 BL 21, BL 22 BL 23, BL 25	Gua sha to mid-back BL 13 to BL 25	PC 6, SP 4, ST 36 CV 12, CV 6, ST 25
Flank pain	BL 18, BL 20 BL 23, BL 38 GB 25, BL 47	Gua sha to mid-back, include lateral BL channel and ribs to axillary line	TW 6, GB 34 LIV 3, LIV 14 Dai Mo: GB 41 (left is left sided pain), TW 5 (right if left sided pain) reverse if right sided pain palpate and Tx oblique constriction
Subcostal pain, hepatomegaly, splenomegaly	BL 13, BL 15 BL 38, BL 17 BL 18 BL 20 Pee Gen	Gua sha to upper and mid-back to BL 23 lateral to include areas of pain referred to back	PC 6, SP 4, ST 36 CV 12, LIV 4 LIV 13, ST 21 SP 6, SP 9, SP 10 TW 6, GB 34
Hepatitis/jaundice	BL 13, BL 15 BL 18, BL 19 BL 20, GV 9	Gua sha to upper back, mid- back to low back epigastric to hypchondrial region	PC 6, SP 4, ST 36 CV 12, LIV 13 LIV 14, LIV 3, GB 38, GB 34
Stomach ulcer	BL 13, BL 15 BL 18, BL 20 BL 21, Ah Shi	Gua sha to upper and mid-back Gua sha to epigastric region	PC 6, SP 4, ST 36, LI 11 CV 12, CV 13 ST 21, CV 4, CV 6, ST 25
Nausea with or without vomiting	GV 14, Bl 13, Bl 18	Gua sha to upper and mid back	PC 6, SP 4, ST 36 CV 12
Hiatal hernia	BL 17, BL 18 BL 20, BL 21	Gua sha to upper back, mid-back	PC 6, SP 4, ST 36 CV 12, CV 13 LIV 14, LIV 13 ST 18, ST 21
Bloating, gas distension	BL 13, BL 18 BL 20, BL 25	Gua sha to mid-back, low back, upper, if tender	PC 6, SP 4, ST 36 CV 12, CV 6 CV 4, LIV 13
Hypochlorhydria	BL 18, BL 20 BL 21, BL 23	Gua sha to upper + mid-back	PC 6, SP 4, ST 36 SP 6, LIV 3 CV 12, ST 21
Pancreatitis	BL 18, 19, 20, 21 Yi Shu ('pancreas hollow') aka M-BW-12 between BL 17 and BL 18	Gua sha to upper back, mid-back; Gua sha to epigastric region	LI 4, 11, PC 6 ST 36 CV 4, CV 12, ST 25
Cholecystitis	BL 18, BL 19 BL 20, GV 9	Gua sha to upper back, mid-back epigastric region, hypochondrial region on right	LI 4, PC 6, CV 12, ST 21 rt TW 6, GB 34 extra point M-LE-23 LIV 13, GB 24
Any Phlegm disorder	BL 13, BL 20 BL 23	Gua sha to whole back	ST 36, ST 40, CV 12 SP 5
Deficiency conditions	BL 15, BL 17, BL 23 short needle retention	Gua sha to back area according to palpation and constriction	Yin tang, SP 6, ST 36, CV 6 shorten time of needle retention Continue to rest patient for 30 min

Continued

Table 8.2 Treatment of Middle Jiao disorders—cont'd

Disorder	Needle	Gua sha	Needle
Deficient Blood/anemia	BL 15, BL 20, BL 23	Gua sha to back area according to palpation and constriction	CV 12, PC 6, CV 4 ST 36
Diarrhea, irritable bowel, Crohn's/colitis, Deficient Spleen Yang, collapse of Central Qi	Bai Hui GV 20 BL 13, BL 18 BL 20, BL 23 BL 25, GB 30, BL 50, BL 57	Gua sha to whole back, emphasis on mid- to low back, across hips into GB 30 area Bl 50 area at crease of lower buttock	ST 36, ST 37 CV 12, ST 25 CV 6, CV 4, KI 16 SP 6 Sore anus: BL 57, GV 1 (patient is prone: insert at angle from above the coccyx and toward anus)
Rib pain, intercostal neuralgia	BL 13, BL 17 BL 18 Ah Shi pts Posterior ribs and back	Gua sha to area of back according to ribs affected, – above, below and lateral on ribs to mid axillary line Use small cap to apply Gua sha between ribs, move flesh off of ribs to complete expression of sha.	TW 6, GB 34 PC 6, Yin tang LIV 13, LIV 14 LIV 2, LIV 3 LIV 5 Dai mo: GB 41 (left if left sided pain) TW 5 (right if left sided pain) reverse if pain is at right ribs Palpate and Tx leg GB channel
Rib fractures/dislocation	BL 13, BL 17 BL 18 Ah Shi pts Posterior ribs and back	Gua sha to area of back according to affected ribs and on back above and below. Apply Gua sha up to point of tolerance at axilla. Note: do not Gua sha over acute fracture, sprain, dislocation or contusion	Apply gauze soaked in Zhen Gui Shui to area of trauma unless skin is broken Leave for 20 min TW 6, GB 34 LIV 14, PC 6 ST 18 Consider Dai mo as above
Back pain	BL 60, BL 54 (40) or BL 57 BL 10, BL 11 BL 13, BL 15 BL 17, BL 20 BL 23	Gua sha to back, with sha expressed above, through and below affected area.	TW 5, GB 41, bilateral: if pain is one-sided: Tx GB 41 on affected side, TW 5 opposite to affected side Yin tang, KI 3 ST 36, SP 6 SP 2
Herpes zoster, shingles at mid-body (Treat shingles with acupuncture at initial signs of prodromal pain or outbreak even if patient is on medication. Add Gua sha as soon as lesions have healed to prevent PHN. If patient has PHN within 6 months to a year of an outbreak, emphasize repeated Gua sha treatment at the back and along the dermatome)	GV 14, BL 13 BL38, BL 15 BL 17, BL 18 Huato and BL channel points at the level of the affected dermatome	Gua sha is applied after lesions have healed. Upper back and middle back for mid-body shingles. Follow dermatome to axilla and front of the body (note: while tx is focused on affected side, palpate opposite side at dermatome level and treat if indicated)	LI 4, LIV3, LI 11, SP 10 Yin tang, ST 36, GB 38 'Surround the Dragon' treatment: shallow needle insertion every inch along but outside of lesion scars. Point needles toward lesion. Set for 20–25 min

Lower Jiao disorders (Table 8.3)

For problems located in the Lower Jiao, Gua sha is applied to the back and may also be applied to the front and sides of the body. Treatment must also be considered above and below any area of the lower back. These considerations point to a need to not only treat a specific area of pain but those areas that feed, drain or otherwise associate with a primary area or problem.

For treatment of leg problems Gua sha would always be applied to the mid- to lower back and hip on the affected side, never to the extremity alone. As well, Gua sha can be extended from the body down the affected aspect of the leg, above, below and over a joint directly. The acupuncture points are not intended as a delimiting prescription but are suggested as options for core treatments to be adapted to a patient's specific presentation by the practitioner.

Table 8.3 Treatment of Lower Jiao disorders

Disorder	Needle	Gua sha	Needle
Low back, acute pain	BL 60 BL 54 BL 25 BL 23 GV 14, BL 10 Ah Shi above or below	Gua sha to back, with sha expressed above, through and below affected area	SI 3, BL 62 TW 5, GB 41 ST 36, CV 6 Palpate and Tx constricted obliques and iliopsoas muscles Dai mo, as above with mid-back pain
Chronic back pain	As above + BL 17, 20	As above	As above KI 3, ST 36 SP 6 Dai mo TW 5, GB 41, bilateral or if pain is one-sided: tx GB 41 on affected side, TW 5 opposite to affected side
Lumbar disc herniation	BL 60, BL 54 BL 25, BL 23 GV 14, BL 10 Ah Shi above or below, Huato points associated with disc	As above	KI 3, ST 36 SP 6, TW 5, GB 41 Dai mo as above
Renal colic/kidney pain	GV 14, BL 13 BL 17, BL 18 BL 23, BL 47 GB 25	Gua sha to mid-back, lateral over posterior ribs + low back Back – above, through and below affected area	TW 6, GB 34 LIV 3, LIV 14 SP 6, KI 3 Dai mo as above
Deficient Kidney Yang	GV 14, GV 4 BL 20, BL 23	Gua sha to back, with sha expressed above, through and below affected area.	KI 3, SP 6 ST 36 CV 6, CV 4
Bladder pain	GV 14, BL 15 BL 18, BL 23 BL 28, BL 32, BI 57	Gua sha to mid-back, low back, sacral area and hip	SP 6, SP 9 LIV 8 CV 6, CV 4, CV 3, ST 29, or point between ST 29 and ST 30
Cystitis	GV 14, BL 15, BL 18 BL 23, 27, 28	Gua sha to mid-back, low back, sacral and hip area	SP 6, SP 9 CV 6, CV4 CV 3 ST 29
Urinary retention/incontinence	BL 23, BL 32 BL 33, BL 15 BL 27, BL 28	As above	SP 9, SP 6, CV 6, CV 3 CV 4 to retain, leaking urine CV 2 to release urine
Urinary frequency	As above	As above	SP 6, SP 9 ST 36, BL 57 CV 3, CV 4 CV 6, ST 29+
Prostatitis	BL 17, BL 20 BL 23, BL 25 BL 26, BL 28 BL 57	Gua sha to mid-back, low back, sacrum and lateral	SP 6, SP 9 CV 3, CV ST 27, ST 29 CV 1
Pelvic floor pain	BL15, BL18 BL 20, GB 30 BL50, BL 57	Gua sha to mid- and low back, across top of hips, at BL 50 crease to drain pelvic floor; top of thigh and inguinal area if indicated	Sp 6, SP 10 ST 36, ST 39 Yin tang Tx Ah Shi trigger points at thigh Palpate and Tx constricted obliques and iliopsoas Tx pelvic floor Ah Shi points
Genitals/pain	BL 18, BL 23 BL 32, BL 57, GB 30	Gua sha to mid- to low back, sacrum and lateral to sacrum, across top of hips, at BL 50 crease to drain pelvic floor Top of thigh and inguinal area if indicated	LIV 3, LIV 5 LIV 8 SP 6, SP 10 LIV 11, CV 2 CV 4, ST 28 or ST 29 Palpate and Tx constricted obliques and iliopsoas

Continued

Table 8.3 Treatment of Lower Jiao disorders—cont'd

Disorder	Needle	Gua sha	Needle
Herpes/genital lesions	BL 18, BL 23, BL 25, BL 32, BL 57 GB 30, Ah Shi points	As above	SP 6, SP 9 SP 10 LIV 2, LIV 8, GB 38 LIV 11, CV 4 CV 2, ST 29
Spermatorrhea, premature ejaculation	BL 15, BL 23 BL 47	Gua sha to mid- to low back, sacrum and lateral to sacrum, across top of hips Upper back if indicated	GB 20 Yin tang, Bai hui KI 3, SP 6 ST 36, CV 6 CV 4, CV3 ST 27
Impotence	BL 15, BL 23 GV 4	Gua sha to mid- to low back, sacrum and lateral to sacrum, across top of hips Upper back if indicated	SP 6, KI 3 HT 7, PC 5 CV 4, CV 6, ST 27, Yin tang
Vaginitis/leucorrhea: cold/white/clear	BL 13, BL 20, BL 23, GV 4	Gua sha to mid- to low back, sacrum and lateral to sacrum, across top of hips Upper back if indicated	SP 6, ST 36 LIV 3 CV 4, CV 6 ST 29 warming moxa to abdomen
Vaginitis/leucorrhea: hot/yellow/smelly	BL 18, BL 20 BL 23, BL 32	Gua sha to mid- to low back, sacrum and lateral to sacrum, across top of hips Gua sha to mid- and upper back	SP 6, SP 9 LIV 2 LIV 14 CV 3, CV 4 ST 29, GB 38
Lubrication: too much	BL 20, BL 23, BL 32, GV 4	Gua sha to mid- to low back	SP 6, CV 6 CV 4 ST 36, GB 26
Lubrication: too little	BL 15, BL 22 BL 23	As above	KI 6, KI 3 LIV 3 SP 6, CV 3 CV 4
Colon	BL 20, BL 23 BL 25	Gua sha to mid-back, low back, sacrum and area lateral to sacrum	ST 36, ST 37 ST 39 SP 6 PC 6, SP 4 if Blood Stasis ST 25, CV 6 SP 15, LIV 13 Palpate and treat constricted obliques and iliopsoas muscles
Prolapse of rectum	Bai Hui GV 20 BL 57, BL 25 BL 23, BL 20	Gua sha to mid-back, low back, sacrum and area lateral to sacrum, over coccyx and area lateral to coccyx	SP 6, ST 36, ST 39 CV 6
Hemorrhoids	GV 20 BL 57, BL 25 BL 23, BL 20 BL 30 Points lateral to coccyx GV 1	Gua sha to mid-back, low back, sacrum and area lateral to sacrum, over coccyx and area lateral to coccyx, GB 29 to GB 30 area	SP 6, ST 36 CV 6, KI 16, CV 12, ST 27, CV 3 Extra point Erbai
Uterus/ovaries	BL 15, BL 18 BL 20, BL 23 BL 32, BL 57	Gua sha to mid-back, low back, sacrum and area lateral to sacrum	LI 4, SP 6 CV 3, CV 4 CV 6, GB 26, ST 25, ST 27, ST 28 ST 29 Palpate and release obliques on affected side

Table 8.3 Treatment of Lower Jiao disorders—cont'd

Disorder	Needle	Gua sha	Needle
Irregular menses	BL 15, BL 18 BL 20, BL 23 BL 31 thru BL 34	Gua sha to mid-back, low back, sacrum and area lateral to sacrum	LIV 3, PC 6, SP 4 SP 6, CV 4, CV 6 ST 28, GB 26
Amenorrhea	BL 15, BL 17 BL 18, BL 23 BL 32, BL 57	As above	LI 4, SP 6 SP 10, PC 6, SP 4 CV 6, CV 4 ST 28, ST 29
Dysmenorrhea	BL 57, BL 18 BL 23 BL 31thru BL 34	As above	SP 9, SP 6 ST 44 LIV 3, CV 4 CV 3, ST 28
Menorrhagia	GV 20, BL 15 BL 18, BL 20 BL 23, BL 32	Gua sha to mid-back, low back, sacrum and area lateral to sacrum	HT 5, SP 10 SP 9, SP 6, CV 3, CV 4 Moxa SP 1 and LIV 1
Uterine fibroids/leiomyoma	BL 57, BL 15 BL 17, BL 18 BL 20, BL 32 Pee Gen	As above	SP 10, SP 9 SP 8, SP 6, PC 6, SP 4 CV 3, CV 4, CV 6
Ovarian cyst	BL 17, BL 18 BL 23, BL 25 BL 32, GB 30	Gua sha to mid-back, low back, sacrum and area lateral to sacrum	SP 10, SP 9 SP 6, LI 4 ST 25, ST 29 GB 26 Palpate and treat obliques on affected side
Inducing, treating labor	BL 17 BL 23 BL 31 BL 32 GB 21 across the muscle	Gua sha to whole back, sacrum across buttocks to GB 30 area	LI 4, SP 6 retain and repeatedly rotate and stimulate needles as patient walks around clinic ear Shen men and Uterus point apply ear seeds or ear magnets
Sciatica BL channel	BL 60, BL 54 BL 25, BL 23 BL channel, sacrum + lateral	Gua sha to low back to sacrum, back of leg Patient is prone on table	CV 6, KI 3 Dai mo: GB 41 (left if left-sided pain) TW 5 (right if left-sided pain) Reverse if pain is on right or Tx bilateral TW 5, GB 41
Sciatica GB channel	GB 30, GB 31 GB 34, GB 39 GB 29, GB 26	Gua sha to low back, sacrum GB 30 area in lateral recumbent position GB 31 area on leg	CV 6, LIV 3 Dai mo: GB 41 (left if left sided pain) TW 5 (right if left sided pain) Reverse if right sided sciatica, or Tx bilateral TW 5, GB 41
Hip pain	GB 31, GB 30 GB 29 GB 34 Ah Shi	Gua sha to low back, sacrum and lateral to hip and GB 30 area Hip Ah Shi	Dai mo: GB 41 (left if left sided pain) TW 5 (right if left sided pain) Reverse if right sided sciatica, or Tx bilateral TW 5, GB 41
Strained hamstring/quads	BL 54, BL 25 BL 26, BL 50 at ischium Ah Shi sacrum and lateral to sacrum Ah Shi leg BL 60, BL57	Gua sha to low back, sacrum, back of leg Ah Shi leg area	SP 6, ST 36 SP 10, ST 34

Table 8.3 Treatment of Lower Jiao disorders—cont'd

Disorder	Needle	Gua sha	Needle
Knee injury/Bi	BL 23, BL 25 BL 54, BL 60 Sacral Ah Shi Lateral sacral Ah Shi	Gua sha to low back, sacrum and hip Gua sha to quads	SP 6, SP 9, SP 10 GB 34, GB 31, LIV 8 Eyes of knee Wings of knee Palpate and reduce constriction at thigh For acute sprain apply gauze soaked in Zhen Gu Shui for 20 min
Injury to lower leg	GB 30, GB 31 GB 34, GB39 Ah Shi	Gua sha to sciatica regions (see above)	SP 6, ST 36 BL 57, BL 59 Ah Shi
Ankle sprain/Bi	BL 60, BL 54 BL 25, BL 23 BL 57 and calf points Sacral Ah Shi Lateral sacral Ah Shi	Gua sha to low back, sacrum Lateral sacral area	SP 5, LIV 4 GB 40, SP 6 KI 3, KI 6 Ah Shi For acute sprain apply gauze soaked in Zhen Gu Shui for 20 min Needle distal points then lightly massage over ankle to reduce swelling
Foot/toe injury/Bi	BL 60, 54, 25, 23 GB 30, 31, 34 Sacral Ah Shi Lateral sacral Ah Shi	Gua sha to low back, sacrum Sacral Ah Shi Lateral sacral Ah Shi	BL 34, GB 39, GB 40 ST 36, LIV 3 GB 41 SP 6, KI 3 ST 44, Ah Shi
Heel pain	As above	As above	KI 3, BL 60 KI 7, KI 8 Palpate and Tx BL 57 area, reactive points of the calf
Plantar fasciitis	As above	Gua sha to calf, low back and hip area	K3, BL 60 Palpate and Tx BL 57 area and reactive points of the calf
Any difficulty walking	GB 30, GB 31 GB 34, GB 39, GB 40 BL 60, BL 54 (TCM 40)	Gua sha to low back, sacrum, back of leg, GB 30 area in lateral recumbent position GB 31 area at leg	SP 6, ST 36 LIV 3 Dai mo: GB 41 (left if left sided problem) TW 5 (right if left sided problem) Reverse if right-sided problem; or Tx bilateral TW 5, GB 41
Uneven leg length, long leg syndrome (treat the long leg side)	GB 26, GB 30, GB 31, GB 32, GB 38, BL 60	Lateral recumbent position: Gua sha to: GB 29-30 area GB 31 area	Dai mo: GB 41 (left if left sided problem) TW 5 (right if left sided problem) Reverse if right-sided problem, or Tx bilateral TW 5, GB 41
Herpes zoster, shingles at the lower body (Treat shingles with acupuncture at initial signs of prodrome pain or outbreak even if patient is on medication. Add Gua sha as soon as lesions have healed to prevent PHN. If patient has PHN within 6 months to a year of an outbreak, emphasize repeated Gua sha treatment at the back and along the dermatome)	BL 15, BL 17 BL 18, Huato and BL channel points at the level of the affected dermatome	Gua sha is applied after lesions have healed to the middle back, lower back and hip area for lower body shingles. Follow dermatome around to the front of the body (note: while Tx is focused on affected side, palpate opposite side at dermatome level and treat if indicated)	LI 4, LIV3, LI 11, SP 10 Yin tang ST 36 GB 38 'Surround the Dragon' treatment: shallow needle insertion every inch along but outside of lesion scars. Point needles toward lesion. Set for 20–25 min

Cases

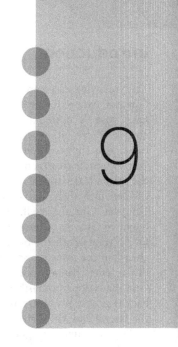

9

CHAPTER CONTENTS

Introduction

The following cases are patients treated by the author using Gua sha, except for the hepatitis case, which is a cited article. Each case is outlined by presenting disorder but includes Tongue, Pulse, other signs and symptoms, and recommendations, as is the tradition in classical Chinese medicine. Rather than list each treatment given in each case, I have compiled the overall treatment approach. The treatment section is divided into three parts: acupuncture points applied before Gua sha, Gua sha itself, and acupuncture points used subsequent to Gua sha. Classical Chinese medicine in the lineage of Dr So treats both the back and the front of the body but not always in the same session. Venting Heat and reducing Excess in the Yang channels is considered first and is the reason why Gua sha is done primarily on the Yang surfaces. Therefore, the back is almost always treated first. Gua sha is applied, and then the lateral and Yin surfaces or front of the body are treated.

The acupuncture point list in each treatment section includes all points used over a period of time. Points for a single treatment were among those listed, not necessarily all those listed. Determination of points was based on location, quality, mutability and association of a problem, application of distal as well as proximal sites, use of palpation and knowledge of previous treatment.

In some cases Gua sha was instrumental in resolution. In others Gua sha was a contributing factor in speeding resolution. Although Gua sha can be done whenever there are the proper indications, in these cases it was not done more frequently than once every one or two weeks.

If you find indications of sha soon after you have done Gua sha, it may indicate low Wei Qi. It can also be a result of repeated alcohol intake, which expands the peripheral capillaries, allowing chill to penetrate.

Where relevant, I noted studies that relate to the case being discussed. Chapter 2 has a complete literature review of studies. Cases here have been arranged by Jiao, beginning with the Upper Jiao. Pinyin names of the points are listed in Appendix B.

Headache, esophagitis, neck and shoulder pain, cervical disc degeneration

Female, 39

Presenting complaint

Patient complained of pain in her neck and shoulders, with numbness, tingling and twitching down her arms. There was loss of mobility in her neck. Headaches ensued from the neck pain. She was diagnosed with arthritis at C4–5, with degenerative disc thinning and cervical disc herniation at C5–6 and bone fusion at C6–7. Magnetic resonance imaging (MRI) showed disc bulge anterior and posterior. Patient received biannual neurological check-ups. It was recommended she have a

discectomy with transplant of the hip bone to fuse cervical vertebrae.

Previous treatment

Patient was under the care of a neurologist and chiropractor.

Tongue

Her tongue was swollen and pale, with pronounced swelling at borders where the flesh was pale and shining. The end of the tongue had tiny raised red dots. An alley down the midline of the tongue was yellow, furry and slightly depressed.

Pulse

Rate 76; Kidney pulses were deep, with Kidney Yin deep and wide. The entire Blood pulse was tight with the Heart pulse also wide.

Other signs and symptoms

Patient had good muscle mass, was a little overweight with slight edema overall. She took Xantac or Tagamet for stomach pain, hiatal hernia, esophagitis and pain in the chest so that she could not swallow her own saliva. She had uterine fibroids with early heavy menses. She had a history of back pain and weakness, frequent urination and sinus problems. Her voice was slightly sing-songy, she preferred talking to feeling or experiencing treatment. She worked as a nurse and was a single mother of three.

Treatment

Back

- GV 14, BL 13, BL 38, TW 15, GB 20, GB 21, alternating Pak Loh, SI 10, Ah Shi trigger points at neck and upper back.
- **Gua sha** was applied to her neck, shoulders, upper and middle back, depending on signs for sha and presenting area of constraint and tenderness.

Front

- LI 4, ST 36, LIV 3, PC 6, LI 13, TW gummy, alternating TW 5, GB 41, neck massage and stretching.

Course of treatment

Five acupuncture treatments for esophagitis, headache, neck and shoulder pain.

Recommendations

Eliminate coffee, cold and sour foods. Keep neck covered to protect from temperature change. Neti pot washes were recommended for sinuses (see Appendix C).

Results

Esophagitis was gone after the first treatment, headaches gone after the second. With each treatment patient experienced increased range of motion with decreasing neck pain. No trajecting pain, tingling or numbness after the fourth session. Off stomach medications by fifth session.

Patient presented again in 6 weeks. A neurological check corroborated her experience of improvement and surgery was cancelled. She had slight neck and shoulder pain, but full range of motion. She received one or two treatments per month (31 total) over the next 2 years for her neck and shoulders, an occasional acute upper respiratory infection and menstrual problems. The improvement in her neck and shoulders continued until it was no longer a chronic problem.

Note: Gua sha has been shown to be effective for neck pain in a randomized controlled trial published in the journal *Pain Medicine* (Braun et al. 2011). Gua sha for neck pain is one of the most studied areas of Gua sha in the Chinese language database (see Chapter 2).

Cluster headaches, post-trauma

Male, 37

Presenting complaint

Patient had attacks of head pain that would completely debilitate him. He carried oxygen with him at all times. His left eye would redden, burn and weep. Diagnosed as cluster headaches, the attacks occurred after an accident where his nose was broken by a baseball. A fragment of bone lacerated an artery and emergency surgery was performed. A piece of metal was left at the site. He had had headaches for 4 years.

Previous treatment

After the emergency surgery, the patient was under the care of neurologists for 4 years. He had been tried on 17 different medications. At one point he was hospitalized and given intravenous antihistamines. Lithium stopped the headaches for 1 year, but he felt weak on the medication. Eventually the headaches returned. The patient wanted to avoid further medication so he was referred by his physician for acupuncture treatment.

Tongue

Bright red and wet with only slight coating at the back center.

Pulse

Deep and slight.

Other signs and symptoms

This patient had a strong muscular build. He worked with computers all day and labored outdoors in his free time. When he first presented he was taking prednisone, 5 mg four times per day, Cardene, 20 mg twice per day, and Zantac. He had severe head pain that would wake him in the night or start in the day. He had to use oxygen to relieve the pain. His urine

was frequent, though he had edema from the prednisone. He felt weak, had no sexual drive and had diarrhea. He was desperate.

The head pain would begin as a burning in the right corner of the eye and nose. The pain would shoot into the eye like fire and then back over the head along the Gallbladder channel, into the occiput, neck and right shoulder.

Treatment

Back

- GV 14, BL 13, GB 20, BL 10. Right side: TW 15, BL 38, SI 14, Pak Loh, GB 12, TW 16.
- **Gua sha** to upper back, concentrating on the right neck and shoulder. Initially sha was dark.

Front

- LI 4, LU 7, GB 40, BL 7, Yin Tang, right LI 11, TW gummy, LI 20, BL 1, BL 2, Yu Yao, Pi Yen, ST 8, Tai Yang, Ah Shi at scar along right nose.
- Bleeding technique applied with small cups around area of trauma. Blood expressed was extremely dark.

Course of treatment

Patient was treated every 10 days for the first 12 treatments, after which the sessions were spaced 2 weeks apart, then 3 weeks, then a month.

Recommendations

Patient was screened for allergens and offensive foods. He was asked to stop all caffeine, alcohol and sugar. This meant he needed to eat a meal for breakfast as opposed to coffee and a Danish. He was eating ice cream before bed each night. All cold, sweet foods were discouraged. Regular meals of nutritious food were encouraged to avoid hypoglycemia.

Yunnan Bai Yao (Yunnan White Medicine) was given for post-trauma congealed Blood. It was recommended to be taken with a shot of rice wine.

Lung Tang Xie Gan (Gentiana Drain the Liver Pill), was given for Shao Yang Heat in the Upper Jiao.

Tien Ma Hu Gan Wan (Gastrodia Tiger Bone Pill) was given initially, with Jiang Ya Pill Pian Hypertension Repressing Tablets subsequently.

Results

His diarrhea stopped with the cessation of all dairy products and was likely due to lactose intolerance. With treatment and other dietary recommendations, his headaches began to diminish in intensity, then in frequency. He was able to reduce and finally stop all medication.

He continued with treatment once every 4–6 weeks. A year after complete recovery he had a recurrence following a neck injury. He resumed treatment every 2 weeks and recovered fully in 6 months. He received a treatment every 4–8 weeks for another year to maintain free flow. It has been over 20 years since he has had treatment and he has had no recurrence.

(Gua sha at the scalp is an essential addition to Gua sha to the upper neck, back and shoulders in cases of migraine or cluster headaches. See Plate 25 as an example).

Cluster headache with allergic rhinitis 'Wind exposure'

Female, 34

Presenting complaint

Patient suffered for years from recurrent fixed and severe head pain diagnosed as 'cluster headache', accompanied by labile allergic rhinitis symptoms that worsened in spring with exposure to pollen. Symptoms worsened if exposed to wind in any season.

Previous treatment

Patient was given migraine medication by her primary care physician to use as needed. Over-the-counter (OTC) analgesics did not relieve her pain. Chinese herbal medicine given by another provider did not address her pain.

Tongue

Tongue was normal pink to pale, with front end and rim of the Tongue redder. No red or white points.

Pulse

Pulse was normal with the exception of a fuller active pulse at the sinus position that is proximal to the first position on both wrists.

Other signs and symptoms

Patient sometimes suffered from constipation that was related to stress, Liver Qi constraint. Her cluster headaches were debilitating when they occurred and frustrating.

Treatment

Back
- GV 14, BL 13, BL 38, TW 15, GB 20, GB 21 BL 10, GB 12, de qi and remove.
- **Gua sha** to upper back and neck, including sides of neck.

Front
- Needle focal fixed area of pain at the scalp.
- **Gua sha** to the scalp at the area of focal fixed head pain.
- LI 4, LU7, TW gummy, LI 20, ST 2 Yin tang ST8.

Additional points
- Liv 2, ST 36, KI3, GB 40.

Course of treatment

Patient had two sessions.

Recommendations

Daily use of Neti wash, which patient began immediately. Eat regular meals of warm cooked food. Avoid fruit during pollen season. Avoid exposure to wind. Patient was already moderate in terms of work and activity.

Results

First treatment resolved cluster headache focal pain. Patient reported for one follow up treatment for allergic rhinitis. Headaches did not recur.

Heachache, chronic sinusitis, food allergies

Female, 45

Presenting complaint

Patient complained of chronic headache at the bridge of the nose, chronic, allergic, inflamed sinuses, postnasal drip alternating with stuffy nose.

Tongue

Thin Tongue body with shallow cross cracks and red tip. Coating was normal and rooted but with thickening at back and overlaid with foamy residue.

Pulse

Fast and wiry. There was a roughness at the Lung pulse and fullness at the sinus positions found distal to the Upper Jiao positions.

Other signs and symptoms

This patient was thin with boundless energy, loud voice and *joie de vivre*. She had normal menses but had premenstrual breast tenderness. Stools were normal and urine frequent. She was allergic to, craved and ate peanut butter, chocolate, wheat, garlic and onions.

Treatment

Back
- GV 14, BL 12, BL 13, GB 20, BL 10, GV 15, BL 38, BL 18, BL 20, BL 23.
- **Gua sha** to upper neck, back and shoulders.

Front
LI 4, LU 7, LI 20, ST 2, BL 2, Yin Tang, ST 8, Tai Yang, BL 7, CV 6, ST 36.

Allergy desensitization[1]

- LI 4, LIV 3, Mu point or Source point of Organ or Organs weakened by allergen (Nambudripod (1989).

Course of treatment

Nineteen treatments in the first year, weekly or every other week; 12 treatments in the second year; four treatments in the third year and one treatment in the fourth year. Gua Sha was done no more than monthly.

Recommendations

Avoid allergies during desensitization process. Use Neti washes daily (see Appendix C).

Results

Patient's sha was initially thin, small and purple. Subsequently, the sha appeared lighter in amount and color. Presenting headache left after the first treatment. Subsequent sessions dealt with sinus pain and blockage and tenderness at the bridge of the nose. Headaches became less intense and less frequent, triggered by eating sugar. Premenstrual symptoms resolved. Eventually sessions included the desensitization to allergens. The outcome was that she no longer craved the offending foods and could eat them occasionally without symptoms.

In the third year she presented with headache and sinus infection producing green mucus. Bi Jen Pian was given following acupuncture and Gua sha with good results.

After that she used the acupuncture sessions to explore the roots of her addictive/allergic behavior. She realized that though the allergic foods caused headaches and sinus problems they also stimulated her high energy state. She liked the power of feeling boundless energy and though the pain was unpleasant it was also a form of self-stimulation, a way to bring attention to herself in the midst of too many projects. As she healed she became less driven in her schedule, created more time for herself and changed her orientation from 'pain as pleasure'.

Neck and shoulder tension pain: Shi Excess condition

Male, 35

Presenting complaint

Patient complained of neck and shoulder pain from overuse of muscles and overwork. His muscles would seize up, causing pain so severe his lips would turn blue. His neck pain extended into his shoulders and down his arms, causing numbness in both hands. He was diagnosed with mild herniations of C4–5 and 5–6, with cervical and thoracic radiculitis.

Previous treatment

This patient had been receiving chiropractic adjustments and had also received a few acupuncture treatments without lasting results.

Tongue

He had a large tongue, damp with a foamy white coating, even throughout in color and texture with occasional red dots at the rim and tendency toward scallops. Coating was varied, greasy in back center. The thickness, greasiness and foaminess of the coating increased or receded depending on the patient's condition.

Pulse

Surprisingly Deficient, thin, deep and weak. This patient's overwork habits severely weakened his Qi allowing concomitant accumulation and stagnation of Qi, Fluids and Blood.

Other signs and symptoms

This patient made fine violins and cellos. He would lose himself in his craft, sometimes working more than 24 hours without a rest. He also suffered from migraines, possibly occasioned by the resins and finishes. He was extremely allergic to the Urishi resin extracted from the poison ivy plant, which is used to finish the wood of violins. He had bouts of asthma, sinusitis and headaches, allergic dermatitis and heat rash. Physically a large muscular man, a tremendous generator of heat and always slightly sweaty. Stools loose, urine infrequent and sleep erratic.

Treatment

Back

- GV 14, BL 13, BL 38, TW 15, GB 20, BL 10, points lateral to CV 4 and 5. Alternating presenting trigger or Ah Shi points, GB 21.
- **Gua sha** to upper back and neck, including sides of neck, shoulders, upper arms and forearms.

Front

- LI 4, LI 11, TW gummy, LI 15.

Additional points for tonification of Spleen

- BL 20, BL 23, CV 12, ST 36, SP 6, CV 6, alternating ST 40, LIV 13.

---

[1]There is no scientific research to support the use of this technique for desensitization of immune mediated allergies. It does appear to shift a patient's subjective relationship to 'sensitivities'.

Course of treatment

First course for neck, shoulders, arms and hands. Fourteen weekly treatments. Subsequent treatments continued to tonify Spleen. Patient used acupuncture and Gua sha to increase creativity.

Recommendations

Stop coffee or any stimulants. Reduce intake of dairy products as they can increase Damp stagnation internally. Regulate work hours, rest when tired and nap if necessary. Er Chen Tang (Two Cured Pill), given for mucus, Lien Chiao Pai Du Pien (Forsythia Defeat Toxin Tablet), for poison ivy outbreak and Lung Tang Xie Gan (Gentiana Drain Liver Pill), for heat rash in groin.

Results

Neck and shoulders stopped seizing up. Patient described improvement as 'not suffering', where he was able to extend himself in work and recover with rest. Body Heat was reduced, heat rash was gone. All numbness of hands and forearms gone, as were headaches. Tongue, pulse and body signs indicated a strengthening of digestion. As sweat was contained and transport of fluid normalized, the urine frequency increased to normal.

Note: Gua sha for neck and shoulder problems are one of the most studied areas of Gua sha in the Chinese language database (see Chapter 2).

Neck and shoulder tension pain: Xu Deficiency condition

Female, 29

Presenting complaint

Patient complained of chronic neck and shoulder pain, cold all over but especially in hands and feet.

Previous treatment

Patient was on a yeast-free diet, taking nystatin three times a day as prescribed by a physician.

Tongue

Pale pink with white coating.

Pulse

Slow, slightly irregular, with spleen Pulse weak and both Kidney pulses scattered.

Other signs and symptoms

She was thin, tired, cold and reported craving sugar and coffee. Appetite was reduced. She was nauseous from the nystatin. Stools were daily and formed, urine was frequent. Sleep was sound but she woke tired. Menses were regular at 28 days, lasting 5 days. The menstrual flow was light, red, with some small clots and no pain. Her fingernails were thin, pale and lined. She had heart palpitations. Patient was vegetarian, ate lots of grains and vegetables but no animal protein. She was afraid that eating caused weight gain.

Treatment

Back

- GV 14, BL 38, TW 15, GV 4, BL 23, KI 3.
- **Gua sha** neck and shoulders. Indirect moxa to BL 20, BL 23 area. Massage neck and shoulders, slow stretch to neck.

Course of treatment

Patient received three treatments. I used few needles in these first sessions and relied equally on Gua sha, massage, indirect moxa and diet as intervention since this patient was extremely weak.

Recommendations

Increase protein intake to twice per day, preferably at breakfast and lunch. Eat warm cooked food, slowly.

Results

The sha that appeared was distinct, small petechiae, pale in color. Patient experienced marked improvement in body warmth and strength. Urination became less frequent. Neck and shoulder pain was reduced. She came back in 2 months for one neck and shoulder treatment and then moved out of the area.

She returned 6 months later. By this time her strength had increased, her tongue was less pale and more fleshy. The pulse picture was similar but stronger.

Treatment

Back

- GV 14, BL 13, 38, TW 15, SI 15, GB 21, 20 and BL 10. **Gua sha** and slow neck stretching (see Plate 11).

Course of treatment

Two sessions treating neck and shoulders.

Results

The sha appeared less pale than previously, but petechiae were still small and light. Treatment eased the pain in the neck and shoulders, but chronic Deficient ache slowly returned due to the severity of Deficiency, overactivity and nutritional inadequacy. It was clear that increasing nutrient-dense food helped this patient. Eventually she introduced some animal products and her Deficiency resolved.

Chronic earache, draining and loss of hearing

Male, 55

Presenting complaint

Patient complained of a lifetime chronic infection in the right ear subsequent to a punctured eardrum as a child. Had earaches and drainage, some headaches at the back of the head, sinus drainage and a peculiar taste in the mouth.

Tongue

Red with thick white coating, slightly dry and sticky.

Pulse

64; clear and even but for Moving Lung pulse.

Other signs and symptoms

His appetite and stools were normal. Urine normal with some night urine. Sleep was good. History of back problems and occasional hemorrhoids. Had two martinis each evening. Worked outside most of the day.

Treatment

Back
- GV 14, TW 15, GB 20, GB 21.
- **Gua sha** to right neck, shoulder and upper back.

Front
- TW 3, 16, 17, 21, GB 2, SI 19, all on right side. Indirect moxa around ear.
- At the third session, left LI 11 and LI 4 were added.
- **Gua sha** in front of ear, along right SCM and scalenes.

Course of treatment

Nine sessions, eight weekly, with the ninth 5 weeks later.

Recommendations

Avoid cold and sour foods, keep ear covered and warm, even to the point of wearing a light hat indoors.

Results

The day after the first treatment he had a rush of brown and red fluid from the right ear, which abated. The ear was less sensitive and hearing improved.

By the third session he had some pain in the ear with clear fluid draining. By the fourth, the fluid was once again brown, bad smelling and his ear really hurt. By the fifth treatment the ear stopped draining completely for the first time, but remained sensitive to cold and noise. By the sixth session he had no pain and no draining with hearing much improved. His neck was now feeling warm. The last three sessions treated his back, hemorrhoids and his ears secondarily. During this time he had one more discharge of clear fluid from the ear.

He presented 5 years later for a hand injury. His ear remained completely healed.

Pediatric bronchitis, croup

Male, 3

Presenting complaint

This child had a severe cough with abundant phlegm in his chest and head, but no fever. Face was red on right cheek.

Tongue

Pink with Lung area red, greasy wet coating.

Pulse

Fast, slippery, moving in Lung position.

Other signs and symptoms

Stools were normal to loose. He was tired but overactive, not sleeping at night due to cough. Parents were exhausted.

Treatment

Back
- GV 14, BL 13.
- **Gua sha** upper back from BL 11 to BL 17.
- Massage BL 20 area, ST 36 to 40 area.

Front massage
- LU 9, LU 8, LU 7 and intercostal spaces at sternum.

Recommendations

No cold food or fluid of any kind and no dairy or soy products. When the mucus is clear and abundant, avoid fruit juice. If mucus is yellow or green, room temperature fruit juice may be given. Er Chen Wan (Two Cured Pill) and San She Chen Pi Mo (Snake Gallbladder, Tangerine Peel Powder) were given for cough and mucus. A croup tent was recommended several times per day (see Appendix C).

Results

Treatment caused increased expectoration of mucus from chest. Coughing lessened so that all slept through the night. He continued herbs for cough for 5 more days, at which time the mucus was resolved and cough infrequent.

Pediatric reactive airway, wheeze

Female, 6 months

Presenting complaint

Patient had respiratory infection that resulted in wheeze, diagnosed as reactive airway condition. This would previously have been diagnosed as asthma and subjected patient to automatic maintenance on asthma medication. Experience led to caution by primary care physicians to assess individual cases in terms of severity, persistence and recurrence of reactive airways before giving a diagnosis of asthma.

Previous treatment

Mother gave infant homeopathic remedies, was nursing and recently introduced to solid food. Patient was nebulized with bronchial dilation medication and was given a prescription for nebulizer if needed.

Tongue

Tongue was normal healthy baby Tongue. Illness was recent onset and had not yet marked the Tongue. Infant was nursing.

Pulse

Pulse was normal but fast with the exception of fuller pulse associated with the Upper Jiao.

Other signs and symptoms

Otherwise healthy infant, no signs of eczema or other atopic symptoms.

Treatment

Back

Mother supine on the table and held baby to her chest; mother removed babies shirt. In this position the child could nurse if she needed to nurse.

- **Gua sha** to infant's upper back along Hua tuo and Bladder channel just to the point of the first appearance of petechiae and then moved to next area. In this manner, the infant remains comfortable and allows Gua sha to continue. Light Gua sha is very effective for infants and does not need to be applied in the same manner as one would for adults.

Front

- Light **Gua sha** to chest area CV channel.
- Light manual stimulation along Lung channel.

Course of treatment

Patient had one emergency session with one follow up in a week, and then in two weeks for several sessions.

Recommendations

This child had very attentive maternal care, was kept warm, and fed, rested and engaged. Suggested first solids not rice- or grain-based but vegetable-based, e.g. avocado, sweet potato, then cooked fruit and stewed meat. Eventual grain solids to be cooked as thin gruel. Babies have appropriately immature digestion and are challenged by solid food that is difficult to break down. Premature solids or solids that are undercooked can result in production of mucus and phlegm damp mucous according to traditional East Asian medicine (TEAM), and add to food sensitivities.[2]

Recommended to return for treatment at first sign of any respiratory infection to prevent reactive airway.

Results

One session stopped the baby's wheezing. Several follow-up treatments every two weeks maintained her recovery. Child suffered from bronchitis and reactive airways recurrence at 21 months of age. Treatment was repeated and here too wheeze stopped and more serious illness and risk of medication was averted.

Acute asthma

Male, 35

Presenting complaint

Asthma attack of 6 hours duration. Patient got only temporary relief from inhaler.

Previous treatment

He was under the care of a physician who prescribed theophylline orally as well as a bronchodilating inhaler.

Tongue

Red, dry with yellow coating. The coating tended to dry out due to rapid breathing and breathing through the mouth.

Pulse

Rapid, fast and full. Medication increased heart rate. The Lung pulse was also floating.

Other signs and symptoms

When taking medication his pulse was rapid and stools loose. Urine was normal to slightly frequent. Muscles of the chest and upper back were tight and painful. He had difficulty

---

[2]It has been suggested that the high glycemic index of white rice cereal may predispose infants to obesity as children and adults.

breathing in and out, but more with exhalation. He was tired and anxious.

Treatment

Back

- GV 14, Ding Chuan, BL 13, 38, 15, 18, 20, 23, GB 21, 20.
- **Gua sha** to upper back, neck and top of shoulders.

Front

- LI 4, LI 11, ST 40, PC 6, SP 4, CV 22.
- **Gua sha** to sternum and lateral from sternum over first 3–4 ribs.

Course of treatment

For the acute asthma, two sessions.

Recommendations

Avoid cold food and drink as this congeals the mucus in the chest and dampens the Spleen into producing more mucus. This includes dairy products. Avoid hot, spicy food as well as shellfish because they cause the Lungs to overheat.

Qing Fei Yi Huo Pian (Lung Clearing, Fire Eliminating Tablets) were given. This formula treats Heat in the Lungs with Phlegm.

Results

The patient felt immediately better, able to inhale and exhale with much less effort. The Gua sha facilitated bronchodilation and expectoration of mucus. His mucus was abundant, yellow and slightly viscous.

For his chronic asthma controlled by medication, weekly treatment for 3 months allowed him to reduce and finally stop the medication with his physician's guidance. Treatments once to twice per month helped to maintain him for a period of 2 years at which time he moved to a warmer climate. During those 2 years his acute attacks became less frequent and were treated as above.

Emphysema

Male, 65

Presenting complaint

Patient had extreme shortness of breath. He was able to drive a car, but only able to walk two or three steps without stopping to catch his breath.

Previous treatment

Patient was under the care of a physician and also received chiropractic adjustment.

Tongue

The tongue flesh was a burnt red or brownish color. There were many cracks and fissures. The coating was uneven, thick, greasy and not rooted.

Pulse

Rapid, thin, moving at the Lung position.

Other signs and symptoms

He continued to smoke two packs of strong cigarettes per day. His stools were loose, possibly from medication, and his urine was frequent.

Treatment

Back

- GV 14, Ding Chuan, BL 12, 13, 38, GB 21.
- **Gua sha** to upper back and top of shoulders in GB 21 area.

Front

- LI 4, LU 7 or 9, PC 6, SP 4, ST 40, LU 1, CV 22, 17.

Course of treatment

Patient received acupuncture and Gua sha every 2–5 weeks.

Recommendations

Avoid cold food and drink. He did not want to quit smoking.

Results

At the end of the session, he was able to expectorate mucus and breathe more freely. After that he could climb stairs and walk further without losing his breath. This patient died of emphysema a year later, but the regularity of his treatment greatly improved his quality of life in his last year.

Chronic obstructive airway disease (COPD)

Female, 69

Presenting complaint

Severe dyspnea (shortness of breath), unable to walk without use of oxygen; anxiety and insomnia.

Previous treatment

Patient regularly participated in Pulmonary Rehabilitation Clinic and was managed with oxygen, inhaled steroid medication and oral medication. Patient also took antibiotics episodically to prevent and treat respiratory infection.

Tongue

Tongue was red, cracked and peeled with redder front rim. Unrooted coat was present at the Stomach area. Central crack to the Tongue tip.

Pulse

Pulse was irregular, fast and smooth.

Other signs and symptoms

Fatigue from effort to breath, anxiety and insomnia.

Treatment

Back
- GV 14, BL 13, BL 43, GB 20, GB 21 (across muscle), SI 11.
- **Gua sha** to upper back, neck and SI 11 area.

Front
- **Gua sha** to LU 1 pectoralis area and at Lung channel upper arm.
- N to LI 4, left PC 6, right SP 4, right LU 7, left KI 6.
- St 36 Yin tang, CV 21, 22.
- Ear magnets were placed at Shen men in ear and renewed at each session.

Course of treatment

Patient had several weekly sessions over the period of time she attended clinic.

Recommendations

Neti wash daily to prevent postnasal drip and potential respiratory infection. Avoid cold and wind, eat and drink mostly warm cooked food. Practice 'Controlled Pause Breathing' (Butyenko BreathTherapy) as described in the book: *Breathing Free* by Theresa Hale (2000).

Recommended to return for treatment at first sign of any respiratory infection to prevent illness and worsening of symptoms.

Results

Anxiety was reduced and patient's sleep improved. Patient experienced periods of time after treatment where breathing was easier, mobility was facilitated. Patient could walk around home without need for constant oxygen. Patient moved out of the area with the approach of winter.

Sarcoidosis

Female, 65

Presenting complaint

Dyspnea and cough, fatigue and weakness, episodic night sweats and occasional fever, anxiety and insomnia. Diagnosis of sarcoidosis-associated cough and difficulty breathing as well as vulnerability to respiratory infection.

Sarcoidosis is an inflammatory disease producing granulomas in affected tissue, for this patient, her lungs. The progression of the disease over time produced scaring or fibrotic lung tissue.

Previous treatment

Patient was being cared for by a pulmonologist. She was prescribed steroidal anti-inflammatory medication, and inhaler medication as needed. She tried to keep the inhaled medication to two doses a day, using more if needed. Patient saw a nutritionist and was taking probiotics and vitamin supplements to reduce inflammation, including B vitamins, EPA/DHA (docosahexaenoic acid and eicosapentaenoic acid) from fish oil, Vitamin A and Vitamin D3.

Tongue

Pink, swollen at sides, crack at Stomach and Lung area. Varied coat, sometimes red at the front rim of the Tongue.

Pulse

Alternately fast or slow, thready in second and third positions, fuller and moving in Upper Burner.

Treatment

- GV 14, Ding Chuan, BL 12, 13, 38, GB 21 SI 11 TW 13.
- **Gua sha** to upper back and top of shoulders at GB 21 area.
- **Gua sha** to SI 11 area.

Front
- **Gua sha** to the chest and LU 1 area.
- LI 4, LU 7 or 9, PC 6, SP 4, ST 36, ST 40, LU 1, CV 22, CV 17.
- If sinusitis, rhinitis or postnasal drip added: LI 20, ST 2, and BL 7 with warm moist compress over sinuses for 10 minutes.

Recommendations

This patient had been managing sarcoidosis for years and so she let me know what had been working for her and we set goals to improve her breathing and quality of life.

Patient was a great cook and had raised a family on home-cooked food so recommending warm cooked food for meals was agreeable. Avoid drafts, moderate raw food or spicy food. Exercise to tolerance, i.e. pace periods of exercise to not become fatigued. Recommended meditation course to deal with fear related to condition.

Course of treatment

Treatments consisted of weekly sessions for several months using acupuncture and Gua sha. The patient specifically requested Gua sha treatment after experiencing significant benefit to breathing. When able to maintain the improvement for a week following treatment, sessions were then moved to every other week and continued for several years. At the first sign of a cold or return of symptoms of cough or worsening dyspnea, the patient would immediately present for treatment.

Results

Regular treatment with acupuncture and Gua sha relieved the severity of dyspnea and cough, night sweating and anxiety that sometimes resulted in insomnia, greatly improving her ability to be active and her quality of life. Her fatigue improved but never completely resolved. As the sarcoidosis progressed her lungs became fibrotic and the patient became home-bound and eventually passed away. During the term of her illness where she was able to have treatment, she credited acupuncture and Gua sha with helping her to live well.

Hyperthyroidism

Female, 43

Presenting complaint

Graves' disease, multinodular goiter, overactive thyroid. Patient experienced flu-like symptoms, racing pulse, disturbed sleep, extreme fatigue, irritability, headaches at vertex and forehead, elevated temperature by 4 p.m. with flushing, sweats and night sweats. Sometimes she had chills in the evening. Her hair texture had changed. When she woke in the night she woke with a start, describing it as a 'burst of alertness'.

Previous treatment

Medically prescribed Tapazole, which inhibits synthesis of thyroid hormones. Physician recommended radiation treatment of the thyroid to stop all thyroid function. Patient would then have to take thyroid hormones orally for the rest of her life. She wanted to avoid this procedure and the results if possible.

Tongue

Very red, reddish purple tip, back of tongue had deep longitudinal fissure and thick greasy yellow coating. Lips were quite red.

Pulse

She had a Shi pulse, fast and full with Liver pulse full and floating, Heart pulse wide and flat, Kidney Yin pulse deep and tight, Stomach Spleen pulse wiry, Kidney Yang pulse wide and not deep.

Other signs and symptoms

Patient's stools were irregular, perhaps every other day. Urine was frequent. She drank 3–4 cups of coffee daily. Menses were early with cramps. She was hot and jumpy.

Treatment

Back
- BL 13, 15, 18, 20, 23.
- **Gua sha** to upper back, neck and shoulders; cumulatively Gua sha to entire back to vent Heat.

Front
- LI 4, LU 7, CV 22, KI 6.

Course of treatment

Twelve sessions in 18 weeks.

Recommendations

Stop coffee as it stimulates and is, in this case, Heat producing. Reduce activity to allow body to rest. Lung Tang Xie Gan (Gentiana Drain the Liver Pill), Tian Wan Bu Hsin Tang (Heavenly Emperor Benefit the Heart Pill) and Er Chen Wan (Two Cured Pill) given successively in pill form.

Results

By the third session she felt a shift in her condition: calmer, more subdued. By the fourth session the tongue was pink, reflecting a decrease in Heat Excess. Sleep was improving but she still woke early in 'flight or fight mode'. By the sixth session sleep continued to improve as she was now sleeping until 6.40 a.m. Her menses was still early but with no fatigue, no headaches, no cramps or clots. By the sixth session, 7½ weeks since starting treatment with me, she began to lose her hair indicating a need to reevaluate the dosage of Tapazole. Her energy was good, even and relaxed; her sleep was not startled. The flushing, fevers, fatigue and headaches stopped but the stools were still sluggish.

Blood work after the seventh session showed she was now slightly hypothyroid. Her physician reduced and eventually stopped the Tapazole. The tenth session treated a shoulder bursitis. Her menses had come on time. At the eleventh and twelfth sessions it was early fall and she reported face flushing, dry skin, no sweats, no palpitations, but Heat in the head and neck. Her tongue was pink with a red tip. I changed the herbs to Da Bu Yin Wan and Ding Xin Wan which resolved the problem. Her thyroid had normalized and she did not require any further treatment. The thyroid remained normal.

Fibromyalgia, Deficient presentation

Female, 37

Presenting complaint

Patient complained of chronic neck and shoulder pain of many years duration.

Tongue

Swollen at sides, reddish at the tip. Coating foamy and dry.

Pulse

Weak, thin overall, weak in Liver position.

Other signs and symptoms

She was tired all the time, sleep was tense and she woke with muscles cramped and fists clenched. She had recurring pre-menstrual syndrome (PMS) and mid-cycle migraines, sweats near her menses and was cold at night. Her periods were regular and normal. She had phlebitis during pregnancy so she wore support stockings to prevent blood pooling. She drank coffee for breakfast. Had two small sons so ate last, if at all.

Treatment

Back
- GV 14, GB 20, Pak Loh, BL 13, 38, TW 15 right, Ah Shi points for upper body pain.
- **Gua sha** to neck, shoulders and upper back (first and third treatments).

Front
- LI 4, TW gummy, GB 41, massage and slow neck stretch with patient supine.

Course of treatment

Patient received four weekly treatments.

Recommendations

Discontinue coffee. Eat breakfast, lunch, dinner and snack in afternoon of nutritious, warm, cooked food to treat Deficiency through food. Regular eating also stabilizes blood sugar, which helps to normalize muscle metabolism.

Results

Her sha was pale with a purple hue. She experienced reduced pain after the first and second treatments. After the third treatment the patient was sleeping better, no longer waking with her fists clenched. By the fourth treatment the patient looked sturdy and less fragile. She requested treatment for seasonal allergic sinusitis.

Her condition improved markedly in four sessions. When her health insurance refused payment she discontinued treatment with regret.

Shoulder pain

Male, 38

Presenting complaint

Patient complained of pain at the right wrist, elbow and shoulder from an injury 6 months prior.

Previous treatment

Medically diagnosed as a rotator-cuff tear while playing basketball. He received physical therapy prescribed by his doctor.

Tongue

Normal tongue, pink, slightly redder at the end, coating thicker at the rear and white.

Pulse

Normal, firm, Lung pulse was rough.

Other signs and symptoms

Patient was very healthy and active, mostly vegetarian. His stools, urine, sleep and digestion were normal. He showed some strain of knees and other joints from athletic use. His activity was restricted due to arm pain.

Treatment

Back
- GV 14, right side: BL 13, BL 38, TW 14, Ah Shi right shoulder anterior.
- **Gua sha** to upper back, shoulder, neck and top of the arm, front and back.

Front
- HT 3, LU 7, SI 5, LI 4, LI 15, LI 14, LI 11.

Course of treatment

Three sessions 1 week apart, another 3 weeks later, then monthly for 3 months. After that the patient came for a treatment after overuse approximately every 2–4 months.

Recommendations

Avoid cold and sour food to ease pain. Recommended Feldenkreis shoulder exercise to increase range of motion.

Results

Pain greatly improved after the first treatment and became localized to shoulder. After the second treatment he returned to basketball or swimming each day. He regained full range of motion but the shoulder would tire before any other part of his body. Acute pain was gone after initial treatment. Though active, the shoulder felt vulnerable over another year then resolved completely.

Tennis elbow

Female, 33

Presenting complaint

Patient complained of pain at the elbow, shoulder and neck from excessive tennis.

Tongue

Pale, sides very scalloped and pale, wet white coating, tip had pink flat dots.

Pulse

Irregular with stops and starts, fast. Qi pulse was wiry, with the Kidney aspect slightly weaker. The Blood pulse was thin and the Heart pulse thin and weak.

Other signs and symptoms

Patient was vegetarian and ate erratically and very little. Hands were cold even in summer.

Treatment

Back
• GV 14, BL 13, TW 15, BL 38, SI 11, GB 21, 20, BL 10.
• **Gua sha** to upper back, neck and shoulder.

Front
• LI 15, TW 14, LI 13, LI 12, LI 11, TW gummy, HT 3, Ah Shi points around elbow.
• **Gua sha** above and below elbow on Yang skin (Plate 15).

Course of treatment

Eleven sessions over 11 weeks, then monthly for 5 months, then every 2–3 months for 8 months. Gua Sha was applied at the first session and then about once monthly.

Results

Improved after each session. Pain returned with repetitive traumatic arm motion, such as 5 hours of tennis. Over time the pain took longer to return and the sessions were spread out. The tendinitis at the elbow remained a barometer in helping her to judge her limits.

Carpal tunnel syndrome

Female, 41

Presenting complaint

Patient complained of pain in the wrists, hand and up the arm, diagnosed as carpal tunnel syndrome by her physician and chiropractor. Her physician referred her for surgery, but the patient hoped to avoid surgical intervention.

Tongue

Red body, with deep longitudinal midline crack. Coating was greasy, especially in back. Tongue was wet.

Pulse

Clear but thin. Faint at Kidney positions; Liver pulse was wiry and more full.

Other signs and symptoms

Patient drank a lot of coffee and a good amount of alcohol. She was a high energy person and physically strong. Stools were normal and urine frequent. She had regular periods but with marked PMS and dysmenorrhea.

Treatment

Back
• GV 14, TW 15, BL 13, GB 21, LI 16, 15 and 14, TW 14, SI 11, 10.
• **Gua sha** to neck, shoulders, upper back and upper arm.

Front
• LI 4, LI 11, LI 10, TW gummy, PC 6, PC 7, SP 6.

Course of treatment

Four sessions 1 week apart, then three more at 2 weeks apart.

Recommendations

Stop coffee, avoid cold and sour food. Vitamin B6 was given, along with B complex, and vitamins C and E.

Results

After the first sessions the patient had relief from pain but had more tingling, almost like the feeling one gets when the blood returns to a hand that has fallen asleep. Soon after this the tingling and pain left. Activities such as ironing and splitting wood no longer caused pain. She stopped coffee but was aware that when she began to drink it again her pain would slowly return. Over time her hands improved so that she could tolerate some coffee without ill effect. Her problem resolved without the need for surgery.

Hand parasthesia related to repetitive stress in jazz pianist

Male, 40

Presenting complaint

Repetitive stress injury from daily piano rehearsal and performance. Hands were numb with some tingling and some pain. Anxiety related to injury as music was his livelihood. Patient toured in US and Europe and reported vulnerability to respiratory infections related to fatigue and exposure.

Previous treatment

Physical therapy without remedy. Analgesic pain medication.

Tongue

Tongue was normal pink, some redness at the front rim and fluting at the sides reflecting Gan qi, Liver Qi Constraint.

Pulse

Pulse was 78, regular and otherwise unremarkable.

Other signs and symptoms

Anxiety related to injury/condition.

Treatment
Back
- GV 14, BL 13, BL 43, GB 20, GB 21 (across muscle), SI 10 and 11, TW 13.
- **Gua sha** to upper back, neck and SI 11 area.
- **Gua sha** to upper arms.

Front
- **Gua sha** to LU 1 pectoralis area and Lung channel at the upper arm.
- **Gua sha** to forearms at San Jiao, TW channel.
- N to LI4, TW channel points per palpation, TW5, TW3.
- Yin tang.
- ST 36.
- Ear magnets were placed at Shen men in ear and renewed at each session.

Course of treatment

Patient had three sessions a week apart, then every other week for 2 sessions.

Recommendations

For his respiratory vulnerability: Neti wash daily to prevent postnasal drip and potential respiratory infection. Avoid cold and wind, eat and drink mostly warm cooked food and drink. Practice 'Controlled Pause Breathing', (Butyenko Breath

Therapy) as described in the book: *Breathing Free* by Theresa Hale (2000). Recommended to return for treatment at first sign of any respiratory infection to prevent illness and worsening of symptoms. Regarding his forearms and hands, recommended that he take breaks from playing, stretch and relax his arms and hands and engage in other exercise activities to benefit overall health.

Results

Patient exclaimed immediately after Gua sha: 'Now that's what I'm talking about'. He could feel his hands! Anxiety was reduced immediately. He continued to play, record and perform. He reported for treatment over the years at the first sign of any forearm tightening. The symptoms of parasthesia, numbness and tingling never returned.

Acute rib fracture

Female, 34

Presenting complaint

Pain under left breast so severe that she could only take a shallow breath, could barely walk and laughing was unbearable. She remembered hearing a pop while loading a heavy object overhead onto a truck the day before. She consulted with her physician who diagnosed a fracture of the seventh rib and prescribed pain-relieving medication.

Tongue

Pale with wet edges, dry center (maybe from pain medication). This patient's tongue was normally slightly pale and wet, with some swelling and redness at the edges.

Pulse

Wiry, slightly rapid, otherwise not very different from her usual pulse.

Treatment
Back
- Ah Shi points lateral to T5, T6 and T7, BL 13, BL 17 and BL 18.
- **Gua sha** was applied to the back only, where patient could tolerate touch comfortably.

Front
- Zhen Gu Shui (Rectify Bone Liquid) liniment was applied with gauze to the painful site under the left breast, for 20 minutes. Concurrent needling was performed at TW 6 and GB 37 for rib pain.

Course of treatment

This patient had one emergency session.

Recommendations

Further treatment was recommended, with rest from heavy labor and avoidance of cold and sour foods.

Results

The strangling nature of the rib pain subsided immediately with the first treatment. Patient could breathe deeply, walk, get in and out of a car and giggle slightly. She did not continue treatment as she needed to immediately resume a full work schedule. The rib ached until it healed, approximately 5 weeks.

Postacute rib fracture

Female, 65

Presenting complaint

Patient complained of severe pain at the side of the body, over the ribs. She had fallen on the ice 8 weeks before, sustaining a blow to the ribs. The bruising had long subsided but the pain had only slightly reduced. She had been diagnosed with a broken rib and told to limit her activities until it healed.

Tongue

Normally a big tongue, there was a new characteristic of purple color to the tongue material.

Pulse

Rate was 64 and the quality was tight in the middle positions. The Kidney pulses were deep and the Upper Jiao pulses were weak.

Treatment

Back

- Ah Shi points on the back, lateral to thoracic vertebrae 4–10.
- **Gua sha** applied to back.

Side

- In the recumbent position, with the top leg extended and bottom leg bent: TW 6, GB 34 and 37, Ah Shi points at loci of pain, GB 22.
- **Gua sha** to ribs: posterior to and right up to site of pain. Loci of pain withstood touch, but pressure caused too much pain.

Course of treatment

Patient received three treatments with Gua sha applied the first and second session. By the second session, the area of the break itself was treated with Gua sha.

Results

Patient felt 60% better after the first treatment, able to move without pain, and sleep was undisturbed. The area of the trauma remained sensitive to touch, but after the second and third treatment was 95% reduced. Gua sha could be applied to the site of the rib fracture only because the trauma was so old, there was no evidence of contusion or bruising and the patient could withstand some pressure at the site. The fracture healed and pain completely resolved.

Old trauma

Male, 38

Presenting complaint

Patient complained of back pain lateral to thoracic vertebrae 9 and 10.

Tongue

Red with dry, slightly greasy white coating.

Pulse

Tight and fast. Liver pulse wiry and full. Kidney pulses deep and tight.

Other signs and symptoms

Patient was mugged and beaten as a boy of 14. One area that was badly bruised remained tight, tender and restricted. In periods of stress this patient's back pain would begin at this locus, spread and worsen. He also smoked 2–3 packs of cigarettes per day and drank coffee throughout the day.

Treatment

Back

- Needle to Ah Shi point of injury, points above and below along the BL channel. BL 17 added.
- **Gua sha** bilaterally from 3rd thoracic to 2nd lumbar vertebrae.

Course of treatment

Two treatments.

Recommendations

Avoid cold and sour food. Be conscious of the injured area, that is, take periodic breaks to stretch the back and relax from habitual positions.

Results

Patient was reluctant to have area treated as there was fear associated with the trauma. The sha was deep purple, almost black, indicating it was very old congealed Blood. During the second treatment the patient wept as he remembered the pain of the beating. The specific locus of pain resolved and remained clear through subsequent years.

Plum pit throat (globus hystericus, esophageal stenosis or spasm)

Male, 22

Presenting complaint

Patient experienced episodes of difficulty in swallowing, which might begin with vomiting, then 'feels like there is food stuck in my throat'. He became unable to swallow his own saliva, dehydrated and weak.

Tongue

Red with purple area at center. The coating was white and greasy.

Pulse

Fast and wiry. Liver position was full.

Previous treatment

This patient had been hospitalized for previous attacks.

Other signs and symptoms

Patient had a history of food allergies and dyspepsia related to stress. Urine and stool were normal. Sleep was good but he worked until 3 a.m. He liked cold milk and junk food. He reported the plum pit attacks were brought on by stress, marijuana, shellfish and turkey. He also noticed that milk increased mucus in his throat.

Treatment

Back
- GV 14, BL 15, BL 17, BL 18, BL 20.
- **Gua sha** to neck and upper back.

Front
- LI 4, ST 36, CV 12, PC 6, CV 17, LU 9.

Course of treatment

Patient had four acute episodes over 9 years, requiring one to two sessions to clear acute attack. Gua sha was always done at the first treatment with excellent results.

Recommendations

For acute state, relaxation recommended: soft music, dim lights, etc. The aim here was to calm the Liver, which had constrained Qi and Phlegm in the throat. At all other times,

avoid cold or greasy fluids and food, including milk. Eat slowly in a quiet atmosphere. Er chen Wan (Two Cured Pill) given for mucus. Ban Xia Hou Po Tang (Pinellia and Magnolia Bark Decoction) given subsequently.

Results

Acute attack cleared 80% after first treatment. A follow-up was always done within a few days. The first episode I treated was at the end of 1984, with the second 6 months later. He presented 3 years later with the same acute problem and again 5 years later. At the most recent attack the patient expressed interest in correcting precipitating factors using acupuncture, Gua sha, diet and lifestyle change.

Deltoid–pectoralis pain

Female, 41

Presenting complaint

Patient complained of chest pain at the pectoralis major and deltoid muscles. The pain radiated into the lateral ribs and down the arm.

Previous treatment

She had received massage, which gave only temporary relief.

Tongue

Normal color, slightly puffy at edges. There were cracks at the Lung area only.

Pulse

64, unremarkable.

Treatment

Back
- GV 14, BL 12, BL 13, BL 43, TW 15, TW 14, SI 9, SI 10, GB 20, GB 21, LI 16.

Front
- LU 1, Ah Shi on pectoralis major.
- **Gua sha** at upper back, shoulder, chest, anterior upper arm, lateral ribs and at forearm (Plates 12 and 13).
- LI 4, LU 7, LIV 3, PC 6, CV 17, ST 44.

Course of treatment

One session.

Recommendations

Avoid cold and sour food. Keep area warm, including at night, and wear a shirt that covers the muscles. Hydrochloric acid pills were recommended with large meals as pain in these muscles can relate to decreased hydrochloric acid production (hypochlorhydria).

Results

Patient fully recovered after one session.

Arrhythmia

Male, 42

Presenting complaint

Patient had irregularity of heart rhythm. He was unsettled and mildly anxious; 'feels like butterflies in my chest'.

Previous treatment

Patient was under the care of a cardiologist who had prescribed medication to normalize the heart rate and rhythm. If the medication did not remedy the arrhythmia in a few more days the patient was to be hospitalized.

Tongue

Pink, very red at the tip, with thin white coating.

Pulse

76, irregular and strong.

Other signs and symptoms

Patient had a history of cocaine use, which he recently resumed. He drank Coca-Cola and coffee throughout the day and worked like a horse. He also smoked cigars.

Treatment

Back
- BL 13, BL 14, BL 15, BL 23.
- **Gua sha** to upper back, T1 through T7 area.

Front
- PC 6, HT 7, ST 36, CV 14.

Course of treatment

One session.

Recommendations

Relaxed breathing and meditation. Stop cocaine, caffeine and smoking.

Results

Normal heart rhythm resumed approximately 3 hours after treatment with acupuncture and Gua sha.

Fibrocystic breast 'normala'

Female, 30

Presenting complaint

Patient had pain and swelling in right breast, with lumpiness and distinct nodules.

Previous treatment

Patient was being treated by her gynecologist.

Tongue

Large and puffy with scalloped edges. Coating was light yellow and thicker at the rear of the tongue. The tongue tip and edges were red.

Pulse

The rate was normal, the quality was thin and wiry. The Liver pulse was full and wiry.

Other signs and symptoms

Patient's stools and urine were normal. Her sleep was disturbed. At ovulation she felt pain and pressure at her right breast. One week prior to menses her right breast distended. She overworked at a high-stress job.

Treatment

Back
- GV 14, right BL 13, BL 38, GB 21, SI 11, GB 22, BL 18.
- **Gua sha** to right upper back, shoulder and lateral ribs. (Plate 16 shows Gua sha of this patient.)

Front
- SI 1, GB 34, LIV 14, CV 17; right ST 16, ST 18; left GB 38, LIV 3.

Course of treatment

Patient was seen twice.

Recommendations

Patient was already avoiding methylxanthines found in coffee, black tea and chocolate. She did not drink alcohol. As a way of reducing the constraint of Liver Qi it was suggested that she walk daily 'taking large strides and deep breaths', and regulate her work habits to lessen the stress. Seven Forests Chih-ko Circuma and Blue Citrus tablets were given.

Results

The second session was on day 11 of her menstrual cycle. The right breast had reduced to normal size and comfort and was not increasing in size with the approach of ovulation. The herbs were renewed and the patient left to travel for the summer.

Mastitis

Female, 32

Presenting complaint

Patient had fever, breast pain and hardness, more so in right breast.

Previous treatment

Patient was taking antibiotics prescribed by her physician.

Tongue

Pale pink with red tip and sides.

Pulse

Full and wiry.

Other signs and symptoms

Patient was 3 days post-partum. She was tired but otherwise healthy.

Treatment

Back
- BL 38, BL 13, GB 21, GB 22.
- **Gua sha** to upper back and mid-back.

Front
- SI 1 indirect moxa, CV 17, GB 22, ST 16, ST 18, LIV 14, ST 30.

Course of treatment

Three sessions – the second was 2 days after the first, the third a week later. Gua sha at first session only.

Results

The patient experienced 60% relief of pain immediately. By the third session she was healed and nursing without discomfort.

Note: Gua sha has been shown to be effective in the treatment of breast distension/mastitis in a randomized controlled trial published in the *Journal of Nursing Research* (Chiu et al. 2010).

Postmastectomy pain

Female, 47

Presenting complaint

Patient complained of pain at her chest around and through to upper back, 1 year after mastectomy.

Previous treatment

Physical therapy after surgery.

Tongue

Big, red at borders and end, some slices on the body of the tongue. The coating was light yellow and thicker at the back.

Pulse

Tight at both Middle Jiao positions. The Lung pulse was slightly moving and the Heart Pulse was weak. Both Kidney pulses were deep.

Treatment

Back
- GV 14, BL 13, BL 38, SI 11, SI 10, SI 9, GB 21.
- **Gua sha** to upper back. Left: GB 22, TW 15. Gua sha to ribs under left scapula around to GB 22 area.

Front
- SI 1, TW 5, TW gummy, GB 37, GB 34, PC 6, SP 4, CV 17.

Course of treatment

Five treatments.

Results

Patient felt 70% improved after the first treatment. The remaining sessions helped to increase her range of arm motion without pain. She recovered completely.

Influenza with nausea and diarrhea

Female, 35

Presenting complaint

Acute flu symptoms of headache, fever, body aches, nausea and diarrhea. Patient was in her third day of illness.

Previous treatment

Self-prescribed ginger tea and vitamin C.

Tongue

Red at borders and tip, dry with coating white to light yellow, thicker at back.

Pulse

80, thin, weaker in both Kidney positions.

Other signs and symptoms

Patient was hypothyroid, in the process of increasing Synthroid. When her thyroid was low she got frequent acute illnesses. She would become fatigued, somnolent and edematous, had pressure in her head and a lowered voice. Her menses arrived early.

Treatment

Back
- GV 14, BL 12, BL 13, BL 18, BL 20.
- **Gua sha** to entire back.

Front
- LI 4, TW 5, KI 7, moxa burned on a slice of aconite on salt filling navel at CV 8.

Course of treatment

Two sessions with Gua sha at the first session.

Recommendations

Bedrest. Stop ginger tea that is useful at the initial stages of flu or cold where there is chill and nausea. By this stage the patient was hot with a red tongue and fast pulse and the ginger was countertherapeutic. Drink plenty of fluids at least at room temperature. If unable to eat regular food, start with rice congee (one cup of rice cooked with eight cups of water).

Results

All signs of flu left within 2 days after treatment. A follow-up session was given 1 week after the first session to ensure full recovery.

Shingles, postherpetic neuralgia

Female, 53

Presenting complaint

Shingles: postherpetic neuralgia (PHN), pain along thoracic dermatome 6 months post outbreak.

Previous treatment

Course of antiviral medication at herpes zoster onset, which did not prevent PHN.

Tongue

Tongue was normal, pink with swollen and redder sides and normal thin white coat.

Pulse

Pulse was 64; patient was athletic.

Other signs and symptoms

Nervousness, as she described, not anxiety. Always busy. Persistence of the pain bothered the patient because it reminded her of what she was told by another health care provider at the onset of shingles outbreak: that her immune system was compromised. This notion worried the patient.

Treatment

Back
- Prone position.
- GV 14, BL 12 or BL 13, BL 43, BL 15, to move Qi in area of upper body.
- BL 17, BL 18, BL 20, to move Qi in the middle body.
- **Gua sha** to the upper back and mid-back along the Huato channel and the first and second Bladder channel. Gua sha along the area of the dermatome taking care to cover above and below the dermatome. Gua sha on mirror dermatome area at alternate session.

Front
- **Gua sha** at axilla and around to the front of the body and upper abdomen area following the dermatome path of pain.
- Yin tang.
- LI 4, PC 6, SP 4, TW gummy.
- SP 6, ST 36, CV 4, CV 6, CV, 12, CV 17.
- Treatment of any tender points along dermatome.

Course of treatment

Patient had three treatments.

Recommendations

Avoid spicy and salty food; otherwise eat warm cooked meals. If patient had been treated during acute term would have recommended: Seven Forests Myrrh Tablets and Red Peony Tablet two of each three time per day.

Results

PHN completely resolved without recurrence or any residual sensation. The patient attributed the resolution to Gua sha where she felt immediate change in pain after treatment.

Note: shingles can result in PHN that has a significant impact of functional status and health-related quality of life in older adults (Schmader et al. 2007). Shingles is responsive to acupuncture during the course of the outbreak (Ursini et al. 2011). The technique prescribed by Dr So included treatment of known skin points and to surround the lesions along the dermatome with shallow needling, one needle every inch, resting needles in place for 20–25 minutes (see Chapter 8).

Gua sha is indicated and may be applied after the lesions have healed and the skin is intact (Nielsen 2005). Treatment in these early stages of herpes zoster prevents PHN. It is recommended to treat not only the area of the pain along the dermatome but to treat the mirror trajectory on the opposite side even if there were no lesions present. Studies have shown damage to epidermal nerve fibers in half of the patient who have PHN where pain severity in the apparent affected side correlates significantly with the severity of this contralateral fiber loss (Bennett and Watson 2009).

Splenomegaly/hepatomegaly

Female, 27

Presenting complaint

Patient complained of abdominal pain. There was tenderness and swelling of liver and spleen easily palpated and extreme fatigue with swollen glands of the neck and armpits.

Previous treatment

This patient's medical specialist diagnosed her with Hodgkin's disease (but later retracted this diagnosis after the patient recovered from treatment with me). She had been on Synthroid until 5 years prior to this acute illness. Patient was taking vitamins B, C, A, D and E.

Tongue

Pink, pale, with orange color at the borders and red dotted tip. There were cracks at the center. The coating was unremarkable.

Pulse

Rate of 56, even, clear but thin. The Heart pulse softened and both Middle Jiao pulses were firm.

Other signs and symptoms

Patient's appetite was good, stools were loose with some diarrhea, and urine was frequent with some night urine. Her menses was regular lasting 4–5 days, no clots or pain but the blood tending to darken. She slept a lot but did not feel rested when she woke. She got dizzy, especially if overheated. Both of her knees were weak and bothered her. She had occasional night sweats and her hands and feet turned orange.

Treatment

Back

- BL 13, BL 15, BL 17, BL 18, BL 20, BL 21, BL 38, Pee Gen.
- **Gua sha** to upper back, middle back and lower back: to entire back over time.

Front

- TW 6, GB 34, LIV 3, LIV 13, CV 12, CV 17, CV 6.

Course of treatment

Sixty-five sessions over 33 months. At first the patient received treatment a minimum of three times per month, then twice per month.

Recommendations

Avoid coffee, alcohol and recreational drugs. As the patient was eating very little protein I recommended 2–4 ounces of concentrated protein twice per day to be eaten at the beginning of the meal. Eliminate grape juice as it may be loosening the stool. Nap each afternoon for at least 20 minutes. Chinese patent herbs were given: Yan Hu Suo (Corydalis Pain Pills), Shu Kan Wan (Soothe the Liver pill) and initially Po Chai pills with meals. Later Wu Chi Pai Feng Wan (Black Cock, White Phoenix Pills), in chewable form, or Bazhen Tang (Women's Precious) was given to nourish the Blood.

Results

The symptom of loose stool improved after the first treatment. Within a month of treatment her liver profile improved to normal and the hepatomegaly was reduced, but the liver remained tender and slightly enlarged. The enlargement of the spleen gradually improved over 3 months. Pulse rate increased from 56 to 64–72. After 3 months she was able to return to part-time work, but she was extremely sensitive to chemicals, strong smells and airborne particulates. Exposure would cause sore throats, headaches and liver pain. Treatment and support were aimed at dealing with any acute disorder: sore throats, swollen glands, fever, sinus infection or colds, while she was continuing to recover her health from the chronic lymphatic disorder. Her abdominal pain receded but would return when she was spent. As her health gained, the orange of the hands, feet and tongue turned to a normal pink.

She enrolled in a Masters program in her field and has fully recovered without recurrence.

Chronic active hepatitis B (HBV)

Male, 20

Approximately 17.5% of the 2 billion HBV carriers in the world are chronically infected. The goal of anti-HBV therapy is to prevent the development of progressive disease, specifically cirrhosis and liver failure, as well as hepatocellular carcinoma development and death. Anti-HBV agents are associated with systemic side-effects, including renal toxicity and development of resistance for long-term users (Chan et al. 2011). A case published in the Western journal *Clinica Chimica Acta* by Chan et al. documents a 20-year-old male chronic hepatitis B carrier who presented with abnormally high levels of alanine transaminase (ALT), aspartate transaminase (AST) and alkaline phosphatase (ALP) in liver function test, indicating immune-active phase of hepatitis B infection and inflammatory damage in the liver. Ultrasound examination of liver was normal without fibrotic or cirrhotic changes. He did not have any known dermatological, neurologic, respiratory, cardiovascular, gastrointestinal, urogenital, musculoskeletal, neuropsychological, endocrinologic or vascular diseases. He did not take regular medication that affects the levels of liver function and cytokines, and did not have any antiviral drugs before and during the study period.

Gua sha was applied to the back. Forty-eight hours after receiving Gua sha, the patient showed changes in a number of serum markers: a decline of liver enzymes (ALT and AST) indicating reduced chronic inflammation, an elevated plasma heme oxygenase-1 (HO-1), and a modulation of T-helper (TH)1/Th2 balance. HO-1 has been shown to be hepatoprotective (Xia et al. 2008), and its upregulation is induced by Gua sha (Kwong et al. 2009).

In this case, and in general, Gua sha may be effective in transiently reducing the inflammatory injury to the liver when chronic hepatitis B moves into the immune active phase indicated by liver function test. Further trials are underway to determine the frequency or dosage of the application of Gua sha in cases of HBV and potential hepatitis C (HCV) (Zhu et al. 2008) liver inflammation.

Stomach ulcer

Male, 36

Presenting complaint

Patient complained of sharp epigastric pain, more after eating, and did not like touch or pressure. The complaint was medically diagnosed as a stomach ulcer but the patient refused medication.

Tongue

Red with Stomach crack, yellow greasy coating thicker at the center Stomach area.

Pulse

Wiry and full especially at both Middle Jiao positions.

Other signs and symptoms

Patient worked as a contractor. His job involved physical and mental stress.

Treatment

Back
- BL 13, BL 18, BL 21.
- **Gua sha** to middle back.

Front
- ST 36, PC 6, CV 12, ST 21, Ah Shi left lateral to CV 11.

Course of treatment

Six sessions.

Recommendations

Avoid overheating foods: spicy, greasy and roasted. Avoid alcohol and coffee.

Results

Patient experienced steady improvement over the six sessions. Symptoms resolved completely. There has been no recurrence in the 10 years since.

Cholecystitis

Female, 54

Presenting complaint

Patient had recently had two gall bladder attacks with severe hypochondrial pain and pressure into her abdomen and through to her back. The most recent attack followed a meal of scallops wrapped in bacon, rack of lamb and ice cream. A sonogram ordered by her physician confirmed gallstones.

Tongue

Red and dry. Coating white and foamy.

Pulse

Fast with Qi pulse smooth, wide and full. Wood pulse was flat, full and active.

Other signs and symptoms

Patient had frequent, loose stools. She was overweight with a jovial disposition. She volunteered that she did not like to exercise; she liked to smoke cigarettes and drink coffee. Her sleep was disturbed.

Treatment

Back
- GV 14, BL 13, BL 38, BL 18, GV 9, BL 19, BL 20, BL 23, BL 25.
- **Gua sha** to upper back, especially at BL 38 area of pain, and to middle back BL 18 and BL 19 area.

Front
- GB 34, TW 6 or TW Ah Shi forearm, GB 24 right, M-LE-23 right.

Course of treatment

Fourteen sessions over 7 months. The first three were 1 week apart. The fourth was 3 weeks later and treated an upper respiratory infection. Following this she had treatment every 2–3 weeks.

Recommendations

Avoid fat by eating lean meats, fish and chicken without the skin. Avoid cold food and fluid because of their congealing effect. Avoid coffee, chocolate and alcohol because of their ability to increase Damp-Heat. Increase vegetable and grains in diet. Use raw flax oil on salad alternating with olive oil.

Results

She had no further attacks of pain. During the course of treatment she quit smoking and began exercising for pleasure. She joined a cooking class. At this point her blood sugar elevated. Her doctor wanted her to lose weight to bring her blood sugar down. He recommended Opti-fast, a liquid diet that causes rapid weight loss. It also precipitates gall stones as well as eventual weight gain. At this point the patient informed me she had done this diet before, which may have contributed to her stones. The doctor felt if the stones got worse they would remove them surgically.

Back pain

Male, 35

Presenting complaint

Patient complained of back pain, radiating into the left hip, groin, quad and down to foot. Top of left foot was numb. Disc herniations at L4 and L5.

Previous treatment

Patient was referred by his Rolfing practitioner.

Tongue

Scalloped, white coating, red tip.

Pulse

Overall the pulse was thin. The Blood pulse was weak, the Stomach and Spleen pulse was tight. The sinus pulse on the right was quite full.

Other signs and symptoms

Patient was a skiing, windsurfing, mountain climbing athlete. Though he was in great physical shape, his muscles stiffened and cramped, he tired easily and his extremities were chilled easily. He drank coffee, a lot of fruit juice and smoked marijuana every day. His stools were loose, he had frequent urine, slept well but did not remember his dreams. He was bothered by sinus congestion.

Treatment

Back
- BL 60, 54, GV 14, BL 23, left BL 25, Ah Shi near left BL 20.
- **Gua sha** to back neck and shoulders.

Side
- Left GB 30, 31, 34, 37 in recumbent position.
- **Gua sha** to left GB 30 area.

Front
- KI 3, TW 4, GB 41 alternating SI 3, BL 62.

Course of treatment

Six sessions over 8 weeks.

Recommendations

Here the function of the Kidneys and Spleen had been weakened by marijuana, coffee and fruit juice. As a diuretic, coffee stimulates the function of the Kidney. The overstimulation eventually weakens the Kidney causing frequent urination, night urine, weakened back and knees. Because coffee acts as a stimulant, it disrupts the harmony of Liver Qi. Overall there results an imbalance in the Liver Qi, Deficiency in the Kidney Qi, Kidney Yang, Liver and Kidney Yin.

Marijuana is a herb that depletes the Yin and the Yang. It weakens the Kidneys, eventuating Deficiency of Kidney Yang and Spleen Yang, Kidney Yin and Liver Yin. Patients who smoke marijuana, depending on their constitutional make-up, will present with symptoms of either an imbalance or Deficiency, of Yin or Yang. Chill, cramping and loose stool are typical of Deficient Spleen Yang. Chill, frequent urination, back pain and back injury are typical of Deficient Kidney Yang. Studies have shown that men who use marijuana regularly can also suffer from a decreased sperm count, representing in Chinese medicine a compromise of the Kidney Jing.

Fruit juice is often taken cold and is by nature cooling. This chills and dampens the Spleen, weakening digestion and causing the stool to be loose. It also contributes to congestion and mucus from the nose, since the Spleen owns the nose.

For his back to heal completely, it was recommended this patient stop marijuana and fruit juice. Eventually he might resume occasional coffee and fruit juice with no harmful effect.

Initially, a mix of Jade Pharmacy's Meridian Circulation and Meridian Passage was given for the back, then a modified decoction of Sheng Ling Bai Du San (Ginseng, Poria, Attractylodes Powder) was given to strengthen the Spleen, support the back and the will. This worked so well that he requested to take it long-term while traveling and it was given in powder form.

He was referred back for continuation of Rolfing.

Results

Immediate relief of back pain was felt after the first treatment. The resolution of sha in the back greatly strengthened and warmed him. He was able to reduce, then give up the marijuana, coffee and juice. His cramping and fatigue ended. He reported for the fifth session with slight numbness at the top of the left foot. This was after windsurfing for 5 days in a row. By the sixth session all of his back symptoms were fine and he requested a treatment for his sinuses.

Severe acute back pain: thoracic and lumbar spine fracture, non-small cell lung cancer

Female, 81

Presenting complaint

Severe acute back pain, unable to stand or dress, only able to walk a few steps. Patient was being treated for stage 4 non-small cell carcinoma of the lung with Navilbine and Tarceva®. The chemotherapy created acute loss of bone density. A stumble and fall resulted in fractures to the vertebra and spinous processes at T11, T12, and L1.

Previous treatment

Patient was prescribed pain medication that made her groggy and fearful of another fall. She stopped taking it.

Tongue

Tongue was red, dry with superficial cracks. Slight coat, no leukopenia on the Tongue.

Pulse

The pulse was weak and thready, tight in the Middle Jiao position, and deep in Lower Jiao position.

Treatment

Back

With patient seated in a chair, back to me:
- GV 14, BL13, BL15 for anxiety from pain.
- BL 38, BL 17, BL 18, BL 20, BL 21, Pee gen.
- **Gua sha** from BL 13 area to BL 22 at the back.

Front
- Yin tang, ear magnets at Shen men.

Course of treatment

Patient had two sessions five days apart with acupuncture and Gua sha applied both times.

Recommendations

Suggested to patient to have someone purchase a wrap-around back brace to wear if required to stand or walk. Encouraged patient to move around a bit every day, and to eat meals even if small meals. Suggested that patient have her vitamin D levels

checked by her oncologist at her next bloodwork and they were 0. Pharmaceutical vitamin D was prescribed for 1 month. High doses of vitamin D can also pull calcium out of the bones. Patient was then placed on 4000 IU/day of vitamin D3 supplement.

Results

After the first treatment the patient was immediately able to take a full breath and to walk and stand without severe pain. Her back fatigued easily. She reported she got the back brace. Within a few days she was able to walk around her house and to drive her car, and return to playing bridge. She discarded the back brace after 2 weeks and was able to return to her full activity level.

Treating cancer patients can be a challenge for any provider who is always aware of an inability to cure the patient. In some sense any offering pales. This case turned that notion on its head. This patient lived another year beyond the expectation of her doctors. And while no treatment cured her cancer, acupuncture and Gua sha gave her precious active and pain free months.

Low back pain, Shi presentation, Damp-Heat stagnation

Male, 36

Presenting complaint

Patient had pain shooting down the left leg, sometimes both legs. The pain worsened with use, so by the afternoon he could no longer stand. He had back surgery 2 years before for herniated disc. The surgery paralysed his right leg, which slowly recovered. He reinjured his back a year later, resulting in the current pain.

Previous treatment

Physical therapy and chiropractic adjustment.

Tongue

Big, red, furry and cracked body. Coating was white, sticky and greasy, indicating Damp-Heat. There were red raised bumps at the end of the tongue.

Pulse

Pulse was fast, slippery and wide. The middle positions were especially wide.

Other signs and symptoms

Patient drank coffee, smoked cigarettes, occasionally marijuana, and used alcohol infrequently. He was accustomed to rigorous physical labor. His stools were loose, several times per day. Urine was normal. Sleep was interrupted by leg pain. He had high blood pressure but could not tolerate medication.

Treatment

Back

- BL 62, SI 3, BL 20, BL 23, BL 25, BL 26 left of laminectomy scar, L2, L3 Hua Tuo, Ah Shi points: left hip, top of left thigh and right mid-back trigger point.
- **Gua sha** to back area at first treatment and when needed.

Front

- Shen men, LIV 2, TW 5, GB 41, ST 36, GB 26. Fu Fang Du Zhong Pian.

Course of treatment

Patient had 5 treatments over 5 weeks, then a session every 2–4 weeks as needed.

Recommendations

Eliminate coffee and marijuana due to their depleting effect of the Kidneys. The Kidneys own the back. All back pain, even injury, has its Ben or root in the Kidneys. Recommended quiting cigarettes soon. Keep back covered and warm. Avoid sour and cold foods. Fu Fang Du Zhong (Pian Eucommia tablets) given for back pain and hypertension.

Results

The first treatment provided relief for 4 days. The tongue became more pink, but had white foamy coating (Spleen Deficiency) over the white greasy coating. Red dots at the front remained. After the second treatment the patient was able to do more, with leg pain reduced and he was active in the evening. He quit coffee and eventually cigarettes. Diarrhea changed to semiformed stools. After the fifth session his blood pressure stabilized. Sleep became sound and he needed less of it. Treatments began in February. By summer the patient built a pond on his homestead, requiring considerable physical labor. He sustained a back injury mishandling a large log that necessitated surgery.

Lower back strain

Female, 42

Presenting complaint

Patient complained of straining her low back while using exercise equipment. She also overworks in a standing position.

Previous treatment

Patient was already receiving care for Deficient-Kidney-related fatigue, chill and frequency of urination.

Tongue

Pink, swollen sides, coating thin and dry.

Pulse

Rate 72, overall thin and slightly wiry. Kidney pulses deep and slightly wiry.

Other signs and symptoms

Previous treatment for the Kidneys improved the complaints of urinary frequency, chill and fatigue. Patient ate well and digestion was normal though she had occasional irritable bowel pain. Menses were normal.

Treatment

Back

- BL 60, BL 54, BL 25, BL 23, Ah Shi lateral around psoas muscle.
- **Gua sha** to mid- and low back. Indirect moxa over BL 23 and Kidney area.

Front

- KI 3, TW 5, GB 41.

Course of treatment

Patient had two treatments 1 week apart with Gua sha at the first session.

Recommendations

Moderate activity, take a break from using exercise machines, rest and avoid coffee. Du Huo Ji Sheng Tang given in tincture form as Meridian Circulation.

Results

Pain and lumbar strain resolved completely.

Low back and knee pain from weakened Kidney

Male, 35

Presenting complaint

Patient strained his back shoveling snow. His knee locked and his back stiffened. He stood bent and crooked and he had fear of moving.

Tongue

Pink, pale and wet with white coating.

Pulse

Kidney pulses were deep and weak. Heart pulse was empty.

Other signs and symptoms

Patient dressed in lots of layers and was fearful of cold. Stools and sleep were normal with episodic frequent urine. He officiated at and played basketball a few times a week, which was traumatic to his back. Patient ate regularly but was deficient in protein foods.

Treatment

Back

- BL 60, BL 40, BL 25, BL 17, Ah Shi points of low back and lateral to sacrum and coccyx.
- **Gua sha** to back, low back, sacrum and lateral buttocks for knee, eyes and wings of knee, ST 36, GB 34, LIV 8, massage.

Front

- SI 3, BL 62 or TW 5, GB 41.

Recommendations

Avoid cold and sour foods. Soak in Epsom salts bath. Take calcium and magnesium supplements. Increase protein foods.

Course of treatment and Results

Three sessions at the beginning of 1986 resolved complaint. He hurt himself shoveling in 1987, for which he received four sessions. The knee was operated on subsequent to a basketball injury. Five years later he presented with his crooked back from another basketball trauma. He could still play, but couldn't touch his toes. Four weekly sessions resolved this, at which point I referred him to a practitioner of Feldenkreis to help him develop a back consciousness and strength to prevent further injury.

Knee Bi syndrome – arthritis

Male, 71, retired

Presenting complaint

Patient complained of pain in his left knee, diagnosed as arthritis. Knee replacement recommended by physician. Knee hurt when climbing stairs. It was swollen and painful but not red or hot to the touch.

Previous treatment

Pharmaceutical.

Tongue

Big, pink with red dot at the center. Sides of tongue were slightly purple. Coating was greasy, wet and yellow. There were purple spots under the tongue.

Pulse

Interrupted, rough and wiry in Heart position, with widened pulse at left Kidney Yin and right Lung position. Earth position was wiry, slightly floating.

Other signs and symptoms

Patient had normal appetite and stool. He urinated frequently, but also drank coffee. He had elevated blood pressure. His tongue coat was probably greasy white, stained yellow by the coffee.

Treatment

Back

- BL 60, BL 54, BL 20, BL 25, BL 23, Ah Shi at left gluteus medius for knee, GB 30, 34.
- **Gua sha** to mid- to lower back, left hip and sacrum (see Plate 17).

Front

- Left ST 36, LIV 8, eyes of knee and wings of knee, indirect moxa.
- Massage knee area toward body.
- Wrapped knee to retain heat in the joint.

Course of treatment

Patient received three weekly treatments for his knee. At the first and second treatments, Gua sha was used at different areas of the back. The fourth treatment was for pain and stiffness across shoulders and neck.

Recommendations

Keep knee warm. Eat only warm cooked food. Avoid coffee, cold and sour foods. Du Huo Ji Sheng Tang (Angelica Pubescens and Sangjisheng) decoction given.

Results

After two treatments he was walking round 18 holes of golf. His knee felt great and he felt strong overall. The tongue normalized in color and coat. He continued to play 18 holes of golf. The knee surgery was postponed indefinitely.

Foot pain/Morton's neuroma and plantar fasciitis

Male, 53

Presenting complaint

Patient complained of stabbing pain in both feet. He was an avid runner and downhill skier. The pain did not bother him while running or skiing, but afterward was excruciating. Continued movement and ice helped.

Tongue

Normal color. The front sides were swollen, reddish and wet. The coating was thin, even, rooted and slightly yellow.

Pulse

Slightly rapid, with the Lung pulse fine and weak, Heart pulse flat and wide and Liver pulse very full.

Other signs and symptoms

Took Ventolin for asthma, which was precipitated by cats, dogs and cold weather. He drank 4–5 cups of coffee per day. Appetite, stools and sleep were normal.

Treatment

Back

- BL 59, BL 23, GB 34, GB 30, Ah Shi on right hip.
- **Gua sha** to low back, hip and GB 30 area.

Front

- GB 38, 40, 41. LIV 3, Ah Shi on bottom of foot with moxa burnt on needle.
- Additionally for neuroma: electrical stimulation on needles between ST 44 and Ah Shi at bottom of right foot at 160 cycles/second and 2000 amps.
- Electrical stimulation in 'Chase the Dragon's Tail' method with moist cotton probes from ST 36 to foot Ah Shi points, ST 36 through foot, points between the metatarsals through to bottom of foot, including LIV 3.

Course of treatment

He received three treatments, after which he left on winter vacation where he would be on a boat for 1 month and able to rest the foot.

Recommendations

Stop the coffee. Stretch, massage and, if necessary, ice foot after use. Seven Forests Stephania tablets were given.

Results

After the first treatment the intensity of pain decreased. He was able to run several times with less pain after. Both feet improved significantly by the time he left for vacation.

Long leg treatment

Female, 45

Presenting complaint

Patient complained of back pain into hip, with one leg noticeably longer than the other.

Tongue

A 'baby's' tongue, pink, normally slightly dry from pain medication.

Pulse

Normal if slightly Deficient in Blood aspect, slightly weak in Kidney positions.

Other signs and symptoms

Frequent urination, chronic recurring cystitis, chronic Deficient headache that was low-grade but always there. Stools normal, loose or stuck. Menses normal with some premenstrual exacerbation of symptoms and fatigue.

Treatment

Back

- BL 60, BL 54, BL 20, BL 23, BL 25.
- **Gua sha** to mid- to lower back.

Side

- The following points were treated on the long leg: GB 30, GB 31, GB 32, GB 34, GB 38 in recumbent position with top leg bent, Gua sha around GB 30 and 31–32 area.

Results

One session corrected the long leg imbalance, stabilized the back and eliminated the pain. Patient continued treatment for the other chronic problems over the next year. The long leg imbalance did not return.

Sciatica, chronic, complicated by laceration scar to buttocks

Male, 73

Presenting complaint

Patient complained of pain in left buttock, down leg and concentrated at shin and ankle. Several years earlier, a tractor rolled over on him, lacerating his buttocks. The sciatica dated from the accident.

Previous treatment

He had been evaluated by two neurologists and had received physical therapy. The physical therapist thought his pain was vascular and recommended a vascular specialist. He had taken anti-inflammatory medication prescribed by his neurologist.

Tongue

Pale, wet, slightly puffy and swollen with greasy coating that had a foamy aspect. Pale red dots at tip. Shook slightly.

Pulse

Strong and wiry with Lung pulse slightly moving.

Other signs and symptoms

Patient was thin, active and in good health. His sleep was good but interrupted by night urine. He drank coffee and black tea. He was happily married, ate regularly and was involved in the community.

The sciatica pain compromised his activity and quality of life. When the scar was touched the muscles of the buttocks and upper leg spasmed. Stools were normal. Blood pressure was slightly high, but he was not on medication for it. He had involuntary spasms of muscles in legs and arms.

Treatment

Back

- Left BL 60, BL 54, BL 25, BL 23, BL 20 and Ah Shi at piriformis.
- **Gua sha** to lower back and buttocks.

Side

- Lateral recumbent, GB 30, 31, 34, 39 and 40.
- Scar treatment: points along the scar. **Gua sha** along scar.

Course of treatment

Nine sessions altogether. The first seven were 1 week apart, the eighth then at 2 weeks, the ninth 1 month later.

Recommendations

Avoid coffee and caffeinated tea. Supplement with 500 mg calcium and magnesium for a time. Fu Fang Du Zhung Pian given for blood pressure and to strengthen back. Huo Luo Xiao Ling Dan (Fantastically Effective Pill to Invigorate the Collaterals), modified, given in decoction.

Results

After the first session the Wind spasms began to abate and the leg began to improve slightly. After the third session he was considerably improved and began to work out. Now the pain would come and go, worsening if he stood for a length of time. He resumed fast walking and working out, having pain only with prolonged use. Each treatment to the scar improved his condition. Convinced the scar tissue was the cause of his problem, I referred him back to his neurologist. Four doctors told him that if the scar was involved with the pain, it would be much worse.

I referred him to a physician certified in acupuncture who could inject the scar with medication. Several of these treatments completely cured his chronic sciatica.

Hamstring strain

Male, 46

Presenting complaint

Cramping and pain at the back of right leg. Patient bicycled 3–4 times per week. He rode 35 miles one day, the next day gardened, then biked 16–20 miles. The next day he played softball with leg cramps and sustained an injury. He was unable to affect the pain by movement, stretching, hot or cold application. The leg was contracted, unable to extend fully without pain.

Previous treatment

Patient had received no other treatment for his injury.

Tongue

Normal, unremarkable.

Pulse

Normal, slightly wiry.

Treatment

Back

- BL 60, BL 57, BL 54, BL 36 and Ah Shi lateral to BL 36. Ah Shi points on mid area, back of leg.
- **Gua sha** to back and buttocks while prone; then **Gua sha** to ischium and hamstring muscles with patient on hands and knees, in 'dog' position.

Course of treatment

Patient received two treatments.

Recommendations

Stop coffee because of its pro-inflammatory effect. Take calcium and magnesium supplement. Keep area warm, postpone rigorous physical activity. Stretch the leg with care.

Results

Patient was 95% improved a few days after the first treatment. He recovered fully a short time after the second treatment, returning to his usual schedule of activity.

Chill, chillphobia, knee pain and swelling

Female, 33

Presenting complaint

Patient felt very cold, had knee pain and swelling and mild low-back pain.

Tongue

Flat, pale pink, slightly pinker at the tip. Coating at the rear of the tongue was slightly yellow.

Pulse

Slow, weak overall with Middle Jiao showing more strength.

Treatment

Back
- BL 60, BL 54, BL 25, BL 23, Ah Shi on lateral gluteus medius trigger point for knee.
- **Gua sha** to whole back (see Plate 8) and lateral gluteus medius.

Front
- ST 36, SP 10, ST 34, eyes of knee, medial wing of knee.

Course of treatment

Two sessions 8 days apart, then a third session 4 months later.

Results

After the first session she felt warm all over. Her knees were no longer swollen or painful, but weak. Four months later she asked to be treated again for knee weakness. She reported that the sensation of warmth had remained.

Leg pain, quads

Male, 56

Presenting complaint

Patient complained of pain from inguinal region down the top of both legs.

Tongue

Thick, red, with dry, pasty, dirty white coating. Crack along the midline.

Pulse

Slow and leathery, Kidney pulses deeper and weaker. Lung pulse was tight.

Other signs and symptoms

He smoked two packs of cigarettes per day, drank lots of coffee. His job involved many hours of driving. He did not exercise beyond walking to and from the car. His stools were stuck, urine was frequent, sleep was disturbed.

Recommendations

Stop coffee and cigarettes. Walk daily, especially on days that involve long drives.

Treatment

Back
- BL 17, BL 18, BL 23, BL 25, BL 57.
- **Gua sha** to mid- to low back.

Front
- ST 36, ST 34, three Ah Shi points at the top of thigh.
- **Gua sha** to top of thigh.

Course of treatment

Three sessions.

Results

The leg pain and restriction were relieved immediately. The follow-up treatments cleared remnants of discomfort and served to destagnate the Qi and Blood in the pelvis. He did not alter the habits that contributed to his problem and presented 2 years later with the same problem caused by long hours of driving and inactivity. The same treatment was applied successfully.

Constipation

Female, 28

Presenting complaint

Patient complained of constipation with abdominal distension and fatigue. She also had pain at the back of the ears extending to the occiput. Her ears felt stuffy and hearing was obstructed.

Tongue

Pale with a red tip. The coating was light yellow, thick and greasy at the back. The front of the tongue was wet. The sides were pale and wet.

Pulse

Rate 76–80, weak in both Kidney positions. Blood pulse was thin and weak. Liver pulse was thin and wiry.

Other signs and symptoms

Menses regular and normal, but with prolonged premenstrual symptoms of breast distension and mood swings. Stools were every 5 days and passed with difficulty. Patient drank coffee, which helped stimulate bowel movements. Her job was stressful, she ate erratically and forgot to drink fluid. She was cold, with colder hands and feet.

Treatment

Back
- BL 57, BL 25, BL 23, BL 20 for bowels, BL 13, GV 14, GB 20, GB 12, TW 16 for ears and temporomandibular joint.
- **Gua sha** to upper back, neck and shoulders for ears and to middle and lower back for bowels.

Front
- LI 4, TW 6, ST 36, CV 6, ST 25 for bowels, TW 17, GB 2, ST 7 for ear and temporomandibular joint (TMJ).

Course of treatment

Patient was treated three times per month for 3 months.

Recommendations

Stop the coffee as it depletes fluids and increases Heat and obstruction in the Shao Yang, affecting the ears. Drink fluid throughout the day. Referred to dental specialist to be fitted for TMJ appliance.

Seven Forests Asarum 14 was given for ear pain and Bao He Wan (Passive Harmony Pill) for stool, changed to Modified Ji Chuan Wan, (Benefit the River Flow decoction) for constipation due to Deficient Kidney Yang and Kidney Qi.

Results

The stuffiness in her ears cleared and the pain resolved, specifically after Gua sha. The pain gradually returned though not as severe. She agreed to see a dentist who could evaluate her jaw and fit her for an appliance.

The constipation resolved at first, then returned after a business trip. She was very distended, uncomfortable and tired. Ju Chuan Wan was given with excellent results.

Diarrhea

Female, 52

Presenting complaint

Frequent loose stool and diarrhea for 5 months. Patient associates onset with drinking water from a bottle of water she left in her car for weeks. Weight loss, burning stool, fatigue and stress due to urgency and bowel incontinence.

Previous treatment

Antibiotic therapy, Flagyl and Lomotil to slow stool frequency. No response.

Tongue

Tongue was pale, with fluted borders and thin white coat.

Pulse

Pulse was 72 but could race to 88 with stress in the short term.

Other signs and symptoms

Anxiety and fatigue.

Treatment

Back
Prone position:
- BL 60, BL 57, BL 18, BL 20, BL 25, BL 26, BL 31, GB 30.

- **Gua sha** to mid-back, low back, sacrum, lateral to sacrum and across gluteus medius.
- **Gua sha** to upper back for anxiety and Blood stasis constraining internal organ function.

Front
- Yin tang.
- LI 4, PC 6, SP 4, TW 9.
- SP 6, ST 36, CV 4, CV 6, KI 16 or ST 25.
- Pressure manipulation applied to iliacus to stimulate and close Houstonian 'valve' on left, iliocecal 'valve' on right.

Course of treatment

Patient had one treatment.

Recommendations

Eat mainly warm cooked food and fluid in the form of regular meals. Chew food at least 50 times before swallowing. Reduce or eliminate raw food, nuts and seeds until stools normalize. Soak feet in hot water at night for 10 minutes, then cover. Keep feet warm.

Results

Patient was shocked that her unrelenting diarrhea from which she suffered for months stopped completely after one treatment.

Hemorrhoids

Female, 36

Presenting complaint

Patient had prolonged severe pain during and after defecation, with some bright red blood at end of stool or on toilet paper.

Previous treatment

Patient was under the care of a physician who prescribed ointment and time.

Tongue

Large with scalloped edges. Slightly dry in center, cracked with edges more wet and pale. Tip slightly red.

Pulse

Normal rate. Kidney pulses deep. Middle Jiao pulses full and wiry. Overall slightly slippery.

Other signs and symptoms

Her activities were limited by pain. She had fear of defecation. Stools were twice per day. Urine normal. Sleep altered due to pain.

Treatment

Back

- BL 57, BL 25, BL 23, BL 20, BL 18, GV 1, points bilateral to the coccyx.
- **Gua sha** to mid-to lower back, lateral to sacrum and coccyx.

Front

- Bai Hui, ST 36, ST 25, CV 6, PC 4.

Course of treatment

Five weekly sessions. Each session treated hemorrhoids and tonified Spleen. The focus on hemorrhoids was primary in the first four sessions, the Spleen primary in the fifth session.

Recommendations

Avoid sitting on cold surfaces. Daily sitz baths recommended. Take psyllium husk powder to bulk and soften stool. Patent herbal formula Qiang Li Hua Zhi Ling (Fargelin for Piles) given.

Results

This patient had 75% relief within 2 days of the first session, no bleeding and only slight discomfort with the stool. Successive treatments built on this improvement. The Spleen Qi is said to hold things in place. Ptosis in a channel or organ is a sign of weakness in the Spleen. Therefore, tonification of the Spleen stabilizes the resolution of the hemorrhoids and prevents their recurrence.

Acute urinary tract infection, frequent urination

Female, 28

Presenting complaint

Burning urine, pelvic pain over bladder area. Anxiety related to acute pain. Insomnia due to frequent urination. Patient had history of urinary tract infection for which she was treated by antibiotic therapy.

Previous treatment

Antibiotics in past for urinary tract infection. Analgesic pain medication.

Tongue

Tongue slightly red with thicker coat at the back.

Pulse

Pulse was 78 and wiry.

Other signs and symptoms

Cold feet, stress at work, lack of water intake, irregular meals, irregular stools.

Treatment

Back

Prone position:

- BL 60, BL 57, BL 23, BL 28, BL 31, GB 30.
- **Gua sha** to mid-back, low back, sacrum, lateral to sacrum and across gluteus medius.

Front

- Yin tang.
- LI 4, LU 7, KI 6.
- SP 6, SP 9, ST 36, CV 2, CV 3, CV 4, CV 6, ST 29+ (point between ST 29 and ST 30 specific for urinary problems).
- Ear magnets at Shen men in ear.

Course of treatment

Patient had a urine dip to rule out infection. Urine had small number of leukocytes but no blood; sample was sent out for culture. Patient was given prescription for D-mannose[3] and for antibiotics if needed. It was suggested to try the D-mannose first while waiting for the results of the culture. Patient had two treatments with acupuncture and Gua sha.

Recommendations

In addition to the D-mannose, eat mainly warm cooked food and fluid in the form of regular meals. Soak feet in hot water at night for 10 minutes, then cover. Keep feet warm (which supports normal flow of Qi and Blood in pelvis).

Results

Note: acupuncture is effective in treatment and prevention of uncomplicated recurrent lower urinary tract infections (Alraek et al 2002; Aune et al. 1998). Acupuncture also improves urge- and mixed-type incontinence in women after 12 treatments with improvement maintained even at 3 months after the last treatment (Bergstrom et al. 2000).

With Gua sha, acupuncture and D-mannose this patient's frequent and burning urine resolved completely in a much shorter time. Patient kept D-mannose handy to take at the earliest sign of any urinary discomfort and before or just after intercourse (¼ tsp in water).

---

[3]D-mannose is the sugar extracted from cranberries that has been shown to treat and prevent urinary tract infection, not by killing bacteria but by preventing *Escherichia coli* from adhering to the mucosa. *E. coli* is responsible for 90% of urinary tract infections (UTI). In practice, I have found D-mannose to be soothing to patients with a history of urinary problems and I prescribe a therapeutic dose if symptoms are acute. A preventive dose may be taken just before or just after intercourse for patients who experience UTI symptoms after sex.

Frequent urination, prostatitis

Male, 56

Presenting complaint

Burning urine, pelvic pain over bladder area. Anxiety related to acute pain. Insomnia due to frequent urination. Patient had history of urinary tract infection for which he was prescribed antibiotic therapy.

Previous treatment

No previous treatment for frequent urination. Patient was advised that his urinary frequency might persist for months or years.

Tongue

Tongue red, thick, swollen with thick coat.

Pulse

Pulse was 76 and smooth, coinciding with complications of dampness seen on the Tongue.

Other signs and symptoms

Lethargic, depressed and anxious. Sleep apnea. Occasional pain at pelvic floor. Aversion to water to avoid urination.

Treatment

Back

Prone position:
- GV 14, BL 13, BL 38, BL 15, BL 17.
- BL 60, BL 57, BL 23, BL 28, BL 31, BL 32, GB 30.
- **Gua sha** to upper back, mid-back, low back, sacrum, lateral to sacrum and across gluteus medius.

Front
- Yin tang.
- LI, 4 LU 7, KI 6.
- SP 6, SP 9, ST 36, CV 2, CV 3, CV 4, CV 6, ST 29+ (point between ST 29 and ST 30 specific for urinary problems).
- PC 6, SP 4.
- Release trigger points at obliques for lateral lower abdominal pain.
- Ear magnets at Shen men in ear and at prostate point.

Course of treatment

Patient had weeky treatment over 6 months.

Recommendations

Eat mainly warm cooked food and fluid in the form of regular meals. Soak feet in hot water at night for 10 minutes, then cover. Keep feet warm (which supports normal flow of Qi and Blood in pelvis). Recommend D-mannose for any sign of urinary burning.

Patient's oncologist discouraged him from taking herbal medicine.

Results

Reduced anxiety and improved sleep. Frequency of urination abated gradually over time. Sudden sensation of urgency when he was about to urinate still bothered him. Referred for sleep study that confirmed sleep apnea and use of a continuous positive airway pressure (CPAP) machine resulted in much better sleep, energy and mood.

Note: Honjo et al. (2004) demonstrated that acupuncture caused a significant decrease in non-inflammatory pelvic pain with improvement in intrapelvic venous congestion in men. Capodice et al (2007) demonstrated a therapeutic effect of acupuncture in the treatment of the symptoms of chronic prostatitis including urinary frequency and chronic pelvic pain syndrome.

Testicular pain

Male, 45

Presenting complaint

Patient complained of episodic pain in the left testicle, with slight swelling after a trauma to the area. For a short time, the ejaculate had pink streaks of blood. No pain with ejaculation, no change in urine. The injury seemed to have healed but then he took a long hike and sat on some cold rocks. After this the pain came back.

Tongue

Pink, slightly scalloped at sides, coating white and dripping, crack in middle of tongue that extended longitudinally but not to end. Slightly purple at center.

Pulse

Normal; right Kidney pulse was tight indicating possible stagnation.

Other signs and symptoms

Normal urine, sleep and appetite. Stool occasionally loose.

Treatment

Back
- BL 57 for perineum, BL 17, BL 18, BL 23, BL 25, BL 36, GB 30.
- **Gua sha** to mid- to lower back and lateral gluteus medius to GB 30 area.

Front
- CV 1, SP 10, LIV 5, CV 4, ST 27.
- Indirect moxa to lower abdomen and at perineum.

Course of treatment

Two sessions 1 week apart.

Recommendations

Avoid sitting on cold surfaces and avoid intake of cold or sour food. A decoction of Ju He Wan (Tangerine Seed Pill) was given for the pain.

Results

After the first session and Bao of herbs, the pain in the testicle left. There was sensation in the perineum that resolved after the second treatment.

Vulvodynia

Female, 36

Presenting complaint

Conditions of vulvodynia are unique to each patient who experiences them. By necessity, approaches must vary based on the history and response to intervention. This patient had vaginal pain, pain with intercourse, burning pain with urination and no inflammatory signs. Infection ruled out by gynecologist.

Previous treatment

Analgesic pain medication, antibiotics in past for urinary tract infection.

Tongue

Tongue was unremarkable: normal flesh color, slightly redder at the tip with normal coat. Red tip may have related to vexed Heart.

Pulse

Pulse was 72, unremarkable.

Other signs and symptoms

Anxiety related to pain and impact on relationship because of pain during sex. Some aversion to drinking water to avoid urination and emotion associated with the signal of burning urine. Cold hands and feet; patient was thin and focused on maintaining reduced food intake.

Treatment

Back

Prone position:

- BL 60, BL 57, BL 23, BL 25, BL 28.
- **Gua sha** to mid-back, low back, sacrum, lateral to sacrum and across gluteus medius.

Dog position (on all fours):

- **Gua sha** to ischium and medial ischium area.

Front

- Yin tang.
- LI 4, LU 7, KI 6.
- SP 6, SP 9, ST 36, CV 2, CV 3, CV 4, CV 6, ST 29+ (point between ST 29 and ST 30 specific for urinary problems).
- Ear magnets at Shen men in ear.

Course of treatment

Patient had six sessions 1 week apart, with Gua sha at the first, third session, and fifth session.

Recommendations

Eat mainly warm cooked food and fluid in the form of regular meals. Soak feet in hot water at night for 10 minutes, then cover. Keep feet warm (which supports normal flow of Qi and Blood in pelvis).

Referred to a physical therapist who specializes in pelvic floor dysfunction; she had physical therapy (PT) sessions concurrently with acupuncture and Gua sha. PT consisted of releasing pelvic floor muscles through vaginal and rectal manipulation and fascial pressure.

Prescribed D-mannose[4] powder: ¼ tsp four times a day with water.

Results

Burning urine reduced by 80% after the first treatment. Patient was able to have intercourse after the second treatment with only mild tenderness. After the third treatment she was able to have intercourse regularly with no problem. Remaining sessions focused equally on hip pain. Maintenance sessions are given whenever patient experiences any early sign of recurrence. One or two sessions resolves.

Spermatorrhea, premature ejaculation

Male, 40

Presenting complaint

Patient complained of involuntary loss of semen during long periods of sitting meditation. The loss of semen is referred to as Tsa Lung, 'disease of the winds', in Tibetan Buddhism. There was occasional burning urine.

Tongue

Red, with yellow coating, thinner in the middle.

---

[4]D-mannose is the sugar extracted from cranberries that has been shown to treat and prevent urinary tract infection, not by killing bacteria but by preventing *Escherichia coli* from adhering to the mucosa. *E. coli* is responsible for 90% of urinary tract infections (UTI). In practice, I have found D-mannose to be soothing to patients with a history of urinary problems and I prescribe a therapeutic dose if symptoms are acute.

Pulse

Slightly fast at 80. Lung pulse was moving, Kidney pulses were deep, Kidney Yin pulse soft. The Spleen pulse was scattered.

Other signs and symptoms

Occasional hemorrhoids, normal stool. Appetite was excellent, sleep good. Had occasional night sweats in addition to burning urine and chronic dry cough. He showered only once a week. He practiced celibacy and wanted to use treatment sessions to improve his meditation.

Treatment

Back

- BL 15, BL 18, BL 23, BL 27, BL 28, BL 52, GV 4, Bai Hui.
- **Gua sha** to entire back.

Front

- SP 9, SP 6, CV 4, CV 3, ST 29 or ST 27, KI 3.

Recommendations

Stop all caffeine beverages including kukicha tea. Shower daily or every other day. Patient was encouraged to cultivate a sense of surrender and self-acceptance rather than judge the loss of semen as a measure of inferior meditation practice.

Course of treatment and results

This patient received almost weekly treatments for a year. Early on his symptoms changed from acute to episodic burning urine, loss of semen or night sweats. His coughing resolved. Over time his pulse rate fell to 68 and his tongue became less red overall. He achieved greater meditative concentration from acupuncture treatment. Eventually he got married and then received treatment for the Tantric practice of orgasm without ejaculation.

Dysmenorrhea, uterine fibroids

Female, 49

Presenting complaint

Patient complained of pain and heavy bleeding with menses that was regular every 25 days. She was anemic, weak and tired.

Previous treatment

Patient was also seeing her gynecologist. A sonogram revealed multiple fibroids 3 cm in size. She was prescribed Progest cream, then 10% Progest oil.

Tongue

Short tongue body, swollen at the borders, furry, wet, with peeled areas. Color was pale with some areas pale brown/red as opposed to bright red.

Pulse

Rapid, from 92 to 125, and thin. Kidney pulses were deep.

Other signs and symptoms

Patient was extremely anxious and easily frightened. She was weak and anemic from months of menorrhagia. She had heart palpitations, chest pains and insomnia, loose stools or constipation, stomach pain, abdominal pain and lower back pain. She had episodes of near-fainting fatigue while at work. Her urine was frequent and she was chilled easily. She was vegetarian.

Treatment

Back

- Massage and palpate entire back and legs. GV 14, BL 13, BL 15, BL 17, BL 18, BL 20, BL 23, BL 25, BL 32, BL 57.
- **Gua sha** to entire back or mid- and lower back to sacrum.

Front

- LI 4, SP 4, PC 6 opens Chong Mai for treatment of uterus, fibroids and chest/heart; SP 6, SP 8, SP 10, ST 36, CV 3, CV 4, CV 6, CV 17, CV 12, ST 30, ST 29, ST 28, ST 25, Pee Gen, TW 5, GB 41 for back.
- For heavy bleeding, indirect moxa to both feet at SP 1 and LIV 1, five times at each site, to the point of pain. Patient was taught this method to use at home.

An example treatment was:

- GV 14, BL 15, BL 20, BL 23, BL 32.
- **Gua sha** to back.
- SP 4, PC 6, CV 17, CV 12, CV 6.

Course of treatment

Patient was seen biweekly for 2 years.

Recommendations

Avoid cold and sour foods to comfort pain. No stimulants or alcohol. Eat 3–5 small meals per day with attention to increasing protein.

Yunnan Bai Yao (Yunnan White Medicine) given for heavy bleeding, Ba Zhan Tang (Women's Precious) for anemia (as well as iron prescribed by physician). Changed to Seven Forests Restorative Tablets for chaotic menopausal symptoms of Heat and chill.

Xiao Liu Pian (Tumor Reducing Tablet) in granules given for fibroids, Ding Xin Wan (Calm the Heart Pill) for heart palpitations and anxiety. She took Po Chai when traveling.

Results

Treatment and Gua sha helped to resolve the external aspects of her back pain. Her periods became regular at 26–28 days and after a year the flow became normal. The palpitations stopped and anxiety became infrequent. The fibroids initially decreased in size and then stabilized. The patient eventually had a hysterectomy.

References

Alraek, T., Soedal, L., Fagerheim, S., et al., 2002 (October). Acupuncture treatment in the prevention of uncomplicated recurrent lower urinary tract infections in adult women. Am J Pub Health 92 (10), 1609–1611.

Aune, A., Alraek, T., LiHua, H., et al., 1998 (March). Acupuncture in the prophylaxis of recurrent lower urinary tract infection in adult women. Scand J Prim Health Care 16 (1), 37–39.

Bennett, G.J., Watson, C.P.N., 2009 (August). Herpes zoster and postherpetic neuralgia: past, present and future. Pain Res Manag 14 (4), 275–282.

Bergstrom, K., Carlsson, C.P., Lindholm, C., et al., 2000 (March 15). Improvement of urge- and mixed-type incontinence after acupuncture treatment. J Auton Nerv Syst 79 (2–3).

Chan, S., Yuen, J., Gohel, M., et al., 2011 (May 13). Guasha-induced hepatoprotection in chronic active hepatitis B: A case study. Clin Chim Acta in press.

Braun, M., Schwickert, M., Nielsen, A., et al., 2011 January 28. Effectiveness of Traditional Chinese 'Gua Sha' Therapy in Patients with Chronic Neck Pain; A Randomized Controlled Trial. Pain Med.

Capodice, J., Jin, Z., Bemis, D., et al., 2007. A pilot study on acupuncture for lower urinary tract symptoms elated to chronic prostatis/chronic pelvic pain. Chin Med 6 (2), 1.

Chiu, J.-Y., Gau, M.-L., Kuo, S.-Y., et al., 2010 (March). Effects of Gua-Sha therapy on breast engorgement: a randomized controlled trial. J Nurs Res 18 (1), 1–10.

Hale, T., Breathing Free. Three Rivers Press, New York, NY, 2000.

Honjo, H., Kamoi, K., Naya, Y., et al. Effects of acupuncture for chronic pelvic pain syndrome with intrapelvic venous congestion: preliminary results. Int J Urol 2004;11(8):607–612.

Kwong, K.K., Kloetzer, L., Wong, K.K., et al., 2009. Bioluminescence imaging of heme oxygenase-1 upregulation in the Gua Sha procedure. J Vis Exp 30 (August 28), 1385.

Nambudripod, D., 1989. Unsolved Health Problems Solved. Singer Publishing, Rancho Mirage, CA.

Nielsen, A., 2005 (January). Postherpetic neuralgia in the left buttock after a case of shingles. Explore (NY) 1 (1), 74.

Schmader, K.E., Sloane, R., Pieper, C., et al., 2007 (August). The impact of acute herpes zoster pain and discomfort on functional status and Quality of LIfe in Older Adults. Clin J Pain 23 (6), 490–496.

Ursini, T., Tontodonati, M., Manzoli, L., et al., 2011. Acupuncture for the treatment of severe acute pain in herpes zoster: results of a nested, open-label, randomized trial in the VZV Pain Study. BMC Complement Altern Med 11, 46.

Xia, Z.W., Zhong, W.W., Meyrowitz, J.S., et al., 2008. The role of heme oxygenase-1 in T cell-mediated immunity: the all encompassing enzyme. Curr Pharm Des 14 (5), 454–464.

Zhu, Z., Wilson, A.T., Mathahs, M.M., et al., 2008. Heme oxygenase-1 suppresses hepatitis C virus replication and increases. Hepatology 48, 1430–1439.

Gua sha handout

It is strongly recommended to give each patient a handout after applying Gua sha, even if you have provided it on a prior occasion. On the following page is a handout in simple language and format required by our hospital's education and information board (Beth Israel Medical Center, New York, NY).

WHAT IS GUA SHA?

Gua sha is an important hands-on medical treatment that has been used throughout Asia for centuries. *Gua* means 'to rub' or 'press-stroke.' *Sha* is a term that describes the blood congestion in surface tissue that accumulates in areas where the patient may experience stiffness and pain; *sha* is also the term for the little red dots that are raised from applying *Gua sha* (Nielsen 2012). When *Gua* press-stroking is applied in repeated even strokes, *sha* appears as small red dots called 'petechiae' and the pain immediately shifts. In minutes the small red dots fade into blended reddishness. The *sha* disappears totally in two to three days after treatment. The color of *sha* and rate of fading can indicate important information about a patient's condition. Pain relief lasts even after the *sha* is completely gone.

The benefits of *Gua sha* are numerous. It resolves spasms and pain, and promotes normal circulation to the muscles, tissues, and organs directly beneath the area that is treated, as seen in *Gua sha's* immediate effect on coughing and wheezing. Research has shown that *Gua sha* causes a four-fold increase in microcirculation of surface tissue (Nielsen et al. 2007) and can reduce inflammation (Braun et al. 2011; Chan et al. 2011).

The patient experiences immediate changes in stiffness and pain with increased mobility. Because *Gua sha* mimics sweating, it can help to resolve fever. *Gua sha* cools the patient who feels too warm, warms the patient who feels too cold, while relaxing tension and reducing anxiety. Acupuncturists and practitioners of traditional East Asian medicine consider *Gua sha* for any illness or condition where there is pain or discomfort, for upper respiratory and digestive problems, and any condition where touch palpation indicates there is *sha*. *Gua sha* is often done in combination with acupuncture for problems that acupuncture alone cannot address.

After treatment the patient is advised to keep the area protected from wind, cold and direct sun until the *sha* fades. They are also encouraged to drink plenty of water and eat moderately.

References

Braun, M., Schwickert, M., Nielsen, A., et al., 2011. Effectiveness of Traditional Chinese 'Gua Sha' Therapy in Patients with Chronic Neck Pain; A Randomized Controlled Trial. Pain Med 12 (3), 362–369.

Chan, S., Yuen, J., Gohel, M., et al., 2011. Guasha-induced hepatoprotection in chronic active hepatitis B: A case study. Clin Chim Acta 412 (17–18), 1686–1688.

Nielsen, A., 2012. Gua Sha. A Traditional Technique for Modern Practice, second ed. Elsevier, Edinburgh.

Nielsen, A., Knoblauch, N.T.M., Dobos, G.J., et al., 2007. The Effect of *Gua Sha* Treatment on the Microcirculation of Surface Tissue: A Pilot Study in Healthy Subjects. Explore (NY) 3 (5), 456–466.

List of common acupuncture points by number and name

Governing vessel (Du mai)

GV 1 Changqiang
GV 2 Yaoshu
GV 4 Mingmen
GV 9 Zhiyang
GV 11 Shendao
GV 12 Shenzhu
GV 13 Taodao
GV 14 Dazhui
GV 15 Yamen
GV 16 Fengfu
GV 20 Baihui
GV 24 Shenting
GV 26 Renshong

Conception vessel (Ren mai)

CV 1 Huiyin
CV 2 Qugu
CV 3 Zhongji
CV 4 Guanyuan
CV 5 Shimen
CV 6 Qihai
CV 7 Yinjiao
CV 8 Shenque
CV 9 Shuifen
CV 10 Xiawan
CV 11 Jianli
CV 12 Zhongwan
CV 13 Taodao
CV 14 Juque
CV 15 Jiuwei

CV 17 Shanzhong
CV 21 Xuanji
CV 22 Tiantu
CV 23 Lianquan
CV 24 Chengjiang

Bladder channel

BL 1 Jingming
BL 2 Zanzhu
BL 7 Tongtian
BL 10 Tianzhu
BL 11 Dazhu
BL 12 Fengmen
BL 13 Feishu
BL 14 Jueyinshu
BL 15 Xinshu
BL 16 Dushu
BL 17 Geshu
BL 18 Ganshu
BL 19 Danshu
BL 20 Pishu
BL 21 Weishu
BL 22 Sanjiaoshu
BL 23 Shenshu
BL 24 Qihaishu
BL 25 Dachangshu
BL 26 Guanyuanshu
BL 27 Xiaochangshu
BL 28 Pangguanshu
BL 30 Baihuanshu
BL 31 Shangliao
BL 32 Ciliao

BL 33 Zhongliao
BL 34 Xialiao
BL 36 Chengfu (classical BL 50)
BL 43 Gaohuangshu (classical BL 38)
BL 40 Weizhong (classical BL 54)
BL 50 Chengfu
BL 52 Zhishi (classical BL 47)
BL 57 Chengshan
BL 58 Feiyang
BL 59 Fuyang
BL 60 Kunlun
BL 62 Shenmai
BL 63 Jinmen
BL 67 Zhiyin

Kidney channel

KI 1 Yongquan
KI 2 Rangu
KI 3 Taixi
KI 4 Dazhong
KI 5 Shuiquan
KI 6 Zhaohai
KI 7 Fuliu
KI 8 Jiaoxin
KI 9 Zhubin
KI 10 Yingu
KI 16 Huangshu
KI 23 Shenfeng
KI 27 Shufu

Small intestine channel

SI 1 Shaoze
SI 2 Qiangu
SI 3 Houxi
SI 4 Wanggu
SI 5 Yanggu
SI 6 Yanglao
SI 7 Zhisheng
SI 8 Xiaohai
SI 9 Jianzhen
SI 10 Naoshu
SI 11 Tianzhong
SI 12 Bingfen
SI 13 Quyuan
SI 14 Jianwaishu
SI 15 Jianzhongshu
SI 17 Tianrong
SI 18 Quanliao
SI 19 Tinggong

Heart channel

HT 1 Jiquan
HT 3 Shaohai
HT 4 Lingdao
HT 5 Tongli
HT 6 Yinxi
HT 7 Shenmen
HT 8 Shaofu
HT 9 Shaochang

San Jiao (Triple Burner) channel

TB 1 Guanchong
TB 2 Yemen
TB 3 Zhongzhu
TB 4 Yangchi
TB 5 Waiguan
TB 6 Zhigou
TB 7 Huizhong
TB 10 Tianjing
TB 13 Naohui
TB 14 Jianliao
TB 15 Tianliao
TB 17 Yifeng
TB 21 Ermen
TB 23 Sizhukong

Pericardium channel

PC 1 Tianchi
PC 4 Ximen
PC 5 Jianshu
PC 6 Neiguan
PC 7 Daling
PC 8 Laogong
PC 9 Zhongchong

Gall bladder channel

GB 1 Tongziliao
GB 2 Tinghui
GB 12 Wangu
GB 14 Yangbai
GB 15 Linqi
GB 20 Fengqi
GB 21 Jianjing
GB 24 Riyue
GB 25 Jingmen
GB 26 Daimai

GB 27 Wushu
GB 28 Weidao
GB 29 Juliao
GB 30 Huantiao
GB 31 Fengshi
GB 32 Zhongdu
GB 34 Yanglingquan
GB 37 Guangming
GB 38 Yangfu
GB 39 Xuanzhong
GB 40 Qiuxu
GB 41 Zulingqi
GB 42 Diwuhui
GB 43 Xiaxi
GB 44 Zuqiaoyin

Liver channel

LIV 1 Dadun
LIV 2 Xingjian
LIV 3 Taichong
LIV 4 Zhongfeng
LIV 5 Ligou
LIV 6 Zhongdu
LIV 7 Xiguan
LIV 8 Ququan
LIV 11 Yinlian
LIV 13 Zhangmen
LIV 14 Qimen

Stomach channel

ST 2 Sibai
ST 4 Dicang
ST 6 Jiache
ST 7 Xiaguan
ST 8 Touwei
ST 9 Renwing
ST 12 Quepen
ST 18 Rugen
ST 21 Liangmen
ST 25 Tianshu
ST 27 Daju
ST 28 Shuidao
ST 29 Guilai
ST 30 Qichong
ST 34 Liangqiu
ST 35 Dubi
ST 36 Zusanli

ST 37 Shanjuxu
ST 38 Tiaokou
ST 39 Xiajuxu
ST 40 Fenglong
ST 41 Jiexi
ST 42 Chongyang
ST 43 Xiangu
ST 44 Neiting
ST 45 Lidui

Spleen channel

SP 1 Yinbai
SP 2 Dadu
SP 3 Taibai
SP 4 Gongsun
SP 5 Shanqiu
SP 6 Sanyinjiao
SP 8 Diji
SP 9 Yinlingquan
SP 10 Xuehai
SP 15 Daheng
SP 21 Dabao

Large intestine channel

LI 1 Shangyang
LI 4 Hegu
LI 5 Yangxi
LI 10 Shousanli
LI 11 Quchi
LI 12 Zhouliao
LI 14 Binao
LI 15 Jianyu
LI 16 Jugu
LI 20 Yingxiang

Lung channel

LU 1 Zhongfu
LU 3 Tianfu
LU 5 Chize
LU 7 Lieque
LU 8 Jingqu
LU 9 Taiyuan
LU 10 Yuji
LU 11 Shaoshang

Extra points

Yintang
Taiyang
Yuyao
Huatuojiaji
Dingchuan
Jianeiling
Pakloh
Tukyin
Eyes of knee
Wings of knee
Dannangxue M-LE 23
Erbai M-UE-29
TB gummy (palpate for tight or fasciculation point
between TW 9 and TW 10)
Yi shu 'pancreas hollow' M-BW-12

Directions for Neti wash and Croup tent

Neti wash

Neti washing comes from the yogic practice of nasal rinsing.

It is recommended to Neti wash daily when you bathe or shower. It is beneficial to be more consistent during the winter months, if exposed to dust or air pollutants, and during nasal, sinus or upper respiratory events. Fill the Neti pot (also called naso-cup) with warm water and ¼ **to ⅓ teaspoon sea salt or kosher salt that is fine, not coarse. Stir to dissolve the salt.**

Place the spout of the pot in one nostril with your head tilted up, that is, slightly back and slightly to the opposite side. Not too far back … not too far to the side.

Let the water flow into the nose, over the septum and out the other nostril. Some will also travel **over the nasopharynx into the back of the throat**. Catch it there and spit it out rather than swallow.

You do not need to suck the water into your nose or blow it out with vigor. The pressure created from blowing the nose while pinching the nostrils drives some of the mucus and fluid back into the sinuses. Just let the water fall out, blowing gently without pinching the nostrils. In the beginning, to be completely relaxed, it is a good idea to Neti wash in private. The saline solution **will burn if there is too much salt, or not enough salt (happens more often)**.

It is not recommended to Neti over the sink tilting the head forward or to the side. Aside from missing the nasopharynx area, you risk infiltrating the Eustachian tube. If the nostrils are completely swollen so that none of the water can get through, then follow the directions for a croup tent.

Neti washes are excellent in the treatment and prevention of sinus conditions, colds and stuffiness. The head not only feels better but thinking becomes clearer. Neti pots may be obtained from health food stores, pharmacies, health care practitioners or ordered online.

Croup tent

A croup tent is an age-old home care treatment for sinus infections, sinus headaches, colds and coughs. Simple steam can be used, but relief is more pronounced if done in the following manner, adapted from the Native American tradition of my ancestors.

Break off 8–10 end branches from a white pine tree. White pine needles are soft and thin. An end branch might have five needle bunches. Thank the tree. Place these end branches in a soup pot, cover with water and bring to the boil. Simmer for a few minutes and then turn it off. If you do not have access to white pine branches, essential oil of eucalyptus with a drop or two of tea tree oil will do. If none of these are available, simply use water.

Let it cool a little; you do not want it too hot, but you want it still to be steamy. Now sitting at a table, set the pot in front of you and with the lid off place a towel over it and over your head. You are now in a croup tent.

Alternate inhaling the vapor through your mouth and nose. You can adjust the amount of steam by lifting an edge of the towel. The steam will penetrate the sinuses through your nostrils and face. White pine is very high in vitamin C and the vapors help open and soothe the nasal passages. Stay under for 5 or 10 minutes. Take a break and do it again if you like. This pot of pine needle soup can be reheated and reused for several days but don't reuse if it has begun to ferment or grow mold.

Children can use croup tents too but it is best done with an adult in the tent to adjust the steam. Use especially before going to bed. A croup tent will not only shorten a cold, cough or sinus problem but also decrease the discomfort that accompanies these syndromes.

Croup tents are not recommended for 'reactive airways', wheezing or asthma in children.

Tabled articles and studies with full citations: Gua sha literature review

Tables for different categories of papers (Tables 2.3–2.10)

As discussed in Chapter 2, Tables 2.3 to 2.10 (below) are grouped according to kind of article or study, from clinical recommendations to case series to clinical trials of Gua sha treatment alone or in combination with other modalities for specific conditions. Tables 2.1 and 2.2 are found in Chapter 2. The full citations are grouped for each table and follow the Tables below. For studies and discussion on Gua sha biomechanisms, see Chapter 3.

Table 2.3 Gua sha alone: descriptive clinical recommendations for specific conditions (121 articles)

Condition	Authors and date
Cervical spondylosis, spondylopathy	Jiang 2005; Zhang 2010; Zhen and Bai 2007
Cervical tendon lesions	Deng et al. 2009
Cervical spondylosis or pain at waist and lower extremities	Kang 2004
Neck + low back pain	Kang 2003
Head and facial neuralgia	Ge 2008
Soft tissue injury rehabilitation	Chen 2004; Gui 1994
Frozen shoulder	Yu 1998
Tennis elbow	Gao 1999; ('Gua sha' Scraping) 2001
Acute symptoms	Li and Liu 2002
Traumatology disease	Liang 2001b
Fever, 'sha syndrome'	Bai et al. 2007; Bao 2002; Fan 2005; Huang and Guo 2009; Ji and Zheng 2008; Li et al. 2001; Min 2007; Tan and He 2000; Wu 2001; Yang et al. 2007a; Yang et al. 2007b; Zhao 2007; Zhao et al. 2008
Fever, cholera	Zhao et al. 2008
Heatstroke	Ruan and Cui 2005
Upper respiratory infection: cold	(Fingers Gua sha) 2010; (Head and Upper) 2010; Ruan 2008a; Wang and Tang 2001
Relapsing respiratory infection	Pang et al. 2008

Continued

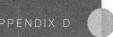

Table 2.3 Gua sha alone: descriptive clinical recommendations for specific conditions (121 articles)—cont'd

Condition	Authors and date
Cough	Gao 2002
Eye diseases	Liang 2001a
Pseudomyopia	Zou et al. 2009
Breast carbuncle/mastitis (*Staphylococcus aureus* or *Streptococcus*)	Wang 2002b
Infant diarrhea	Qu 2010
Stomach problems: constipation	Yang 2010
Epigastric pain	Wang 1996
Ascites due to cirrhosis	Wang 2000
Cardiovascular disease	He 2010
Hyperlipidemia	Du 2003
Hypertension + coronary artery disease	Hu and Zuo 2005
Stroke	Dong 1998
Cerebellar Atrophy	Zhang and Jiang 1999
Acne	Lin and Chen 2000
Chloasma	Wang 1997; Yao 2009
Urticaria	Mao 2009
Neurodermatitis; lichen simplex	Liao et al. 2010
Stress	Liu 2010b
Fatigue, athletic	Fang et al. 2008
Chronic fatigue	Ruan 2008b; Wang 2002a
Stress, insomnia, neck and shoulder pain	Geng 2010
Insomnia	Hu and Chen 2010; Li and Qi 2007
Sleep quality in patients with diabetes	Zhang 2006
Rheumatoid arthritis	Chen et al. 2006; Cong et al. 2005
Systemic lupus	Geng and Yang 2007
Pain, tropical (Africa)	Zhang 2009
Aesthetic medicine	(Gua sha for) 2008; (Jade Gua sha) 2009; Wang 2008a; Wang 2008b; Zhang and Mo 2000
Foot self-care	Huang 2010; Wang 2010a
Elder health, natural	Lin and Yan 2006
Sub-health	Ke 2007
Pain and health	Zhang 2008a; Zhang 2008b
Self-treatment: sleep and headaches	Peng and Liao 2010a; Peng and Liao 2010b
Self-treatment	Wei 2002; Yang and Liu 2007
Obesity	Li 2007
Improve cost-effectiveness	Hai 2007
General guidelines	Cui et al. 2009; (Gua sha is) 2008; (Gua sha Ten) 2009; (Gua sha the) 2004; (Gua sha Treatment) 2009; Liu 2010a; Xu 2008a; Zhang 2009

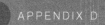

Table 2.3 Gua sha alone: descriptive clinical recommendations for specific conditions (121 articles)—cont'd

Condition	Authors and date
Gua sha commerce	Yin and Qu 2008
How to apply	Liu 2004; Xu 2008b; Yang 2004
To which part of the body	(Human Four) 2000; Liang et al. 2009; Zhang 2008c; Zuo and Wang 2010
Treatment of various illness	Huang 2007; Jiang and Shi 2005; Ruan 2008c; Wang 2010b; Zuo 2010
Oils and tools	Bai and Wu 1998; Chan and Chen 1998; Chen 2008; Chen and Zhang 2001; Sun 2010; Yang 2010
Clinical effect	Wang et al. 2006; Zuo and Wang 2007
As natural medicine	(Simple and natural) 2010; (Traditional Chinese Medicine) 2010
Gua sha as non-toxic, non-drug, natural medicine	Bi 2010; Chen et al. 2010; Dong 2009; (Fu di energy scraping) 2010
History (also related to fever, heatstroke, thermal dysregulation)	Cai 2003; Cao and Dao 2002; Ji 2008; Li et al 2001; Min 2007; Ming 2004; Wu 2010
Gua sha as public health policy	Wu 2010
Misunderstood as abuse in the West	Hu 2002; Xu 2008a

Table 2.4 Gua sha combined with other modalities: descriptive clinical recommendations for specific conditions (62 articles)

Modality combination	Conditions	Authors and date
Gua sha and acupuncture	Stiff neck	Zhang 2010
	Scapulohumeral periarthritis	Chen 2000
	Emotional insomnia	Fan et al. 2009
	Fever	Bai and Lu 2003
	Acute contagious conjunctivitis	Tong and Chen 1999
	Influenza	Shan et al. 2003
Gua sha, acupuncture and massage	Cervical spondylosis	Chen 2002b
	Lumbar muscle strain	Zhou 2000
Gua sha, acupuncture and cupping	Soft tissue injury shoulder	Liu 2008
Gua sha, electro-acupuncture (EA) and point injection	Vertigo/cervical spondylosis	Ruan et al. 2006
Gua sha, acupuncture, moxa and herbs	Arthralgia	Ding 2003
Gua sha, acupuncture, moxa, cupping and ear Tx	Aesthetic medicine	(The Five Elements) 2007
Gua sha, acupuncture, cooling herbs and hydration	Heatstroke	Ma 2005
Gua sha, acupuncture, cupping, pak sha and massage: 'dog days' Tx	Osteoarthritis	Yang et al. 2006
Gua sha, acupuncture, reduction practices and herbs	Lumbar disc herniation	Tang and Liu 2006
Gua sha and massage	Migraine	Cui and Wang 2001
	Cervical spondylosis	Zuo et al. 2005
	Cold fever	An et al. 2010
Gua sha and vibration	Obesity, waistline	('Gua sha' Scraping) 2006
Gua sha and/or cupping	Cutaneous nerve entrapment	Dong 2003

Continued

Table 2.4 Gua sha combined with other modalities: descriptive clinical recommendations for specific conditions (62 articles)—cont'd

Modality combination	Conditions	Authors and date
Gua sha and cupping	Ankle injury	Yang and Han 2006
	Frozen shoulder	Ma 2001
Gua sha and prick bloodletting	Cervical disease	Wang and Hou 2010
	Respiratory infection; cold	Tang et al. 2000
Gua sha, bloodletting and cupping	Throat disease	Bai 2006
Gua sha and herbal medicine	Breast hyperplasia	Meng and Si 2002
	Respiratory infection, fever, sore throat	Tian et al. 2010
Gua sha with Shen Jin Dan (single)	Shoulder periarthritis	Bi et al. 2003
Gua sha with methycobalamin	Postherpetic neuralgia	Zuo 2009
Gua sha with glucosamine	Knee osteoarthritis	Yu 2005
Gua sha and moxibustion	Postpartum missing milk	Chen 2006
	Borderline hypertension	Li and Li 2009
Gua sha, Chinese washing and exercise	Periarthritis shoulder	Li 2008
Gua sha with Miao detoxification	Stubborn chronic conditions	Li 2005
Gua sha with wasp/bee venom cream	Facial paralysis	Chen 2002a
	Lumbar disc herniation	Chen and Cheng 2003
Gua sha, apitherapy and heat	Shoulder periarthritis	Chen 2010
Gua sha, traction and needle knife	Cervical spondylopathy	Wu 2001
Gua sha, folk medicine and pharmacy	Intractable disease	Zheng 2005
Gua sha, diet, tai chi and counseling	Sub-health in college students	Pan et al. 2006
Gua sha as part of comprehensive care	General guidelines	Li 2009; Liu 2006a; Xie 2001; Zhang et al. 2007; Zhao et al. 2002
	General meridian theory	Yang 2005
	Asthma	Ni et al. 2001
	Pediatric dyspepsia	Zhang 2006
	Brain diseases	Zhao and Du 2010
	Nose problems	Wu 2003
	Postsurgical pain control	Wu and Bong 2008
	Cervical disease	Pu and Li 2008
	Shoulder periarthritis	Tang et al. 2008
	Sciatica	Wei 2000
	Difficult diseases Dx and Tx	Guo and Liu 2003
	Cerebral blood pressure	(Cerebral Blood Pressure) 2001
	Aesthetic medicine, beauty	Wang 2004
Gua sha as part of integrative medicine	Cervical spondylosis	Chen and Wang 1999
Gua sha in combinations as non-toxic, non-drug, natural medicine	General	Li 2006
	Sub-health	Liu 2006b
General discussion of risks of infection: acupuncture, physiotherapy, massage, Gua sha and cupping	General	Zhou et al. 2005

Table 2.5 Case series: Gua sha alone for specific conditions (100 articles)

Condition	Number of cases and authors	Condition	Number of cases and authors
Cervical spondylosis, spondylopathy	40 cases (Jia and Li 2000) 58 cases (Leng 1997) 35 cases (Liu 2003) 97 cases (Qiu et al. 2009) 186 cases (Sun et al. 2003) 68 cases (Tong 1999) 30 cases (Wang 2000)	Pain syndromes	70 cases (Pan 2007) 102 cases (Wang 1999) 44 cases (20 neck, 10 shoulder, 8 lumbar, 6 sciatica: Liu 2008) 123 cases (65 cervical spondylosis, 43 shoulder periarthritis, 15 lumbar fibrositis: Zhang and Li 2009) 32 cases (18 neck, 9 periarthritis shoulder, 5 low back: Qing 2001) 57 cases (neck, shoulder, sciatica: Qiao et al. 2006)
Vertigo, related to cervical problem	48 cases (Jia 2003)	Postsurgical adhesions with intestinal obstruction	24 cases (Xie 2000)
Stiff neck	19 cases (Xiao and Tian 2002) 50 cases (Liu 2001) 40 cases (Ma 2004) 50 cases (Xiao et al. 2001) 90 cases (Song and Zhang 2002) 100 cases (Zhao 2001) 28 cases (Zhou and Yang 2002)	Renal colic	40 cases (Cai 2001)
		Acne	14 cases (Hou 1996)
		Eczema	36 cases (Hu 2009)
Neck + shoulder pain	130 cases (Xing and An 2006)	Herpes zoster	70 cases (Qiao and Zuo 2006)
Shoulder periarthritis	69 cases (He 2007) 150 cases (Liu and He 2003)	Postherpetic neuralgia	68 cases (Gao and Chen 2003)
Frozen shoulder	25 cases (Chen 2000) 80 cases (Hu 2001) 52 cases (Tan 2001) 32 cases (Wang et al. 1998b)	Facial paralysis	42 cases (Chen 2003) 36 cases (Xu 1999)
		Migraine	18 cases (Jia and Zhang 2000)
Scalpulohumeral periarthritis	36 cases (Wang and Mei 2003) 82 cases (Zhao 2006)	Headache, functional	300 cases (Wang et al 1998a)
		Headache and dizziness	100 cases (Liu et al. 2003)
Shoulder coagulation disorder	58 cases (Ma 2009)	Headache related to common cold	45 cases (Ding et al. 2009)
Rotator cuff injury	12 cases (Yu 2007)	Upper respiratory infection	90 cases (Qiao and Liu 2000) 50 cases (Song et al. 2000) 100 cases (Wu and Wu 2003)
Shoulder and back myofascitis	124 cases (Shi and Zou 2001) 106 cases (Shi et al. 2000)		
Muscle spasm	3 cases (Gong 2002)	Chronic pharyngitis	20 cases (Hu et al. 2003)
Lumbar myofibrositis	36 cases (Peng 1999a)	Cold with bronchitis	28 cases (Lu et al 2001)
Lumbar disc herniation	186 cases (Song 2002)	Pediatric susceptible to cold	28 cases (Zhou and Xu 2001)
Acute lumbar sprain	10 cases (Wu and Li 2004) 256 cases (Wu et al. 2001)	Bronchial pneumonia, pediatric	30 cases (Liu and Zhang 2001)
Lumbar pain	64 cases (Bao et al. 2003)	Pediatric cold food stagnation	10 cases (Wu and Zhang 2001)
Inpatient back pain	50 cases (Liu and Li 2009)	Pediatric diarrhea	66 cases (Zhao et al. 2002)
Ankylosing spondylitis	36 cases (Liu and Sun 2001)	Cold and influenza	100 cases (Cai 2005); 90 cases (Li 2009)
Epicondylitis	65 cases (Dong 2003)	Fever	60 cases (Chen and Wei 2010)
Sprained ankle	32 cases (Yang 2006)	Chronic sinusitis	34 cases (Zeng 2000)

Continued

129

Table 2.5 Case series: Gua sha alone for specific conditions (100 articles)—cont'd

Condition	Number of cases and authors	Condition	Number of cases and authors
Tx and prevention: asthma	38 cases (Fan 2009)	Insomnia	60 cases (Qi and Li 1999)
Prevention asthma: 'dog days' Tx	38 cases (Yang et al. 2006)		28 cases (Yang 2004)
			24 cases (Jia et al. 2000)
Asthma	30 cases (Men and Wu 1999)	Neurasthenia in students	36 cases (Yang 2005)
Acute mastitis	50 cases (Dong 2002)	Neurasthenia	56 cases (Fan 2000)
Adolescent breast hyperplasia	86 cases (Luo and Liu 2007)	Primary dysmenorrhea	52 cases (Zheng 2000)
Breast disease	38 cases (Liu 2010)	Enuresis, pediatric	32 cases (Mo 2006)
Recovery from induced abortion	30 cases (Ran and Shi 2009)	Internal hemorrhoids	200 cases (Ma 2002)
Chronic hepatitis B	12 cases (Qin 2009)	Stye	37 cases (Wu and Lin 2000)
Jaundice/chronic hepatitis B	38 cases (Wang 2004)	Trachoma	107 cases (Song 2010)
Acute first aid	30 cases (Li and Liu 2002)	**Thermal dysregulation**	
Hiccup in stroke patients	41 cases (Cong 1998)	Cold	32 cases (Li 2004)
Hypertension	50 cases (Xiong and Min 2008)	Cold Sx at back; chillphobia	25 cases (Wang 2002)
	52 cases (Zhong 1994)	Heatstroke	39 cases (Xu 2010)
			50 cases (Tian 1999)
		Severe heatstroke	34 cases (Peng 1999b)

Table 2.6 Case series: Gua sha paired with another modality for specific conditions (106 articles)

Therapies	Condition	Number of cases, and authors
Gua sha + acupuncture	Peripheral facial paralysis, pediatric	126 cases (Guo 2005)
	Peripheral facial paralysis	39 cases (Zhang and Li 2006a)
		39 cases (Zhang and Li 2006b)
	Refractory facial paralysis	30 cases (Guo and Wu 2005)
		30 cases (Ma 2010)
	Trigeminal neuralgia	20 cases (Tu 2000)
	Pediatric cerebral palsy	24 cases (Wang 2002)
	Cervical spondylosis	68 cases (Yang and Zuo 2005)
		86 cases (Feng 2008)
		120 cases (Li 2000)
		60 cases (Wang and Ge 2009)
	Cervical spondylopathy	76 cases (Xing 2003)
	Stiff neck	56 cases (Han and Yang 2006)
		48 cases (Huang 2001)
	Cervical vertigo	43 cases (Wang 2001)
	Occipital neuralgia	86 cases (Wang 2005a)
	Shoulder periarthritis	57 cases (Fan 2010)
	Lumbar back sprain	38 cases (Liu et al. 1999)
	Fasciitis of back	68 cases (Wang 2004)
	Turberositae tibiae epiphysitis	16 cases (Lu and Li 2005)
	Juvenile chronic sinusitis	62 cases (Cui et al. 2008)
	Student sub-health	40 cases (Yang 2006)

Table 2.6 Case series: Gua sha paired with another modality for specific conditions (106 articles)—cont'd

Therapies	Condition	Number of cases, and authors
Gua sha + Jiaji acupuncture	Recurrent mastitis	62 cases (Wu and Wu 2003b, 2006)
Gua sha + warm-needle acupuncture	Epicondylitis	30 cases (Cheng 2008)
	Knee osteoarthritis	48 cases (Wang 2005b)
Gua sha + needle knife therapy	Cervical spondylosis	150 cases (Li 2005a)
	Lumbar disc herniation	30 cases (Li 2005b)
Gua sha + electro-acupuncture EA	Cervical spondylosis	87 cases (Fan 2001)
	Sciatica	66 cases (Li 2001)
	Ankle injury, soft tissue, old	52 cases (Wu 2010)
Gua sha and ear electro-acupuncture	Simple obesity	107 cases (Yin and Bai 2008)
Gua sha and ear acupuncture	Chloasma	50 cases (Wei and Pi 2003)
Gua sha and ear acupressure	Common migraine	60 cases (Zhang et al. 2009)
	ADHD	30 cases (Sun 2003)
Gua sha + acupressure	Pediatric asthma	60 cases (Huang et al. 2002)
Gua sha + massage	Upper respiratory infection, cold	115 cases (Dang 2005)
		50 cases (Wang and Tang 2001)
	Headache	45 cases (Wang and Guan 2009)
	Migraine	54 cases (Guo 2001)
	Cervical spondylosis (X-ray evaluation)	100 cases (Xin et al. 2004)
	Cervical curvature	120 cases (Sun and Wang 1999)
	Periarthritis shoulder	20 cases (Zhang and Jiang 2005)
	Frozen shoulder	54 cases (Ling 2008)
	Lumbar syndrome	66 cases (Chen 2004)
	Lumbar strain	84 cases (Ding 2001)
	Lumbar disc herniation	32 cases (Zou et al. 2002)
	L3 transverse process syndrome	108 cases (Yuan and Huang 2000)
	Cold Bi arthralgia	118 cases (Li 2004)
	Chronic insomnia	78 cases (Tang et al. 2010)
Gua sha + tui na kneading	Soft-tissue injury	560 cases (Chen and Zhang 2009)
	Lumbar transverse process syndrome	64 cases (Lu et al. 2008)
Gua sha (face) + foot reflexology	Chloasma	26 cases (Wang and Wang 2008)
Gua sha + point embedding	Epigastralgia	60 cases (Zhang 2003)
Gua sha + trigger-point injection	Cervical spondylopathy	83 cases (Ma et al 2003)
	Piriformis syndrome sciatica	23 cases (Xiao and Qin 2010)
Gua sha + TDP irradiation	Levator scapulae injury	86 cases (Ren and Wang 2007)
	Stiff neck	115 cases (Wu and Xie 1998)
Gua sha + manual reduction	Cervical disease	78 cases (Gao 2008)
Gua sha + traction	Cervical vertigo	60 cases (Qi and Li 2001)
Gua sha + segmental manipulation	Cervical spondylotic radiculopathy	53 cases (Qian 2009)
	Lumbar disc herniation	250 cases (Tan et al. 1998)
Gua sha + block therapy	Scapula humeral periarthritis	178 cases (Ma et al. 2005)

Continued

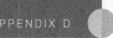

Table 2.6 Case series: Gua sha paired with another modality for specific conditions (106 articles)—cont'd

Therapies	Condition	Number of cases, and authors
Gua sha and cupping	Cervical disease	68 cases (Yang 2004a)
	3rd vertebral process disorder	28 cases (Yang 2004b)
	Shoulder periarthritis	25 cases (Chen 2000)
		36 cases (Yang et al. 2005)
	Thoracic facet-joint disorder	56 cases (Zhao 2006a)
	Supraorbital neuralgia	21 (Liu 2002)
	Menopausal tinnitus	24 cases (Pan et al. 2006)
	Upper respiratory tract infection	100 cases (Wu and Wu 2003a)
	Recurrent respiratory infection, pediatric	100 cases (Shi and Li 2002)
	Acute/chronic gastroenteritis	56 (Yang and Zhang 2006)
	Gastrointestinal dysfunction	26 cases (Twenty-six Patients 2005)
	Influenza	60 cases (Wang and Qi 2001)
	Lumbar strain	51 cases (Ge and Liu 2002)
		38 cases (Xiao et al. 2006)
	Ankylosing spondylitis	35 cases (Qu 2001)
	Dysmenorrhea	42 cases (Xia and Shi 2006)
	Neurodermatitis	80 cases (Wang 2009)
	Lateral femoral cutaneous neuritis	32 cases (Xing et al. 2000)
Gua sha + moxibustion	Lateral femoral cutaneous neuritis	28 cases (Hu 2001)
	Ankylosing spondylitis	52 cases (Zhang 2010)
Gua sha + venom cream	Facial paralysis	42 cases (Chen 2003)
	Frozen shoulder	37 cases (Cheng et al. 2000)
Gua sha with Fulin cream	Cold rheumatoid arthritis	50 cases (Liu et al. 2003)
Gua sha + herbal medicine	Acne	56 cases (Jiang 2005)
	Facial chloasma	38 cases (Kong and Zhou 2005)
	Chloasma	65 cases (Zhang et al. 2010)
	Primary hypothyroidism	30 cases (Zhu 2009)
	Cervical spondylosis	150 cases (Liu and Cui 2006)
	Breast hyperplasia	286 cases (Luo and Liu 2007)
	Acute stomach cramps	18 cases (Miao and Zhou 2005)
	Chronic hepatitis B	27 cases (Zhao et al. 1998)
	Knee osteoarthritis	46 cases (Li and Guo 2002)
Gua sha + bupleurum powder	Refractory insomnia	80 cases (Sun 2002)
	Vertigo	52 cases (Wang et al. 2005)
Gua sha + Dang gui tablets	Dysmenorrhea, student	28 cases (Lu et al. 2006)
Gua sha + Buzhongyiqi pill	Sub-health, college students	78 cases (Ma et al. 2006)
Gua sha + Huoxiang Zhengqi Liquid	Heatstroke	48 cases (Lan 1999)
Gua sha + herbal retention enema	Ulcerative colitis	61 cases (Ya 2003)
		62 cases (Ya 2008)
Gua sha + medication	Chronic prostatitis	150 cases (Zhang and Wang 2006)
	Insomnia in cancer patients	42 cases (Jia et al. 2007)
	Trachoma	100 cases (Liu et al. 2003)
Gua sha + interferon	Chronic hepatitis B	46 cases (Wang 2010)

Table 2.7 Case series: Gua sha combined with two or more other modalities for specific conditions (38 articles)

Therapies	Condition	Number of cases, and authors
Gua sha, acupuncture and massage	Cervical spondylosis	60 cases (Li 1999) 150 cases (Xia 2006) 15 cases (Li et al. 2006)
Gua sha, acupuncture and herbs	Pseudomyopia, student	400 cases (Yue et al. 2004)
Gua sha, acupuncture and cupping	Facial paralysis	30 cases (Cui and Li 2007) 129 cases (Ma 2009)
	Shoulder periarthritis	64 cases (Hu 2001)
Gua sha, acupuncture and bloodletting	Recurrent stye	89 cases (Wu 2006)
Gua sha, acupuncture, cupping and physiotherapy	Knee osteoarthritis	132 cases (Cheng et al. 2007)
	Lumbar disc herniation	210 cases (Cheng 2008)
Gua sha, acupuncture, cupping and massage	Rheumatism	1000 cases (Liu et al. 2001)
Gua sha, cupping and massage	Acute/chronic periarthritis shoulder	25 cases (Yang 2005a)
	Frozen shoulder	104 cases (Zhang 1998b)
Gua sha, cupping, massage and herbs	Neck and shoulder pain	410 cases (Li 2002)
Gua sha, cupping and pressure points	Hiccup	30 cases (Lu et al. 2006)
	Allergic rhinitis	20 cases (Yang 2005b)
Gua sha, cupping and bloodletting	Acute mastitis	89 cases (Wang 2005)
	Facial melasma	120 cases (Liu 2008)
	Soft tissue shoulder disorder	40 cases (Zhou et al. 2006)
Gua sha, cupping, tai chi and aerobics	Sub-health status	59 cases (Yang et al. 2007)
Gua sha, cupping, and rehab exercise	Bi syndrome joint pain	366 cases (Wang 2004)
Gua sha, massage and Tongluo plaster	Shoulder periarthritis	150 cases (Lin et al. 2007)
Gua sha, massage and laser	Cervical spondylopathy	72 cases (Li 2003)
Gua sha, massage, traction and TENS	Stiff neck	200 cases (Cheng 2005)
Gua sha, exercise and herbs	Shoulder periarthritis	120 cases (Geng et al. 2006)
Gua sha, herbs and local injection	Shoulder periarthritis	176 cases (Hou et al 2005)
Gua sha, acupuncture, moxa, cupping, massage and TENS	Shoulder periarthritis	120 cases (Cheng 2004)
Gua sha, ear pressure, diet and exercise	Obesity	67 cases (Li et al. 2001)
Gua sha as part of comprehensive therapy	Acne	44 cases (Li et al. 2007)
	Cervical spondylosis	130 cases (Yang 2003)
	Frozen shoulder	89 cases (Nie and Peng 2000)
	Shoulder–neck pain	410 cases (Zhang 1998a)
	Food addiction	33 cases (Yang 2003)
	Obesity	56 cases (Xin et al. 2003)
	Radiohumeral epicondylitis	148 cases (Ma 2010)
	Acute viral hepatitis	45 cases (Chi et al. 2006)
Gua sha as part of integrative medicine	Heatstroke	62 cases (Yan et al. 2008)
	Fibrositis	26 cases (Gu and Li 2003)

Table 2.8 Gua sha case studies of $n = 1$ (12 articles: 9 Chinese, 2 English, 1 German)

Therapy or combination	Condition	Authors
Gua sha	Chronic active hepatitis B	Chan et al. 2011 (English)
Gua sha	Breast engorgement/mastitis	Chiu et al. 2008
Gua sha	Postherpetic neuralgia, buttock	Nielsen 2005 (English)
Gua sha	Migraine	Schwickert et al. 2007 (German)
Gua sha	Misdiagnosed as syphilis	Wang et al. 2003
Gua sha	Health approach for youth rehabilitation	Wei 2002
Gua sha and cupping	Hypertension and cerebral arteriosclerosis	Fang 2002
Gua sha, bloodletting and herbs	Priapism	Jin et al. 2005
Gua sha and foot reflexology	Shoulder periarthritis	Xue and Chen 2001
Gua sha with fitness exercise	Weakness from congenital heart disease	Zhang 2005
Gua sha with foot acupuncture	Pelvic inflammatory disease	Zhang and Wang 2010
Integrative treatment	Guillain–Barré with respiratory paralysis	Zuo 2005

Table 2.9 Gua sha in clinical trials: comparative, controlled, and/or randomized controlled (55 articles: 53 Chinese, 2 English)

Intervention/controls	n (total/intervention/control)	Condition	Authors
Gua sha + acupuncture vs. medication orlistat	208/108/100	Obesity	(Acupuncture with Gua sha) 2006
Gua sha vs. usual care	200/100/100	Insomnia with COPD patients	Chen et al. 2008
Gua sha vs. electro-acupuncture (EA) vs. Gua sha + EA	90/30/30/30	Lobular hyperplasia of breast	Chen 2008
Gua sha + massage vs. massage alone	48/24/24	Shoulder periarthritis	Ji and Wang 2010
Gua sha + cupping vs. acupuncture + herbs	80/40/40	Stroke sequelae	Li 2008
Gua sha + psychotherapy vs. oral estazolam	60/30/30	Insomnia	Li 2007
Gua sha + interferon vs. interferon alone	71/33/38	Chronic hepatitis B	Li and Huang 2003
Gua sha + Dang gui formula vs. Gua sha vs. Dang gui	56/28/14/14	Dysmenorrhea	Li et al. 2006
Gua sha + acupuncture vinegar iontophoresis vs. frequency current therapy	180/90/90	Cervical spondylosis (nerve root type)	Li et al. 2008
Gua sha + cupping vs. ?	65/39/26	Cervical spondylosis	Liao et al. 2004
Gua sha + moxibustion vs. frequency iontophoresis	60/30/30	Cervical spondylosis	Lin 2009
Gua sha + herbs Zhi Sou San vs. amoxicillin plus licorice tablets	76/42/34	Cough/upper respiratory infection	Liu and He 2008
Gua sha + point injection (HCL DL anisodamine) vs. drug therapy	83/43/40	Cervical vertigo	Liu et al 2010
Gua sha + seton* vs. oral tagamet	100/50/50	Peptic ulcer	Liu et al. 2007; same results but half relapse rate
Gua sha + herbs vs. herbs alone (Qingrejiedu Sanjie)	172/86/86	Acute mastitis	Luo and Liu 2007; combination better

*Seton is an early Western medicine and early Chinese medicine technique of embedding a kind of thread under the skin and allowing it to produce a response. Also known as catgut embedding

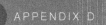

Table 2.9 Gua sha in clinical trials: comparative, controlled, and/or randomized controlled (55 articles: 53 Chinese, 2 English)—cont'd

Intervention/controls	n (total/intervention/control)	Condition	Authors
Gua sha + herbs vs. herbs alone (Qingrejiedu Sanjie)	172/86/86	Acute mastitis	Luo and Liu 2008; combination better
Gua sha + point injection vs. point injection	166/83/83	Cervical spondylosis	Ma et al. 2003
Gua sha + acupuncture vs. oral pills	120/60/60	Pediatric stagnant heat: indigestion syndrome	Mi 2010
Gua sha + acupuncture + diet & health education vs. education alone	70/35/35	Obesity: phlegm damp type	Peng et al. 2009
Gua sha + cupping vs. ibuprofen or other pain medicine	156/72/84	Primary dysmenorrhea	Qiao et al. 2007
Gua sha + EA + cupping vs. EA + infrared Tx	70/35/35	Cervical spondylosis neck pain	Sha 2007a
Gua sha + EA + cupping vs. EA + infrared Tx	70/35/35	Cervical spondylosis neck pain	Sha 2007b (same study different journal)
Gua sha vs. oral medication	304/176/128	Mastitis	Shang and Zhang 2009
Gua sha, herbs + point injection vs. pain pills Voltaren + warming	106/60/46	Shoulder myofascitis	Shi, Bai and Xiong 2000
Gua sha + liquid vs. liquid alone	150/79/71	Recurrent respiratory infection, pediatric	Sun and Wang 2010
Gua sha, acupuncture with moxa vs. acupuncture alone	100/50/50	Back fasciitis	Wang 2006
Gua sha + bloodletting with cupping vs. acupuncture	123/82/41	Acute mastitis	Wang and Li 2006
Gua sha + massage vs. herb brain Ning pills	90/45/45	Headache	Wang and Wei 2009
Gua sha vs. control	88/48/40	Ascites from liver cirrhosis	Wang 2000
Gua sha vs. control	98/50/48	Chronic hepatitis B	Wang 2007
Gua sha + acupuncture vs. usual care conventional medicine	72/42/30	Facial paralysis	Wang 2009a
Gua sha, acupuncture + traction vs. intravenous TMP Tx	86/46/40	Cervical spondylosis pain and cerebral blood flow/ cervical vertebral artery	Wang 2009b
Gua sha, acupuncture + moxa vs. acupuncture + moxa	104/?	Scapulohumeral periarthritis	Wang and Li 2004
Gua sha vs. acupuncture	240/160/80	Lumbar disc herniation	Wang et al. 2004
Gua sha + cupping vs. blood circulating 'drugs'	120/60/60	Low back pain	Wei 2008
Gua sha + qi gong vs. acupuncture	216/160/56	Simple obesity	Wei et al. 2003
Gua sha + Zhuang medicine vs. oral pill group vs. all three	250/?	Chronic colitis	Ya 2009a
Gua sha + Zhuang medicine vs. oral pill group vs. all three	231/?	chronic colitis	Ya 2009b
Gua sha vs. conventional symptomatic Tx	89/45/44	'Autumn diarrhea', hospitalized pediatric patients	Yao and Guo 2009

Continued

Table 2.9 Gua sha in clinical trials: comparative, controlled, and/or randomized controlled (55 articles: 53 Chinese, 2 English)—cont'd

Intervention/controls	n (total/intervention/control)	Condition	Authors
Gua sha vs. Western medicine	?/20/control?	Rheumatoid arthritis	Yu 2005
Gua sha + acupuncture vs. acupuncture alone	96/48/48	Cervical spondylosis	Zhang 2007
Gua sha vs. usual care	128/64/64	Sleep disorders in diabetic patients	Zhang 2006
Gua sha + plum blossom vs. control	99/45/44	Neurodermatitis	Zhang and Wang 2006
Gua sha + plaster vs. herbal medicine	80/40/40	Cervical spondylosis	Zhang and Yang 2008
Gua sha, cupping + analgesic cream vs. gua sha cupping + vaseline	356/180/176	Cold Bi syndrome arthralgia	Zhang et al. 2009
Gua sha + acupuncture vs. acupuncture	85/45/40	Intractable hiccup	Zhong 2006
Gua sha + Tonbi ointment vs. medicine	894/447/447	Lumbar disc herniation	Zhou 2008
Gua sha vs. control?	136/68/68	Prevention and treatment of pediatric influenza	Zhou and Xu 2001
Gua sha vs. cupping vs. EA	127/?/?	Head cold	Zhu et al. 2010
Gua sha + B12 vs. oral B12	48/24/24	Postherpetic neuralgia	Zou 2009
Gua sha vs. drug control	72	Internal injuries, pain	Liu et al. 2002
Gua sha vs. control usual care	44/24/20	Intestinal obstruction after stomach cancer surgery	Xie 2000
Gua sha + pak sha + cupping vs. cupping alone	49	Insomnia	Yang et al. 2006
Gua sha vs. hot packs and massage usual care	81/54/27	Breast engorgement	Chiu et al. 2010 (English)
Gua sha vs. thermal	48/24/24	Neck pain	Braun et al. 2011 (English)

Table 2.10 Gua sha reviews

Type of review	Authors
Research review	Liang and Yuan 2009; Luo 2008; Wang et al. 2006
Literature review	Wang and Yang 2009
Systematic review for pain	Lee et al. 2010 (English)

References for literature searches detailed in tables

References for Table 2.1: terms and complications (see Chapter 2)

Aliye, U.C., Bishop, W., Sanders, K., 2000. Camphor hepatotoxicity. South Med J 93, 596–598.

Amshel, C.E., Caruso, D.M., 2000. Vietnamese 'coining': a burn case report and literature review. J Burn Care Rehabil 21 (2) (Mar-Apr), 112–114.

Anh, T.H., 1976. 'Pseudo-battered child' syndrome. JAMA 236 (20) (Nov 15), 2288.

Ashworth, M., 1993. Child abuse – true or false? Practitioner 237 (1523) (Feb), 108–109.

Bays, J., 2001. Conditions mistaken for child abuse. In: Reece, R.M. (Ed.), Child Abuse: Medical Diagnosis and Management. Lea & Febiger, Philadelphia, 05/12/21 (1994), pp. 358.

Buchwald, D., Panwala, S., Hooton, T.M., 1992. Use of traditional health practices by Southeast Asian refugees in a primary care clinic. West J Med 156 (5) (May), 507–511.

Campbell, W.W., Sartori, R.J., 2003. Nummular erythema in a patient with chronic daily headache. Headache 43 (10) (November), 1112.

Crutchfield, C.E., Bisig, T.J., 1995. Images in clinical medicine. Coining. N Engl J Med 332 (23) (Jun 8), 1552.

D'Allesandro, D.M., D'Allesandro, M.P., 2005. What Are Some of the Presentations for Child Abuse and Neglect? In: PediatricEducation.Org; A Pediatric Digital Library and Learning Collaborative.

David, A., Mechinaud, F., Roze, J.C., et al., 1986. [A case of Cao-Gio. Possible confusion with abuse]. Arch Fr Pediatr (ne observation de 'Cao-Gio.' Confusion possible avec des sevices.) 43 (2) (Feb), 147.

Davis, R.E., 2000. Cultural health care or child abuse? The Southeast Asian practice of cao gio. J Am Acad Nurse Pract 12 (3) (Mar), 89–95.

de Luna, G., Rodriquez, M.F., de Trabajo, G., 2003. Atencion al nino de origin extranjero. Rev Pediatr Aten Primaria 5, 115–142.

Dinulos, J.G., Graham, E.A., 1999. Category 5: Skin manifestations of Cultural Practices: Photo 35: Coining in a Child. In: Self Teaching Module for the Influence of Culture and Pigment on Skin Conditions in Children. Harborview Medical Center, University of Washington. Accessed January 22, 2007. http://ethnomed.org/ethnomed/clin_topics/dermatology/pigment35.html

Du, J.N., 1980. Pseudobattered child syndrome in Vietnamese immigrant children. Can Med Assoc J 122 (4) (Feb 23), 394–395.

Gellis, S., Feingold, M., 1976. Pseudo-battering in Vietnamese children. Am J Dis Child 130, 857–858.

Golden, S., Duster, M., 1977. Hazards of misdiagnosis due to Vietnamese folk medicine. Clin. Pediatr. (Phila). 16, 949–950.

Graham, EA. Chitnarong, J., 1997. 'Ethnographic Study Among Seattle Cambodians: Wind Illness'. In Ethnomed. org. Harborview Medical Center, University of Washington. http://ethnomed.org/ethnomed/clin_topics/cambodian/ethno_wind.html Accessed March 3, 2007.

Habif, T., 2004. Clinical Dermatology: A Color Guide to Diagnosis and Therapy, Fourth ed. Mosby, New York, pp. 64–65.

Halder, R., Nootheti, P., Richards, G., 2002. Dermatological Disorders and Cultural Practices: Understanding practices that cause skin conditions in non-Caucasian populations. Skin and Aging 10 (8), 46–50.

Halder, R.M., Nootheti, P., 2003. Ethnic Skin Disorders Overview. J Am Ac Derm 48 (6), S143–S148.

Hefner, M.E., Kempe, R.S., Krugman, R.D., 1997. The Battered Child. fifth ed. Univ. of Chicago Press, Chicago.

Heyman, W., 2005. Cutaneous signs of child abuse. J Am Acad Derm 53 (1523), 138–139.

Hoffman, J.M., 2005. A case of shaken baby syndrome after discharge form the newborn intensive care unit. Adv Neonatal Care 5 (3), 135–146.

Hulewicz, B.S., 1994. Coin-rubbing injuries. Am J Forensic Med Pathol 15 (3) (Sep), 257–260.

Kaplan, J., 1986. Pseudoabuse–the misdiagnosis of child abuse. J Forensic Sci 1986 (ne observation de 'Cao-Gio.' Confusion possible avec des sevices.) 31, 1420.

Keller E., Apthorp, J., 1977. Folk remedies vs. child battering. Am J Dis Child 131 (10) (Oct), 1173.

Kemp, C., 1985. Cambodian refugee health care beliefs and practices. J Comm Health Nurs 2 (1), 41–52. 45.

Mevorah, B., Orion, E., Matz, H., et al., 2003. Cutaneous side effects of alternative therapy. Dermatologic Therapy 160 (27), 141.

Lachapelle, J.M., Bataille, A.C., Tennstedt, D., et al., 1994. Pseudo-factitial dermatitis: a useful clinical and/or histopathological. Dermatology 189 (Suppl. 2), 62–64.

Lederman, E.R., Keystone, J.S., 2002. Linear Lesions in Travelers or Recent Immigrants. Canadian Journal of Diagnosis. 2002, 68–72.

Levin, N.R., Levin, D.L., 1982. A folk medical practice mimicking child abuse. Hosp Pract (Off Ed) 17 (7) (Jul), 17.

Leung, A.K., 1986. Ecchymosis from spoon scratching simulating child abuse. Clin. Pediatr. (Phila). 25, 98.

Leung, A.K., Chan, K.W., 2001. Evaluating the Child with Purpura. Am Fam Phys 64 (30), 419–428.

Look, K.M., Look, R.M., 1997. Skin scraping, cupping, and moxibustion that may mimic physical abuse. J Forensic Sci 42 (1) (Jan), 103–105.

Mevorah, B., Orion, E., Matz, H., et al., 2003. Cutaneous side effects of alternative therapy. Dermatologic Therapy 160 (27), 141.

Morrone, A., Valenzano, M., Franco, G., et al., 2003. Ethnodermatology: cutaneous lesions cultural practices-related. Journal of the European Academy of Dermatology & Venereology Supplement 17 (Supplement: 3: 311) (November).

Mudd, S.S., Findlay, J.S., 2004. The cutaneous manifestations and common mimickers of physical child abuse. J Pediatr Health Care 18, 123–129: 128.

Ngo-Metzer, Q., Massagli, M.P., Clarridge, B.R., et al., 2003. Linguistic and Cultural Barriers to Care: Perspectives of Chinese and Vietnamese Immigrants. J Gen Intern Med 18, 44–52.

Overbosch, D., Fibbe, W.E., Stuiver, P.C., 1984. Pseudo-bleeding disorder due to coin rubbing. Neth J Med 27 (1), 16–17.

Ponder, A., Lehman, L.B., 1994. 'Coining' and 'coning': an unusual complication of unconventional medicine. Neurology 44, 774–775.

Primack, W.A., Person, J.R., 1985. Nummular purpura: Letter. Arch Dermatol 121 (3) (Mar), 309–310.

Primosch, R.E., Young, S.K., 1980. Pseudobattering of Vietnamese children (cao gio). J Am Dent Assoc 101 (1) (Jul), 47–48.

Rampini, S., Schneemann, M., Rentsch, K., et al., 2002 Camphor intoxication after cao gio (coin rubbing). JAMA 288 (12) (Sept 25), 1471.

Roberts, J.R., 1988. Beware: Vietnamese coin rubbing. Ann Emerg Med 17 (4), Apr, 384.

Rosenblat H., Hong P., 1989. Coin rolling misdiagnosed as child abuse. CMAJ 140 (4) (Feb 15), 417.

Saulsbury, F.T., Hayden, G.F., 1985. Skin conditions simulating child abuse. Pediatr Emerg Care 1 (3) (Sep), 147–150.

Scales, J.W., Fleischer, A.B., Sinal, S.H., et al., 1999. Skin lesions that mimic abuse. Contemp Pediatr 16 (1), 1 Jan, 137–145.

Shah, K.N., Fried R.G., 2006. Factitial Dermatoses in children: Dermatology. Curr. Opin. Pediatr. 18 (4 Pt 2) (Aug), 403–409.

Silfen, E., Wyre, H.W.J., 1981. Factitial Dermatitis–Cao Gio. Cutis 28, 399–400.

Stauffer, W.M., Maroushek, S., Kamat, D., 2003. Medical Screening of Immigrant Children. Clin Pediatr (Phila) 42 (9), 763–773.

Sullivan, T.M., Trahan, A., 2007. Coining. In: Creighton University Medical Center, Complementary and Alternative Medicine. Creighton University Medical School, Omaha, Nebraska, http://altmed.creighton.edu/coining/references.htm. Accessed January 22, 2007.

Tuncez, F., Bagci, Y., Kurtipek, GS., et al., 2005. Skin trauma due to cultural practices: cupping and coin rubbing. London; :P04.30. 14th Congress of the European Academy of Dermatology and Venereology.

Walsh, S., Boisvert, C., Kamitsuru, S., et al., 2004 Formulation of a Plan of Care for Culturally Diverse Patients. Elaboration d'un plan de soin pour des patients de cultures différentes. Int J Nurs Terminol Classif 15 (1), 17–26.

Westby, C., 2007. Child Maltreatment: A Global Issue. Lang Speech Hear Serv Sch 38 (2), 140–148.

Willgerodt, M.A., Killien, M.G., 2004. Family Nursing Research with Asian Families. Journal of Family Nursing 10 (2), 149–172.

Wong, H.C., Wong, J.K., Wong, N.Y., 1999. Signs of physical abuse or evidence of moxibustion, cupping or coining? [comment] on CMAJ 1998. CMAJ 160 (6) (Mar 23), 785–786.

Yeatman, G.W., Shaw, C., Barlow, M.J., et al., 1976. Pseudobattering in Vietnamese children. Pediatrics 58, 616–618.

Yoo, S.S., Tausk, F., 2004 Cupping: East meets West. Int J Dermatol 43 (9), 664.

Zuijlmans, C.W., Winterberg, D.H., 1996. Rubbing with a coin is not abuse. (Untwrijven is geen mishandeling.). Ned Tijdschr Geneeskd 140 (51) (Dec 21), 2552–2554.

References for Table 2.3: Gua sha alone: descriptive clinical recommendations for specific conditions (121)

Bai, L., Ban, L., Fan, L., et al., 2007. Holographic Meridian Scraping in clinical use: Overview. J Military Surgeon in Southwest China 6, 108–109.

Bai, S., Wu, N., 1998. The development and application of oil for Gua sha scraping. China Journal of Orthopaedics and Traumatology 1, 60.

Bao L., 2002. [Fever syndrome interpretation] Discussion on 'sha' condition. Shangai Journal of Traditional Chinese Medicine 36 (12), 36–37.

Bi, G., 2010. Gua sha green therapy. Window of the Northeast Z1, 112–113.

Cai, Y., 2003. Tsai Ting Shubing experience of Old Chinese therapy. New Journal of Traditional Chinese Medicine 35 (3), 7–8.

Cao, Z., Dao, Y., 2002. Overview of Dai medical Gua sha scraping therapy. Journal of Medicine and Pharmacy of Chinese Minorities 8 (3), 22.

Chan, H., Chen, R., 1998. Development and clinical study of the emulsions used in Guasha. Northwest Pharmaceutical Journal 13 (1), 30–31.

Chen, C., 2004. Gua sha in the treatment of soft tissue injury rehabilitation application. Clinical Journal of Traditional Chinese Medicine 16 (6).

Chen, Q., 2008. Gua sha with 'bone million flower oil.' Family & Traditional Chinese Medicine 10, 61.

Chen, Y., Chen, F., Ban, X., et al., 2010. Gua sha therapy and nursing. China Medical Herald 16, 203.

Chen, Y., Zhang, H., 2001. 'Gua sha' scrape lubricant efficacy research and clinical application. Tianjin Journal of Traditional Chinese Medicine Tianjin Zhong Yi 18 (4), 43.

Chen, Z.-h., Shen, Y., Huang Q.-c., 2006. Application of extrinsic therapies in the treatment of patients with rheumatoid arthritis. Chinese Journal of Clinical Rehabilitation 10 (27).

Cong, R., Li, S., Gu, J., 2005. Gua sha of Rheumatoid Arthritis. China's Naturopathy 13 (7), 17.

Cui, X., Dan, T., Yang, X., 2009. Research progress of Gua sha (scraping) therapy. China's Naturopathy 7, 64–65.

Deng, S., Bin, L., Wang, T., et al., 2009. Gua sha treatment of cervical tendon lesions. Chinese Journal of Ethnomedicine and Ethnopharmacy 6, 34–36.

Dong, L., 2009. Gua sha therapy and nursing. China's Naturopathy 2, 58.

Dong, Q., 1998. Therapeutic effects of Gua Sha on patients with stroke. Chinese Manipulation & Qigong Therapy 1, 10–12.

Du, Z., 2003. Using Gua sha holographic meridian scraping in the treatment of hyperlipidemia. Chinese Reflexology Journal 3 (5), 24–25.

Fan, Y., 2005. Gua sha therapy and nursing points. Occupation and Health 21 (10), 1594–1596.

Fang, L., Fang, M., Liu Y.-c., 2008. Research advances of traditional Chinese medicine therapy in treating sports fatigue. Journal of Chinese Integrative Medicine 12, 1305–1310.

2010. Fingers Gua sha a cold. Home Medicine 6, 59.

2010. Fudi energy scraping therapy. China Direct 7, 36.

Gao, C., 1999. Preliminary Investigation on the Rule of Differentiation and Treatment of External Humeral Epicondylitis. Chinese Journal of Information on Traditional Chinese Medicine 6 (3), 50–51.

Gao, Y., 2002. 'Gua sha' Scraping treatment of cough. China's Naturopathy 10 (2), 36.

Ge, C., 2008. Gua sha of the head, face, neuralgia wonders. Chinese Acupuncture & Moxibustion 6, 455.

Geng, L., Yang, M., 2007. Scraping Example 1 Treatment of Systemic Lupus Erythematosus. Modern Health (Medicine Innovation Research) 4 (26), 158.

Geng, Y., 2010. Gua sha conditioning three kinds of sub-health symptoms: fatigue, insomnia and neck and shoulder pain. Zhonghua Yangsheng Baojian 1, 18.

2008. Gua sha for health and beauty. Health Care Today 10, 3–4.

2008. Gua sha is not the more pain the more effective. Jiankang Bidu 6, 29.

2001. 'Gua sha' Scraping for injury (tennis elbow). Journal of Chinese Physician 29 (1).

2009. Gua sha ten errors. China Healthcare & Nutrition 11, 108–109.

2004. Gua sha the common folk therapy. Monthly PF Medical Knowledge 11, 60.

2009. Gua sha treatment overview. Chinese Practical Journal of Rural Doctor 1, 22–23.

Gui, Y., 1994. Gua sha scraping in the treatment of soft tissue injury. Chinese Journal of Sports Medicine 13 (2), 124.

Hai, C., 2007. Gua sha treatment of disease to facilitate cost-effective. Family Medicine (New Health) 4, 61.

He, Z., 2010. Gua sha in the health care and treatment of cardiovascular disease. Zhonghua Yangsheng Baojian 1, 16.

2010. Head and upper back trilogy, the family Gua sha treatment of a cold. Zhonghua Yangsheng Baojian 1, 5.

Hu, G., Chen, M., 2010. Clinical observation of Gua sha treatment of back shu points for Sleep Disorders. J. Tradit. Chin. Med. 3, 517–518.

Hu, J., Zuo, C., 2005. Gua sha for hypertension and coronary artery disease. Chinese Healthcare (Zonghua Yangsheng Baojian) 8, 25–26.

Hu M., 2002. Why is the United States selling Chinese medicine in the food store? – Talk about China and the West (drug food) and cultural exchanges. Food and Health 6, 4–6.

Huang, D., 2010. Gua sha foot self-care a good way. Medpharm & Health 1, 64.

Huang, Q., 2007. Examples of clinical application of Gua sha therapy. Journal of Medicine & Pharmacy of Chinese Minorities. 13 (5), 23–24.

Huang, X., Guo, Z.-s., 2009. Gua sha scraping treatment expert of Qing Dynasty and Shazhangyuheng. Journal of Clinical Acupuncture and Moxibustion 10, 41–42.

2000. Human four People's Liberation Army Health (Jie Fang Jun Jian Kang). 6.

2009. Jade Gua sha Firming Massage Therapy Magic. Medical Aesthetics & Cosmetology 6, 62.

Ji, Z.-H., Zheng, J.-S., 2008. Research on Sha in Ancient China. Universitatis Traditiobnis Medicalis Sinensis Pharmoacologiaeque act Shanghai 6, 19–22.

Ji, Z.-H., 2008. Research on Sha: a complete book for Sha disease. Chinese J of Medical History 3, 170–175.

Jiang, J., 2005. Gua sha of soft tissue loss therapy for cervical spondylotic changes clinical reports. Chinese Journal of Traditional Medical Traumatology & Orthopedics 13 (5), 58–60.

Jiang, Q., Shi, Y., 2005. Gua sha therapy and disease treatment. Journal of Liaoning College of Traditional Chinese Medicine 7 (3), 228–229.

Kang, Y., 2003. Gua sha for cervical disease and low back pain. China's Naturopathy 11 (4), 21–22.

Kang, Y., 2004. Treatment of cervical spondylosis or pain of the waist and lower extremities with 'Guasha.'. Chinese Journal of Ethnomedicine and Ethnopharmacy (Chinese Journal of Folk Medicine) 1, 31–32.

Ke, A., 2007. Traditional Chinese medicine Gua sha therapy effective in improving sub-health. Medical and Health Care Instruments 1, 70.

Li, G., 2007. Scraping Qingzhi solution to observe the effect of the treatment of simple obesity. Lishizhen Medicine and Materia Medica Research 18 (11), 2807–2808.

Li X.-s., Qi L.-Z., 2007. Treatment of Insomnia with Gua sha (Scraping). J Acup and Tuina Science 5 (6), 368–371.

Li, Y., Chen, Z., He, W., Wang, Z., 2001. A survey of traditional medicine of Naxi nationality in Yunnan Province. Chinese Journal of Ethnomedicine and Ethnopharmacy (Chinese Journal of Folk Medicine) 3, 128–130.

Li Y., Liu H., 2002. Application of Guasha in the treatment of acute symptoms. Journal of External Therapy of Traditional Chinese Medicine 11 (4), 55.

Liang, J., Zhang, M., Duan, Q., 2009. Application of bioholographic laws to Gua sha. Yunnan Journal of Traditional Chinese Medicine and Materia Medica 2, 78–79.

Liang, Z., 2001a. 'Gua sha' Scraping therapy for eye diseases. Journal of Chinese Physician 29 (2), 38–41.

Liang, Z., 2001b. Gua sha scraping therapy in traumatology disease. Journal of Chinese Physician 1, 34–36.

Liao, R., He, Y., Tang, D., 2010. Gua sha treatment mechanism of neurodermatitis. J. Tradit. Chin. Med. 6, 1124–1125.

Lin, H., Chen, M., 2000. Clinical study of treatment of acne with Guasha. China Journal of Traditional Chinese Medicine and Pharmacy 15 (1), 75–76.

Lin S.h., Yan L., 2006. Natural therapy in health care for elderly. Chinese Journal of Convalescent Medicine 15 (3).

Liu, J., 2010a. Approach to painless gua sha. Fujian Journal of Traditional Chinese Medicine 3, 56.

Liu, N., 2004. Gua Sha (scraping therapy) in nursing. Journal of Occupational Health and Damage 19 (1), 63–64.

Liu, W., 2010b. Head, face Gua sha with stress. Zhonghua Yangsheng Baojian 1, 4.

Mao, L., 2009. Urticaria treated by Gua sha. China's Naturopathy 9, 13.

Min, O.Y., 2007. Gua sha: the principles of this Chinese Medicine Treatment. Jiangxi J Trad Chinese Med 38 (12).

Ming, Z., 2004. Gua sha law origin. Chinese Journal of Medical History 34 (3), 152.

Pang, J., Liu, Z., Tang, H., et al., 2008. Treating Relapsing Respiratory Tract Infection by Gua sha on Meridians (channels). Guangxi Journal of Traditional Chinese Medicine 5, 48–49.

Peng, M., Liao, Y., 2010a. From head to toe Gua sha self treatment. China Territory Today 6, 47.

Peng, M., Liao, Y., 2010b. From head to toe Gua sha self treatment. World Health (Health Review) 6, 20.

Qu, J., 2010. Gua sha your baby to say goodbye to diarrhea. Zhonghua Yangsheng Baojian 1, 19.

Ruan, J., 2008a. Cold Gua sha therapy. Family Doctor 11, 46.

Ruan, J., 2008b. Gua sha treatment of chronic fatigue. Family Doctor 15, 39.

Ruan, J., 2008c. In the Department of Gua sha therapy. Family Doctor 2, 43.

Ruan, Z.-q., Cui Y.-n.-z., 2005. Gua sha treatment for sunstroke. Journal of Ningde Teachers College (Natural Science) 17 (4), 410–411.

2010. Simple and Natural, the Gua sha. Zhonghua Yangsheng Baojian 1, 1.

Sun, Z., 2010. Gua sha tools, there are doorways. Zhonghua Yangsheng Baojian 1, 8–9.

Tan, J., He, L., 2000. Nursing in the application of Guasha in the treatment of exogenous fever. Guangxi Journal of Traditional Chinese Medicine 23 (6), 40.

2010. Traditional Chinese Medicine Gua sha return to nature. Zhonghua Yangsheng Baojian 1, 4.

Wang, H., 2008a. Gua sha for health and beauty. Jiating Keji 2, 29–30.

Wang, J., 2010a. Benefits of Gua sha foot massage. Zhonghua Yangsheng Baojian 1, 14–15.

Wang, L., Dang, H., Xu, L., et al., 2006. Analysis of efficacy of Gua sha Scraping Therapy. China's Naturopathy 14 (6), 55.

Wang, L., 2000. Application of meridian All-Information Scraping in treatment of ascites due to Cirrhosis (Application of Guasha with holographic meridian in treatment of ascites of cirrhosis. China's Naturopathy 8 (7), 15.

Wang, W., Tang, C., 2001. Treatment of common cold with massage combined with Guasha. Chinese Manipulation & Qigong Therapy 17 (3), 24–25.

Wang, X., 1996. Gua sha Scraping for acute epigastric pain. Henan Traditional Chinese Medicine 16 (6), 369.

Wang, X., 1997. Gua sha therapy chloasma. China's Naturopathy 5, 6–7.

Wang, Y., 2010b. Gua sha taboo. Zhonghua Yangsheng Baojian 1, 17.

Wang, Y., 2008b. On the function of Gua sha treatment in TCM cosmetic. Traditional Chinese Medicinal Research 9, 1–2.

Wang, Z., 2002a. Chronic fatigue nemesis: gua sha holographic scraping of foot. Medicine and Health Care 10 (5), 17.

Wang, Z., 2002b. Holographic Meridian Scraping 'Gua sha' for breast carbuncle 'mastitis.' Medicine and Health Care 10 (8), 119–121.

Wei, J., 2002. 'Gua sha' back to my youth rehabilitation. Zhonghua Yangsheng Baojian Zazhi 8, 40.

Wu, J., 2010. Gua sha therapy exotic supplements. Jiangxi J Trad Chinese Med 4, 70–71.

Wu, L., 2001. 'Gua sha' Scraping therapy. International Medicine and Health Guidance 1, 32.

Xu, L., 2008a. Gua sha, left behind people's health prescription. Home Medicine 22, 36.

Xu, X., 2008b. Probe into Gua sha therapy. China's Naturopathy 11, 6.

Yang, J., Wang, Y., Zhao, M., et al., 2007a. Basic Concept of Sha (Exanthema) and Historical Changes and Developments of Sha-Scraping. Chinese Journal of Basic Medicine in Traditional Chinese Medicine 13 (2), 104–106.

Yang, J.-s., Zhao, M.-l., Wang, Y.-y., et al., 2007b. [Studies on treatment based on differentiation of syndromes of SHA syndrome in Sha Zhang Yu Heng]. Zhonghua Yi Shi Za Zhi 37 (2) (April), 76–79.

Yang, J., 2010. Gua sha in essence, when the three methods combined. Zhonghua Yangsheng Baojian 20–21.

Yang, J., 2004. Gua sha and applications of methods commonly used. J. Tradit. Chin. Med. 45 (11), 875–876.

Yang, L., Liu, Y., 2007. Teach Gua sha scraping, you learn to be your own family physician. Family Medicine (New Health) 4, 59–60.

Yang, L., 2010. By Gua sha a vacation to the stomach. Zhonghua Yangsheng Baojian 1, 11.

Yao, H., 2009. Experience on the treatment for chloasma with Gua sha therapy. China's Naturopathy 3, 11–12.

Yin, S., Qu, S., 2008. I started Gua sha community store. 75.

Yu, J., 1998. Treatment of frozen shoulder with Guasha along meridian. Chinese Journal of the Practical Chinese with Modern Medicine 11 (5). 456–457.

Zhang, F., 2008b. Gua sha for pain and health. Journal for Beneficial Veadings Drug Informations & Medical Advices 5, 25.

Zhang, F., 2008a. Gua sha for pain and health. Medicine and Health Care 16 (2), 54.

Zhang, F., 2008c. Which parts of the body may have Gua sha. Chemists 8, 45.

Zhang, G., Jiang, B., 1999. Clinical study of treatment of cerebellar atrophy with Guasha. Heilongjiang Journal of Traditional Chinese Medicine. 6, 49.

Zhang, J., 2006. Gua sha scraping therapy observed to improve the quality of sleep in patients with diabetes. Tianjin Journal of Nursing 14 (3), 159.

Zhang, J., 2009. Gua sha in Africa. J. Tradit. Chin. Med. 4, 703.

Zhang, S., 2010. Seven Cervical Gua sha to Help. Zhonghua Yangsheng Baojian 1, 12–13.

Zhang, X., Mo, L., 2000. 'Gua sha' Scraping therapy for facial beauty and health care. Chinese Journal of Aesthetic Medicine 9 (1), 15–16.

Zhang, Y., 2009. Gua sha is not the more pain the more effective the more black.

Zhao, M.-l., Li X.-Q., Zhang Y., 2008. Ancient fever diagnosis and differential diagnosis. Chinese J of Basic Med in Trad Chinese Med 11, 859–861.

Zhao, Y. 2007. Experience of Diagnosis and Treatment for Exanthematology. Henan Traditional Chinese Medicine 27 (1), 42–43.

Zhen, Z., Bai, S., 2007. Chinese medicine Gua sha acupoint application effect in treatment of cervical spondylosis. Chinese Journal of Traditional Medical Traumatology & Orthopedics 15 (7), 70–71.

Zou, W., Hu, Y., Hong, W., 2009. Gua sha meridian points in treatment of clinical pseudomyopia. Practical Clinical Journal of Integrated Traditional Chinese and Western Medicine 4, 76.

Zuo, J., Wang, F., 2007. Clinical effect of treatment of Tujia medical Gua sha scraping. Journal of Medicine & Pharmacy of Chinese Minorities 13 (2), 28–29.

Zuo, X., Wang, J., 2010. Gua sha: the basic approach chart. Zhonghua Yangsheng Baojian 1, 1.

Zuo, Z., 2010. Gua sha can play any role. Friends of Farmers 7, 42.

References for Table 2.4: Gua sha combined with other modalities: descriptive clinical recommendations for specific conditions (62)

An, H., Fan, B., Yang, S., 2010. Gua sha plus massage in the treatment and care of cold fever patients. Journal of Emergency in Traditional Chinese Medicine 5, 886–887.

Bai, X., Lu, F., 2003. Treatment of fever with Gua sha and acupuncture. Chinese Acupuncture & Moxibustion 23 (8), 467.

Bai, Y., 2006. Bloodletting, Cupping and Gua Sha comprehensive treatment of throat diseases. China's Naturopathy 14 (7), 59–60.

Bi, S., Shang, Y., Pan, X., 2003. Gua sha combination treatment of periarthritis of shoulder (Treatment of frozen shoulder with Guasha combined with Shen Jin Dan (TM)).

Chinese Journal of Rural Medicine and Pharmacy 10 (10), 29.

2001. Cerebral blood pressure treatment and health care functions. Biomagnetism 1 (2).

Chen, C., Cheng, L., 2003. Venom Preparation Gua sha treatment of lumbar disc herniation. Chinese Journal of Clinical Rehabilitation 7 (29), 4008.

Chen, C., 2002a. Treatment of facial peripheral paralysis with wasp cream Guasha in 42 cases. Chinese Journal of Clinical Rehabilitation 16 (19), 2975.

Chen, J., 2000. Scapulohumeral periarthritis treated by contralateral needling and scraping sha (Treatment of frozen shoulder with contralateral needling and Guasha. Journal of Clinical Acupuncture and Moxibustion. 16 (4), 40.

Chen, J., 2010. TCM Apitherapy Gua sha with the heat treatment of shoulder periarthritis. Apiculture of China. 5, 34–35.

Chen, M., 2002b. Application of 'Gua sha' massage and acupuncture therapy in the rehabilitation of cervical spondylosis. Chinese Journal of Clinical Rehabilitation 6 (14), 2140–2141.

Chen, M., 2006. Gua Sha and Moxibustion treatment of postpartum missing milk (queru). J Clin Acup and Moxibust 22 (11), 17.

Chen, W., Wang, C., Clinical study of treatment of cervical spondylosis with integrated traditional and western medicine. Tianjin Journal of Traditional Chinese Medicine 16 (3), 17–18, 1999.

Cui, X., Wang, J.-p., 2001. Treatment of Migraine with Guasha scraping combined with Massage. China's Naturopathy 9, 45.

Ding, X., 2003. Arthralgia Treatment. Journal of Guiyang College of Traditional Chinese Medicine 25 (3), 61–62.

Dong, F., 2003. Treatment of cutaneous nerve entrapment syndrome. China Journal of Orthopaedics and Traumatology (Chinese Bone-setting) 16 (5).

Fan, R.-G., Li, X.-X., Li, K.-f., 2009. Dialectical acupoint selection combined with Gua sha scraping in the treatment and care of emotional insomnia. Journal of Practical Traditional Chinese Internal Medicine 7, 94–95.

2006. Gua sha scraping and vibration reduces fat, waist change become slim. Medical Aesthetics and Cosmetology 11, 24–25.

Guo, X., Liu, Z., 2003. Diagnosis and treatment of difficult diseases: ideas and methods. Forum on Traditional Chinese Medicine 18 (1).

Li, X., Li, C., 2009. Gua sha moxibustion treatment of borderline hypertension. China's Naturopathy 9, 23–24.

Li, X.-p., 2006. Several Questions to be Solved in Developing TCM at present. Xinjiang Journal of Traditional Chinese Medicine 24 (5), 1–5.

Li, Y., 2009. Application of Chinese medicine in community health services. J. Tradit. Chin. Med. 10, 2005–2006.

Li, Z., 2008. Combined triple treatment of periarthritis with Chinese washing, gua sha and functional exercises. Chinese Journal of Medical Traumatology & Orthopedics 6, 53, 56.

Li, Z., 2005. Miao-detoxification technique, then Gua sha. Health Care Today 11, 32–33.

Liu, F., 2006b. Appropriate technology in medicine and health services in the community experience in the application of. Journal of Community Medicine 4 (16), 62–63.

Liu, F., 2006a. Overcome sub-health. Zhonghua Yangsheng Baojian 11, 25–26.

Liu, Q., 2008. Acupuncture with Gua sha and cupping for soft tissue injury shoulder strain. Chinese Journal of the Practical Chinese with Mode 4, 317.

Ma, B., 2001. Treatment of frozen shoulder with cupping therapy combined with Guasha. Hubei Journal of Traditional Chinese Medicine 23 (1), 46.

Ma, Z., 2005. Care for the prevention of heat-stroke. Fam. Med. 8, 34–35.

Meng, L., Si, J., 2002. 'Gua sha' 'scraping' with Chinese medicine treatment of hyperplasia of mammary gland. Chinese Journal of Information on Traditional Chinese Medicine 9 (11), 43.

Ni, W., Yu, S., Wang, H., et al., 2001. The treatment of asthma due to cold with point application therapy. (Acupuncture 'therapy' treatment of bronchial asthma). Shanghai Journal of Acupuncture & Moxibustion 20 (3), 10–11.

Pan, L., Li, Y., Ma, Y., et al., 2006. An integrated approach to the sub-health status of college students. Health Vocational Education 24 (23), 68.

Pu, G., Li, P., 2008. Chinese medicine for cervical disease, diagnosis, treatment research. Gansu J Trad Chinese Med 21 (5), 5–7.

Ruan, J., Hu, Y., Wen, M., et al., 2006. Electro-acupuncture, Gua Sha, injection integrated treatment of vertigo symptoms in cervical spondylosis. Chinese Journal of Rehabilitation Medicine 21 (6), 548–549.

Shan, G., Li, F., Wang, S., 2003. Clinical study of treatment of influenza with acupuncture and Gua sha. Shanghai Journal of Acupuncture and Moxibustion 22 (4), 26.

Tang, C., Liu, Q.R., 2006. Quadruple therapy experience treatment of lumbar disc herniation. Guangming Journal of Chinese Medicine 21 (8), 66–67.

Tang, S.M., Liu, E.L., Liu, Z.W., 2008. Sequential therapy of shoulder periarthritis. Journal of Sichuan Traditional Chinese Medicine 26, 108–109.

Tang, Y., Zhang, J., Zhang, D., 2000. Treatment of cold with Guasha combined with blood-letting puncturing. Chinese Acupuncture & Moxibustion 20 (2), 128.

2007. The five elements can lose weight magnetic meridian qi technology. Medical Aesthetics and Cosmetology 3, 54.

Tian, L., Chen, Z., Wang H., et al., 2010. Experience of Gua sha treatment of cold with Traditional Chinese Medicine. Tianjin Journal of Traditional Chinese Medicine 2, 109.

Tong, L., Chen, G., 1999. Treatment of acute contagious conjunctivitis with acupuncture and Guasha. Chinese Acupuncture & Moxibustion 19 (9), 576.

Wang, C., Hou, S., 2010. Gua sha with prick blood treatment of cervical disease. Heilongjiang Journal of Traditional Chinese Medicine 1, 37–38.

Wang, Y., 2004. Shaving make you more beautiful. Medical Ethics and Cosmetology 5, 112–113.

Wei, J., 2000. Treatment of sciatica with non-drug combination therapy. Chinese Manipulation & Qigong Therapy 16 (6), 47.

Wu, J., 2001. Cervical Spondylopathy Treated Comprehensively with Stretching (traction) Scraping (Guasha) and Needle-knife (needle-scalpel therapy). J Clin Acup and Moxibust 11, 9.

Wu, Y., Li, F., 2008. Post surgical pain control in patients with new initiative. Chinese J of Modern Drug Application 222 (11), 79–80.

Wu, Z., 2003. References to external treatment for nose (problems). Journal of External Therapy of Traditional Chinese Medicine 12 (5), 32–33.

Xie, Z., 2001. Application of Chinese medicine theory and technology-rich content of the profile of clinical nursing. Tianjin Journal of Nursing 9 (1), 46–48.

Yang, J., 2005. Chinese medicine principles of point selection in the application of physical therapy. Chinese Journal of Rehabilitation Theory and Practice 11 (1), 20.

Yang, X., Han, G., 2006. Cupping Gua Sha Treatment of ankle injury. Modern Traditional Chinese Medicine 26 (1), 24.

Yang, X., Zhang G., Wang Y., et al., 2006. Treatment Based in Differentiation of Symptoms and Signs on Dog–days in Summer and Osteoarthritis. Journal of External Therapy of Traditional Chinese Medicine 15 (1), 23.

Yu, R., 2005. Gua sha with glucosamine hydrochloride capsule treatment of knee osteoarthritis. Chinese Manipulation & Qi Gong Therapy 21 (5), 37–38.

Zhang, C., 2010. Acupuncture, gua sha rubbing method and the examples of treatment of stiff neck. Journal of Clinical Acupuncture and Moxibustion 2, 23.

Zhang, L., Yang, J.-s., Zhu B., et al., 2007. Brief talk about the main cultural quintessence and diagnostic and therapeutic techniques of acupuncture and moxibustion protection. Chinese Acup and Moxibustion 27 (2).

Zhang, Y., 2006. Dyspepsia Diagnosis and Treatment of Children??? Nine laws – Xing-Bo Zhao experience in treatment of children with dyspepsia. Chinese Community Doctors 22 (19), 33.

Zhao, N., Zhao, J., Hu, C., 2002. Some Kinds of Unique External Therapies of Gelao Nationality Medicine. Chinese Journal of Ethnomedicine and Ethnopharmacy 6. 323.

Zhao, S., Du, T., 2010. Acupuncture, gua sha, knocking through points quadruple therapy by different diseases and the effectiveness of specific operation expression. Modern Journal of Integrated Traditional Chinese and Western medicine 16, 2032–2034.

Zheng, K., 2005. Case Report on the Treatment of Intractable Disease by Folk Traditional Medicine and Pharmacy. China's Naturopathy 13 (11), 7–8.

Zhou, J.-y., He, Q., Li, X.-l., et al., 2005. Hospital infection in Traditional Chinese medicine diseases: supervision and data analysis. Chinese Journal of Nosocomiology 15 (12), 1403–1404, 1389.

Zhou, X., 2000. Treatment of lumbar muscle strain with massage, acupuncture and Gua sha. China's Naturopathy 8 (5), 27.

Zuo, J., 2009. Methylcobalamin and Gua sha combined treatment of postherpetic neuralgia. Zhejiang Journal of Integrated Traditional Chinese and Western Medicine 10, 639–640.

Zuo, S., Lu, G., Lu, X., 2005. Gua sha manipulation treatment for cervical spondylosis. Chinese Manipulation & Qi Gong Therapy 21 (5), 19.

References for Table 2.5: Case series: Gua sha alone for specific conditions (100)

Bao, D., Liu X.Q., 2003. Gua sha treatment of 64 cases of low back pain. People's Military Surgeon 46 (10), 617.

Cai, H., 2001. 40 cases of renal colic treated with Guasha. China's Naturopathy 9 (10), 18.

Cai, W., 2005. Gua sha treatment of cold and fever influenza A in 100 patients. Chinese Community Doctors 21 (15), 36.

Chen, C., 2003. 42 cases of treatment of peripheral facial paralysis with Guasha assisted by Shen Feng Jing (TM). Traditional Chinese Medicine Journal 2 (1), 62.

Chen, H., Wei, S., 2010. Antipyretic effect of Gua sha therapy. Journal of Practical Traditional Chinese Internal Medicine 8, 95–96.

Chen, X., 2000. 25 cases of treatment of frozen shoulder with Guasha and cupping therapy. Journal of Practical traditional Chinese Internal Medicine 14 (1), 46–47.

Cong, T., 1998. 41 cases of treatment of hiccup of apoplexy patients with Guasha. China's Naturopathy 1, 24.

Ding, Li, Xiao-ping, X., Ping, Z., 2009. Clinical observation of the effects of Gua sha therapy for headache due to common cold. Journal of Acupuncture and Tuina Science 5, 283–285.

Dong, K., 2003. Point scraping treatment of external humeral epicondylitis 65 cases. People's Military Surgeon 11, 681.

Dong, L., 2002. Holographic Meridian Scraping Therapy 'Gua sha' in 50 cases of acute mastitis. Modern Medicine Health 18 (8), 696.

Fan, S., 2000. 56 cases of treatment of neurasthenia with Guasha. Journal of Changchun College of Traditional Chinese Medicine 16 (2), 32.

Fan, Y., 2009. Clinical observation of Gua sha treatment of the Bladder channel for prevention and treatment of bronchial asthma. Journal of Acupuncture and Tuina Science 5, 278–279.

Gao, Y., Chen, Z., 2003. Gua sha therapy of 68 cases of herpes zoster (post herpetic) neuralgia. Chinese Community Doctors 19 (7), 36.

Gong, Y., 2002. Report of 3 cases of individualized treatment of muscle spasm based on Liver Theory. Liaoning Journal of Traditional Chinese Medicine 29 (7), 436–437.

He, W., 2007. Gua sha, scraping the treatment of 69 cases of scapulohumeral (shoulder) periarthritis. J Practical Traditional Chinese Medicine 23 (11), 720–721.

Hou, B., 1996. Gua sha scraping treatment of 14 cases of acne. China's Naturopathy 6, 29–30.

Hu, B., 2001. 80 cases of treatment of frozen shoulder with Guasha along meridian. Henan Traditional Chinese Medicine 21 (6), 51.

Hu, J., 2009. Gua sha treatment of 36 cases of hand and foot eczema. Journal of Sichuan Traditional Chinese Medicine 6, 118–119.

Hu, Y., Tian, Z., Tian, Q., 2003. Gua sha treatment of 20 cases of chronic pharyngitis. Journal of Hebei Traditional Chinese Medicine and Pharmacology 18 (1), 38.

Jia, Y., Li, H., Zhang, W., 2000. [Guasha (Sand Scraping) Therapy in Treatment of 24 Cases with Obstinate Insomnia 24 cases of treatment of refractory insomnia with Guasha. Journal of Clinical Acupuncture and Moxibustion 16 (3), 39–40.

Jia, Y., Li, H., 2000. 40 cases of treatment of cervical spondylosis with Guasha. China's Naturopathy 8 (3), 5–6.

Jia, Y., Zhang, W., 2000. 18 Cases of treatment of migraines with Guasha. Journal of Clinical Acupuncture and Moxibustion 16 (2), 36–37.

Jia, Y., 2003. Gua sha treatment of 48 cases of vertigo. Journal of Traditional Chinese Medicine and Chinese Materia Medica of Jilin (Jilin Journal of Traditional Chinese Medicine) 23 (11), 42.

Leng, M., 1997. Gua sha scraping treatment of 58 cases of cervical spondylosis. Anhui Medical University 3, 51.

Li, J., 2004. 32 cases of cold treated with gua sha. China's Naturopathy 12 (11), 21.

Li, X., 2009. Gua sha treatment of 90 cases of cold/flu. Family Nurse 20, 1831.

Li, Y., Liu, H., 2002. The use of 'Gua sha' Scraping therapy in acute first-aid. Journal of External Therapy of Traditional Chinese Medicine 11 (4), 55.

Liu, A., 2003. Thirty-five patients with cervical spondylopathy treated with Gua sha. China's Naturopathy 11 (5), 20.

Liu, G.-x., Sun, X.-h., 2001. 36 cases of treatment of ankylosing spondylitis with Guasha. Journal of Research in Chinese Traditional Medicine 17 (1), 27–28.

Liu, J., Li, F., 2009. The clinical application of the Gua sha (scraping) Health Act (50 cases). China Contemporary Medicine 15, 155.

Liu, J., Wang, J., Zhang, H., 2003. Clinical study of 100 cases of treatment of headache and dizziness with Guasha. Heilongjiang Journal of Traditional Chinese Medicine 1, 45–46.

Liu, S., 2008. Gua sha for treatment and nursing of pain syndrome. China's Naturopathy 16 (2).

Liu, W., Zhang, S., 2001. Treatment of 30 cases of bronchial pneumonia in children with Guasha (cutaneous scraping therapy). Shanxi Journal of Traditional Chinese Medicine 22 (12), 750.

Liu, Z., He, L., 2003. Gua sha treatment of periarthritis of shoulder -clinical report of 150 cases. Modern Traditional Chinese Medicine 4, 61–62.

Liu, Z., 2001. 'Gua sha' scraping treatment in 50 cases of stiff neck. China's Naturopathy 9 (2), 29.

Liu, Z., 2010. Gua sha treatment of thirty-eight cases of mammary glands. Shanghai Journal of Acupuncture and Moxibustion 2, 116.

Lu, Y., Zhang, R., Du, M., 2001. 28 cases of treatment of cold complicated with bronchitis using Guasha. China's Naturopathy 9 (11), 11.

Luo, X., Liu, N., 2007. Gua sha scraping the treatment of adolescent breast by clinical observation of 86 cases of illness. Chinese Journal of Information on Traditional Chinese Medicine 14 (7), 61.

Ma, B., 2009. Gua sha treatment of 58 cases of shoulder coagulation disorder. Journal of External Therapy of Traditional Chinese Medicine 4, 15.

Ma, W., 2002. 200 cases of treatment of internal hemorrhoids with Guasha. Chinese Journal of Coloproctology 22 (3), 43.

Ma, X., 2004. Gua sha treatment of 40 cases of stiff neck. Zhejiang Clinical Medical Journal 6 (2), 99;101.

Men, C., Wu, H., 1999. 30 cases of treatment of asthma with Guasha. Journal of Sichuan Traditional Chinese Medicine 17 (5), 53.

Mo, F., 2006. Scraping the treatment of 32 cases of enuresis in children. Guangxi Journal of Traditional Chinese Medicine 29 (3), 46–47.

Pan, S., 2007. Gua sha scraping therapy experience of 70 cases of pain. Guangxi Journal of Traditional Chinese Medicine 30 (3), 40–41.

Peng, G., 1999a. 36 cases of treatment of chronic myofibrositis of lumbar muscle with Guasha. Shaanxi Journal of Traditional Chinese Medicine 20 (3), 129.

Peng, H., 1999b. 34 cases of treatment of severe heatstroke with Guasha. China's Naturopathy 7 (5), 15–16.

Qi, C., Li, Z., 1999. 60 cases of treatment of insomnia with Guasha. Shanxi Journal of Traditional Chinese Medicine 15 (3), 30.

Qiao, Q., Liu, D., 2000. Gua sha scraping in the care and treatment of 90 cases of cold. Changzhi Medical College 14 (1), 73.

Qiao, Q., Zhao, Y., Zuo, Q., 2006. Holographic Meridian Scraping treatment of 57 cases of pain. Journal of Changzhi Medical College 20 (4), 307–308.

Qiao, Q., Zuo, Q., 2006. Gua sha in the treatment of herpes zoster. Journal of Qiqihar Medical College 27 (13), 1585–1586.

Qin, J., 2009. Holographic Meridian Scraping method in 12 cases of chronic hepatitis B. Journal of Yanan University (Medical Science Edition) 40, 106, 108.

Qing, F., 2001. 'Gua sha' scraping treatment of 32 cases of pain. China's Naturopathy 9 (4), 8–9.

Qiu, J., Dong, M., Deng, M., 2009. Gua sha treatment of nerve root cervical spondylosis. Chinese Manipulation & Qigong Therapy 1, 20–21.

Ran, Q., Shi, A., 2009. Study on Shi's Bian stone comprehensive therapy for rehabilitation after induced abortion. Chinese Acupuncture & Moxibustion 25, 103–105.

Shi, X., Bai, S., Xiong, D., 2000. Clinical study of 106 cases of treatment of shoulder and back myofascitis. Chinese Journal of Traditional Medical Traumatology & Orthopedics 8 (5), 51–52.

Shi, X., Zou, J., 2001. 124 cases of treatment of shoulder and back myofascitis with gua sha therapy. Hubei Journal of Traditional Chinese Medicine 22 (7), 47.

Song G., Qi D., Jia, Q., 2000. 50 cases of treatment of cold with Gua sha. JuLin Traditional Chinese Medicine 20 (2), 41.

Song, H., 2010. Cuttlefish bone Gua sha treatment: clinical observation of 107 cases of trachoma. Forum on Traditional Chinese Medicine.

Song, J., Zhang, H., 2002. 'Gua sha' treatment in 90 cases of stiff neck. West China Medical Journal 1, 109.

Song, Q., 2002. Gua sha treatment of 186 cases of lumbar disc herniation observed effect. Henan Journal of Surgery 8 (4), 33.

Sun, Z., Wang, S., Niu, S., Liu, Q., 2003. Holographic meridian scraping therapy report of 186 cases of cervical spondylosis. Central Plains Medical Journal 30 (7), 32.

Tan, H., 2001. 52 cases of treatment of frozen shoulder with 'Gua sha.' Shanghai Journal of Acupuncture & Moxibustion 20 (3), 36.

Tian, H., 1999. 50 Cases of Sunstroke Treated with Gua sha. Chinese Acupuncture & Moxibustion 19 (7), 446.

Tong, Y., 1999. 68 cases of treatment of cervical spondylopathy with Guasha. Shanghai Journal of Acup and Moxibustion 18 (4), 48.

Wang, B., Sun, P., Wang, L., 1998a. Treatment of functional headache with Guasha. Report

of 300 cases. Chinese Journal of the Practical Chinese with Modern Medicine 11 (2), 140.

Wang, L., 2004. Holographic meridian scraping Gua sha therapy for 38 cases of jaundice associated with chronic hepatitis B. China's Naturopathy 12 (11), 21–22.

Wang, L., 2000. Treatment of stiff neck with gua sha and holographic meridian. Chinese Acupuncture & Moxibustion 20 (6), 355.

Wang, P., Mei, B., 2003. Thirty-six patients with scapulohumeral periarthritis (frozen shoulder) treated by gua sha. China's Naturopathy 11 (10), 17–18.

Wang, S., 2002. 'Gua sha' scraping treatment of 25 cases of coldness symptoms back. Hubei Journal of Traditional Chinese Medicine 24 (9), 36.

Wang, W., 1999. 'Gua sha' scraping therapy for 102 cases of pain syndrome. Journal of Nursing Science 14 (2), 97.

Wang, Y., Gao, H., Li, S., 1998b. 32 cases of treatment of frozen shoulder with Guasha along meridian. Chinese Journal of the Practical Chinese with Modern Medicine 11 (10), 941.

Wu, J., Li, H., 2004. Gua sha treatment of acute lumbar sprain. Journal of Henan University of Medical Science 23 (3), 66.

Wu, J., Lin, Z., 2000. Treating stye by Guasha Fa in 37 cases: 37 cases of stye with Guasha. Chinese Journal of the practical Chinese with Modern Medicine 13 (12), 2480.

Wu, N., Zhang, H., Xiao, Q., et al., 2001. 'Gua sha' therapy clinical experience for 256 cases of acute lumbar sprain. Journal of Traditional Chinese Orthopedics and Traumatology 13 (3), 47.

Wu, X., Wu, X., 2003. Gua sha at the back can treat upper respiratory tract infection: 100 cases. Journal of External Therapy of Traditional Chinese Medicine 12 (2), 31.

Wu, Z., Zhang, X., 2001. 'Gua sha' Scraping treatment for pediatric cold 'food stagnation' disease. Sichuan Journal of Physiological Sciences 23 (4), 183.

Xiao, B., Tian, M., 2002. 'Gua sha' scraping the treatment of 19 cases of stiff neck. China's Naturopathy 10 (2), 35–36.

Xiao, Q., Zou, J., Wang, S., 2001. 50 cases of treatment of stiff neck with Guasha. Hubei Journal of Traditional Chinese Medicine 23 (4), 46.

Xiao, Q., Zou, J., Wang, S., 2001. 'Gua sha' scraping treatment for 50 cases of stiff neck. Hubei Journal of Traditional Chinese Medicine 4, 46.

Xie, Z., 2000. Gua Sha Treatment of incomplete adhesions after abdominal cancer, 24 cases of intestinal obstruction – attached to conventional Western medicine treatment of 20 cases of control observation. Zhejiang Journal of Traditional Chinese Medicine 35 (8), 333.

Xing, S., An, G., 2006. Gua sha scraping treatment of 130 cases of neck and shoulder pain. China's Naturopathy 14 (10), 19–20.

Xiong, Y.-p., Min, O.Y., 2008. Gua sha treatment of 50 cases of hypertension. Jiangxi J Trad Chinese Med 5, 60.

Xu, L., 1999. 36 cases of treatment of peripheral facial paralysis with Guasha along meridian. Fujian Journal of Traditional Chinese Medicine 30 (3), 43–44.

Xu, X., 2010. Traditional Chinese acupoint scraping gua sha in treating heatstroke syndrome; clinical observation and care in 39 cases. Nursing Journal of Chinese People's Liberation Army 8, 609–610.

Yang, X., Lu, X., Liu, Y., et al., 2006. Gua sha winter disease in the summer for 38 cases of bronchial asthma. Journal of External Therapy of Traditional Chinese Medicine 15 (2), 22.

Yang, X., 2004. Gua sha treatment of 28 cases of insomnia. Journal of Practical Traditional Chinese Internal Medicine 18 (4), 375.

Yang, X., 2005. Gua sha treatment of 36 cases of neurasthenia students. China's Naturopathy 13 (5), 19–20.

Yang, X., 2006. Treatment analysis of 32 cases of ankle sprain. Chinese Journal of School Health 27 (10), 909.

Yu, S.-m., 2007. Experimental research on the mechanism of scraping 'gua sha' in twelve cases of sports arthropathy injuries. Journal of Beijing Sport University 6, 798–800.

Zeng, Y., 2000. 34 cases of treatment of chronic sinusitis with scraping and eliminating method. Journal of Tianjin College of Traditional Chinese Medicine 19 (2), 12.

Zhang, G., Li, Y., 2009. Gua sha treatment of chronic pain diseases: clinical observation. Hebei Traditional Chinese Journal of Medicine and Pharmacology 4, 41.

Zhao, H., 2001. 'Gua sha' Scraping therapy for 100 cases of stiff neck. Chinese Manipulation & Qigong Therapy 17 (1), 46.

Zhao, Z., Xu, M., Wu, Y., 2002. Clinical study of 66 cases of treatment of non-severe infantile diarrhea with Guasha. Lishizhen Medicine and Materia Medica Research 13 (5), 292.

Zhao, Z., 2006. Gua sha in the treatment of 82 cases of scapulohumeral periarthritis. Hebei Journal of Traditional Chinese Medicine 28 (6), 456.

Zheng, H., 2000. 52 Cases of treatment of primary dysmenorrhea with Guasha. Journal of External Therapy of Traditional Chinese Medicine 9 (4), 25.

Zhong, Y., 1994. Antihypertensive effect of Gua sha scraping therapy in 52 cases of essential hypertension. Inner Mongolia Journal of Chinese Medicine 13 (4), 22–23.

Zhou, P., Xu, Y., 2001. Prevention and treatment of children susceptible to cold with Guasha with holographic meridian (28 cases). China's Naturopathy 9 (1), 24.

Zhou, X., Yang, Z., 2002. 'Gua sha' treatment for 28 cases of stiff neck. China's Naturopathy 10 (8), 17–18.

References for Table 2.6: Case series: Gua sha paired with another modality for specific conditions (106)

Chen, C., 2003. On 42 Cases of Peripheral Facial Paralysis Treated by 'Gua sha' Scraping the Patients' Neck, Chest or Back with Shenfengjing. Traditional Chinese Medicine Journal 2 (1), 626–628.

Chen, J., Zhang, J., 2009. Back, neck and shoulder massage with Gua sha treatment in 560 cases of soft tissue injury. Guangxi Journal of Traditional Chinese Medicine 3, 24–25.

Chen, L., 2004. Treating 66 cases of third lumbar transverse process syndrome with massage. Henan Traditional Chinese Medicine 24 (5), 72–73.

Chen, X., 2000. 25 cases of treatment of frozen shoulder with Guasha and cupping therapy. Journal of Practical traditional Chinese Internal Medicine 14 (1), 46–47.

Cheng, L., Chen, C., Zuo, Z., et al., 2000. Treatment of frozen shoulder by external use and topical scraping of Shen Feng Jing (37 cases). Journal of Fujian Agricultural University 3, 383–385.

Cheng, S., 2008. Combination of warm needling and Gua sha in 30 cases of humeral epicondylitis. Chinese Journal of Nanjing University of Traditional Chinese Medicine (Natural Science) 4, 270–271.

Cui, Z., Xu, Y., Kang, J., 2008. Gua sha, acupuncture treatment of 62 cases of juvenile chronic sinusitis. Hebei Traditional Chinese Journal of Medicine and Pharmacology 10, 1073.

Dang, H., 2005. Gua Sha and massage treatment in 115 cases of cold-type cold. Chinese Manipulation & Qi Gong Therapy 21 (2), 14–15.

Ding, M., 2001. 'Gua sha' scraping and massage therapy treatment of chronic lumbar muscle strain Scraping 84 cases of clinical observation. Chinese Manipulation & Qigong Therapy 17 (2), 49.

Fan, H., 2010. Acupuncture and Gua sha treatment of periarthritis of the shoulder. Shanghai Journal of Acupuncture and Moxibustion 7, 441.

Fan, X., 2001. The role of 'Gua sha' Scraping therapy with electro-acupuncture on rehabilitation cervical spondylosis (87 cases). Modern Rehabilitation 25 (18), 128.

Feng, L., 2008. Eighty six cases of cervical spondylosis treated by acupuncture and Gua sha. Journal of Practical Traditional Chinese Internal Medicine 6, 58–59.

Gao, X., 2008. Gua sha followed by manual reduction treatment of 78 cases of cervical disease. Journal of Practical Traditional Chinese Internal Medicine 4, 87–88.

Ge, Z., Liu, X., 2002. Gua sha and cupping therapy combined with 51 cases of acute lumbar sprain. Xinjiang Journal of Traditional Chinese Medicine 20 (2), 26–27.

Guo, S., 2001. 'Gua sha' Scraping and Massage Treatment of Migraine. China's Naturopathy 9 (9), 42.

Guo, X., 2005. Gua sha with acupuncture treatment in 126 cases of peripheral facial paralysis in children. Shanxi Journal of Traditional Chinese Medicine 21 (1), 35.

Guo, Y., Wu, W., 2005. Puncturing needle traction method combined with facial Gua sha in the treatment of 30 cases of refractory facial paralysis. Journal of Clinical Acupuncture and Moxibustion 21 (11), 28.

Han, W., Yang, M., 2006. Selection treatment identified all the way through 56 cases of stiff neck. Shanghai Journal of Acupuncture and Moxibustion 25 (11), 27.

Hu, Z., 2001. Twenty-eight Cases of Lateral Femoral Cutaneous Neuritis Treated with Combined Therapy of 'Gua sha' scraping and Moxibustion. China's Naturopathy 9 (12), 40–41.

Huang, Y., Sun, Z., Yu, Z., 2002. Gua sha, scrape with finger pressure point treatment of 60 cases of pediatric asthma. Journal of Practical Traditional Chinese Medicine 18 (4), 40–41.

Huang, Y., 2001. Gua sha 'scraping' and acupuncture with 48 cases of stiff neck. China's Naturopathy 9 (9), 42–43.

Jia, Y., Wu, X., Song, C., 2007. General treatment of advanced cancer patients' experience of insomnia. Chinese Primary Health Care 21 (09), 93–94.

Jiang, X., 2005. Gua sha and external application of Chinese medicine in the treatment of acne. Tianjin Journal of Traditional Chinese Medicine 22 (1), 67.

Kong, W., Zhou, Y., 2005. Gua sha and Chinese herbal medicine in the treatment of 38 cases of facial chloasma (melasma). Henan Traditional Chinese Medicine 25 (1), 50–51.

Lan, F., 1999. 48 cases of treatment of heatstroke with Guasha combined with Huoxiang Zhengqi Liquid (TM). China's Naturopathy 7 (12), 23–24.

Li, B., 2004. 118 Cases of cold-type arthralgia treated with massage gua sha (118 cases). China's Naturopathy 12 (4), 26.

Li, C., Guo, B., 2002. Gua sha and traditional Chinese medicine treatment of osteoarthritis of the knee. Hubei Journal of Traditional Chinese Medicine 24 (6), 46.

Li, M., 2000. Cervical spondylosis of nerve type treated by acupuncture and scraping. Report of 120 cases. Henan Journal of Chinese Medicine 20 (4), 64.

Li R., 2001. Sciatica Treated With Electro-Acupuncture And Scraping. Report Of 66 Cases. J Clin Acup and Moxibust 7, 42.

Li, Z., 2005a. Gua sha with needle-knife therapy on cervical spondylosis (150 cases). Journal of External Therapy of Traditional Chinese Medicine 2, 31.

Li, Z., 2005b. Needle-knife with Gua sha scraping in 30 cases of lumbar disc herniation. Liaoning Journal of Traditional Chinese Medicine 32 (2), 150.

Ling, M., 2008. Massage and Gua sha in treating 54 cases of frozen shoulder. Technology Wind 9, 58.

Liu, F., Jin, K., Tan, L., 2003. 100 cases of treatment of trachoma with Guasha and drug therapy. Hunan Journal of Traditional Chinese Medicine 19 (5), 46–47.

Liu, H., Wu, Y., Zhang, H., 1999. 38 cases of treatment of acute lumbar back sprain with acupuncture combined with Guasha. Henan Journal of Traditional Chinese Medicine and Pharmacy 14 (3), 32.

Liu, J., Li, Z., Lin, H., 2003. Clinical observation of 50 cases of Fu Lin Gua sha treatment for cold rheumatoid arthritis. Chinese Manipulation & Qigong Therapy 19 (1), 52–53.

Liu, S., Cui, J., 2006. Gua sha treatment with oral traditional Chinese medicine in the treatment of 150 cases of cervical spondylosis. Henan Traditional Chinese Medicine 26 (2), 61–62.

Liu, Y., 2002. 'Gua sha' and cupping treatment with 21 cases of supraorbital neuralgia. J Clin Acup and Moxibust 18 (6), 10.

Lu, H., Li, J., 2005. Application of acupuncture and gua sha method of massage in treatment of epiphysitis of turberositae tibiae in 16 patients. China's Naturopathy 3, 39–40.

Lu, X., Liu, J., Shi, X., 2008. Sixty four cases third lumbar transverse process syndrome treated with Gua sha and local kneading method. Chinese Manipulation & Qigong Therapy 11, 29–31.

Lu, X., Zheng, L., Liu, Y., et al., 2006. Twenty-eight cases of dysmenorrhea in students treated with Gua sha combined with Danggui tablets. China's Naturopathy 14 (19), 61–62.

Luo, X., Liu, N., 2007. Chinese herbs with Gua sha treatment of 286 cases of mammary glands (breast hyperplasia). Liaoning Journal of Traditional Chinese Medicine 34 (8).

Ma, H., Li, S., Zheng, H., 2003. Clinical study of 83 cases of treatment of cervical spondylopathy with Guasha assisted by injection at acupoint. Journal of Clinical Acupuncture and Moxibustion 19 (2), 27–28.

Ma, J., 2010. Acupuncture and Gua sha treatment of 30 cases of intractable facial paralysis. Journal of Practical Traditional Chinese Medicine 3, 179.

Ma, S., Cao, J., Chen, L., et al., 2005. Summary of 178 Cases of Scapula Humeral Periarthritis Treated by the Block Therapy and the Therapy of Guasha. Gansu Journal of Traditional Chinese Medicine 18 (4), 17.

Ma, Y., Xia, J., Ren, Y., et al., 2006. Effect of Buzhongyiqi pill with Gua sha treatment for college students in poor health (gray state sub-health). China's Naturopathy 14 (11), 60–61.

Miao, G., Zhou, L., 2005. Chinese Medicine Gua sha treatment of 18 cases of acute stomach cramps. Guangming Journal of Chinese Medicine 20 (5), 64–65.

Pan, H., Zhou, J., Shen, Q., 2006. Gua sha cupping and acupuncture treatment of 24 women with menopausal tinnitus. Traditional Chinese Medicine Research 19 (5), 31–32.

Qi, C., Li, Z., 2001. Variable traction and 'Gua sha' scrape the treatment of cervical vertigo summary of 60 Cases. Gansu Journal of Traditional Chinese Medicine 14 (4), 30–31.

Qian, Z., 2009. Segmental manipulation with Gua sha treatment for 53 cases of cervical spondylotic radiculopathy. Jiangxi J Trad Chinese Med 8, 58–59.

Qu, B., 2001. 35 Treatment of Ankylosing spondylitis with Guasha and cupping therapy. New Journal of Traditional Chinese Medicine 33 (10), 49.

Ren, Z., Wang, X., 2007. TDP irradiation treatment combined with Gua sha in 86 cases of levator scapulae injury. Shaanxi Journal of Traditional Chinese Medicine 28 (10).

Shi, L., Li, J., 2002. Gua sha and cupping the back for prevention and treatment of 100 cases of recurrent respiratory tract infection in children. Fujian Journal of Traditional Medicine 33 (2), 48.

Sun, R., Wang, Q., 1999. Clinical study of 120 cases of treatment of straightening of cervical curvature with Guasha combined with massage. Chinese Manipulation & Qigong Therapy 15 (3), 34–35.

Sun, S., 2003. Gua sha ear pressure treatment of 30 cases of ADHD children (30 cases of treatment of hyperkinetic child syndrome with Guasha combined with ear-acupoint pressing. Chinese Acupuncture & Moxibustion 23 (2), 120.

Sun, X., 2002. Clinical observation of bupleurum powder point scraping treatment in 80 cases of refractory insomnia. Chinese Journal of Clinical Rehabilitation 6 (11), 1671.

Tan, F., Hu, Y., Wang, H., et al., 1998. 250 cases of treatment of lumbar disc herniation with Guasha combined with rotary manipulation. Journal of Practical Traditional Chinese Medicine 14 (2), 26.

Tang, H., Yan, S., Huang, L., 2010. Clinical observation of massage and gua sha treatment on sleep quality in chronic insomnia. Guangxi Medical Journal 7, 795–797.

Tu, Q., 2000. Primary Trigeminal Neuralgia treated by acupuncture and scrape therapy. Report of 20 cases. Journal of Clinical Acupuncture and Moxibustion 16 (7), 40–42.

2005. Twenty-six Patients with Gastrointestinal Dysfunction Treated by Gua sha scraping and Cupping. China's Naturopathy 13 (10), 40.

Wang, C., Qi, W., 2001. 60 Cases of treatment of influenza with Guasha and baguan. Journal of Changchun College of Traditional Chinese Medicine 17 (4), 30.

Wang, F., 2009. Baguan and Gua sha in 80 cases of neurodermatitis. Hebei Traditional Chinese Journal of Medicine and 4, 581.

Wang, H., Guan, S., 2009. Gua sha and massage in the treatment of headache, 45 cases. Hunan Journal for Traditional Chinese Medicine 4, 52–53.

Wang, H., 2002. Clinical Observation of Acupuncture and 'Gua sha' treatment on 24 Patients with Cerebral Palsy. Chinese Journal of Basic Medicine in Traditional Chinese Medicine (TCM based on the Chinese Medical Journal) 8 (8), 58–59.

Wang, L., 2005a. Chinese Medicine external treatment of 86 cases of greater occipital neuralgia. Jilin Journal of Traditional Chinese Medicine 25 (5), 45–46.

Wang, L., 2004. Gua sha and acupuncture treatment of 68 cases of fasciitis of the back. Jilin Journal of Traditional Chinese Medicine 24 (5), 46–47.

Wang, L., 2010. Holographic Meridian Scraping method combined with interferon in 46 cases of chronic hepatitis B. Chinese Journal of Ethnomedicine and Ethnopharmacy 12, 189.

Wang, M., 2001. 'Gua sha' scraping treatment with acupuncture and 43 cases of cervical vertigo. Journal of Anhui Traditional Chinese Medical College 20 (5), 37–38.

Wang, R. Li, Wu, J., 2005. Vertigo treated by Gua sha with dai horns and modified Xiaoyaosan: 52 cases. Yunnan Journal of Traditional Chinese Medicine and Materia Medica 26 (6), 42–43.

Wang, X., Wang, Y., 2008. Twenty-six cases of chloasma treated by foot reflexotherapy combined with face gua sha. Journal of External Therapy of Traditional Chinese Medicine 4, 42–43.

Wang, X., 2005b. Warm needle treatment with Gua sha in 48 cases of knee osteoarthritis. Journal of North China Coal Medical College 7 (2), 199.

Wang, Z., Ge, L., 2009. Sixty cases of cervical spondylosis treated by acupuncture combined with gua sha (scraping). Chinese Journal of Convalescent Medicine. 10, 930–931.

Wang, Z., Tang, C., 2001. Treatment of common cold with massage combined with Guasha. Chinese Manipulation & Qi Gong Therapy 17 (3), 24–25.

Wei, D., Pi, L., 2003. Auricular therapy with Gua sha for chloasma (50 cases). Henan Journal of Traditional Chinese Medicine and Pharmacy 23 (2), 53–54.

Wu, J., 2010. Treating of old soft tissue injury of the ankle joint with electroacupuncture and Gua sha: a report of 52 cases. Jiangxi J Trad Chinese Med 7, 54–55.

Wu, X., Wu, X., 2003a. 100 cases of treatment of upper respiratory tract infection with Guasha and moving cupping therapies. Journal of Practical Traditional Chinese Medicine 19 (3), 145.

Wu, X., Wu, X., 2006. Acupuncture plus gua sha of Jiaji for 62 cases of recurrent mastitis. Journal of External Therapy of Traditional Chinese Medicine 15 (3), 57.

Wu, X., Wu, X., 2003b. Gua sha Jiaji acupuncture treatment of recurrent attacks of 62 cases of mastitis. Chinese Acupuncture & Moxibustion 23 (9), 535.

Wu, K., Xie, C., 1998. Gua Sha meridian scraping with TDP treatment efficacy of 115 cases of stiff neck. China's Naturopathy 5, 9.

Xia, J., Shi, L., 2006. Gua sha and cupping in the treatment of dysmenorrhea. Shandong Journal of Traditional Chinese Medicine 25 (3), 195.

Xiao, B., Qin, W., 2010. Gua sha combined with trigger point injection therapy in 23

cases of piriformis syndrome (sciatica). China's Naturopathy 6, 16–17.

Xiao, J., Ma, Y., Zhang, G., et al., 2006. Scraping, Cupping treatment of 38 cases of lumbar muscle strain. Henan Traditional Chinese Medicine 26 (3), 61–62.

Xin, Y., Yu, H., Zhang, C., 2004. X-ray features of cervical spondylosis treated with Chinese medicine. Chinese Journal of Clinical Rehabilitation 8 (11), 2059.

Xing, C., Wang, W., Wang, Y., 2000. 32 cases of treatment of neuritis of the lateral femoral cutaneous nerve with moving cupping therapy combined with Guasha. Journal of Practical Traditional Chinese Medicine 16 (12), 28.

Xing, J., 2003. Seventy-six cases of treatment of cervical spondylopathy with acupuncture combined with Guasha. Hebei Journal of Traditional Chinese Medicine 25 (3), 212–213.

Ya, T., 2008. Sixty-two cases of chronic ulcerative colitis treated with Zhuang medicine detoxification therapy with traditional Chinese medicine Enema and Gua sha treatment. Chinese Journal of Information on Traditional Chinese medicine 3, 60.

Ya, T., 2003. Strong medical detoxification therapy: gua sha and retention enema with Chinese medicine for chronic ulcerative colitis: observation of 61 cases. Chinese Journal of Ethnomedicine and Ethnopharmacy 5, 287–288.

Yang, D., 2006. Gua sha and acupuncture treatment of sub-health state (40 cases). Journal of Sichuan Traditional Chinese Medicine 24 (12), 100–101.

Yang, L., Zuo, J., 2005. Acupuncture and Gua sha treatment of cervical spondylosis (68 cases). Journal of Clinical Acupuncture and Moxibustion 21 (8), 119–121.

Yang, X., Guo, Y., Li, Y., 2005. Traditional treatment methods 36 cases of periarthritis of shoulder. Practical Preventive Medicine 12 (2), 426.

Yang, X., Zhang K., 2006. Fifty-six Patients with Acute and Chronical Gastroenteritis Treated by Scraping Combined with Cupping. China's Naturopathy 14 (8), 56.

Yang, X., 2004a. Gua sha and cupping treatment of 68 cases of cervical disease. China's Naturopathy 12 (11), 35.

Yang, X., 2004b. Twenty-eight Patients with Third Vertebral Transverse Process Syndrome Treated by Gua sha Scraping and Cupping. China's Naturopathy 12 (10), 34.

Yin, T., Bai, Q., 2008. Ear electroacupuncture with Gua sha for 107 cases of simple obesity. Liaoning University Journal of Traditional Chinese Medicine 5, 123–124.

Yuan, J., Huang, W., 2000. Clinical study of 108 cases of treatment of L3 transverse process syndrome with massage therapy and Guasha. Chinese Manipulation & Qigong Therapy 16 (6), 31.

Zhang, J., Wang, Z., 2006. Gua sha treatment of 150 cases of chronic prostatitis. Medical Journal of Chinese People's Health 18 (10), 792.

Zhang, M., Chen, Y., Jing, Z., 2010. Treatment of 65 cases of chloasma with Gua sha skin scraping method and 'qubai meibai decoction.'. Journal of Traditional Chinese Medicine Jiangsu 7, 23–34.

Zhang, M., Jiang, X., 2005. Gua sha and massage treatment of periarthritis of shoulder. Chinese Manipulation & Qi Gong Therapy 21 (3), 22.

Zhang, S., 2010. Fifty-two patients with ankylosing spondylitis treated by Gua sha and moxibustion. China's Naturopath 6, 19–20.

Zhang, X., Hu, L., Zhang, X., 2009. Gua sha with auricular acupressure treatment of common migraine in sixty patients. Chinese Journal of Traditional Medical Science and Technology 2, 143–144.

Zhang, X., Li X., 2006a. Thirty-nine Patients with Peripheral Facial Paralysis Treated by Acupuncture and Gua sha scraping. China's Naturopathy 14 (10), 52.

Zhang, X., 2003. Embedding and Gua sha in the treatment of 60 cases of epigastralgia. Henan Journal of Traditional Chinese Medicine and Pharmacy 23 (3), 21.

Zhang, Z., Li, X., 2006b. Gua sha and acupuncture treatment of 39 cases of peripheral facial paralysis. Journal of Community Medicine 4 (12), 55.

Zhao, G., Chen, Y., Lu, M., et al., 1998. 27 cases of treatment of chronic Hepatitis B with Guasha combined with Jiang Ganling (TM) and Qiang Lining (TM). Chinese Journal of Integrated Traditional and Western Medicine on Liver Diseases 1, 49–50.

Zhao, Y., 2006a. Gua sha and cupping treatment of thoracic facet joint disorder. Chinese Journal of Basic Medicine in Traditional Chinese Medicine (TCM based on the Chinese Medical Journal) 12 (3), 227.

Zhu, H., 2009. Efficacy of and Zhuang medicine (herbs) after Gua sha treatment in 30 cases of primary hypothyroidism. Journal of Medicine & Pharmacy of Chinese Minorities 33–34.

Zou, F., Wang, Y., Zhang, C., 2002. 32 cases of combined treatment of lumbar disc herniation observed. Journal of Ningxai Medical College 24 (1), 34–35.

References for Table 2.7: Case series: Gua sha combined with two or more other modalities for specific conditions (38)

Cheng, L.B., Dai, J.Y., Chen, Y.Q., et al., 2007. Analysis Effect of Synthetical Therapy Mainly Using 'shenfengjing' Scraping For Knee Osteoarthritis (132 cases). Guangming Journal of Chinese Medicine 22 (8), 38–40.

Cheng, L., 2008. Observation of the curative effect of combined therapy mainly with Shenfengjing on lumbar intervertebral disc protrusion (lumbar disc herniation) clinical observation). Modern J Integrated Trad Chinese and Western Medicine 17 (4).

Cheng, X., 2004. Chinese moxibustion, acupuncture, cupping, electrotherapy, scrape, massage therapy, such as an organic integrated efficacy analysis of 120 cases of periarthritis of shoulder. Chinese Manipulation & Qi Gong Therapy 20 (6), 30–31.

Cheng, X., 2005. Clinical observation of electrotherapy, traction and Gua sha comprehensive treatment of 200 cases of stiff neck. Chinese Manipulation & QI Gong Therapy 21 (12), 26–27.

Chi, X., Jiang, J., Xiao, H., 2006. Gua sha with a comprehensive treatment of patients with acute viral hepatitis. Guandong Medical Journal 27 (10), 1576.

Cui, W., Li, Q., 2007. General treatment of 30 cases of refractory facial paralysis. Jilin Journal of Traditional Chinese Medicine 27 (6), 44.

Geng, D., Guo, W., Miao, Z., 2006. Comprehensive treatment of 120 cases of periarthritis of shoulder (frozen shoulder). Journal of External Therapy of Traditional Chinese Medicine 15 (5), 47.

Gu, Z., Li, Y., 2003. 26 cases of treatment of fibrositis with integrated traditional and western medicine. Hebei Journal of Traditional Chinese Medicine 25 (11), 877.

Hou, W., Zhang, R., Li, Y., 2005. Chinese and Western Integrative Medicine for 176 cases of periarthritis of shoulder. Henan Traditional Chinese Medicine 25 (11), 58–59.

Hu, J., 2001. Acupuncture Cupping Gua Sha Treatment A Clinical Observation of 64 cases of periarthritis of shoulder. J Clin Acup and Moxibust 17 (10), 5–6.

Li, B., 2003. 72 cases of treatment of cervical spondylopathy with combination therapy of laser, massage and Gua sha along meridian. Chinese Journal of Information on Traditional Chinese Medicine 20 (4), 91.

Li, D., Sun, L., Gong, H., et al., 2001. 67 Patients with Simple Obesity Treated with Combined Therapy. J Clin Acup and Moxibust 9, 11–12.

Li, J., 2002. Comprehensive treatment of 410 cases of neck and shoulder pain. Practical Clinical Journal of Integrated Chinese and Western Medicine 2 (1), 35–36.

Li, S., 1999. Traditional Chinese medicine acupuncture massage, followed by Gua Sha Treatment of cervical spondylosis. Modern Rehabilitation 3 (7), 73.

Li, X., Wang Y., Wang, J., et al., 2007. Forty-four Patients with Acne Treated by Comprehensive Therapy. China's Naturopathy 15 (4), 54–55.

Li, Z., Cui, F., Yang, X.W., 2006. Gua sha, cupping Massage treatment of 15 cases of cervical spondylosis. Modern Preventative Medicine 33 (12), 2477.

Lin, Z., Jia, J., Lin, K., et al., 2007. Comprehensive treatment of 150 cases of periarthritis of shoulder. Chinese Manipulation & Qi Gong Therapy 23 (9), 29–30.

Liu, J., Cai, S., Jiang, Z., 2001. Integrated traditional Chinese medicine treatment of rheumatism: 'Gua sha' scraping in 1000 cases. Modern Rehabilitation 5 (12), 113.

Liu, W., 2008. Gua sha, bloodletting and cupping of 120 cases of facial chloasma. Chinese Medicine Modern Distance Education of China 6 (4).

Lu, X., Li, Y., Yang, X., 2006. Bamboo save point pressure point hiccup treatment of 30 cases of hiccup. Journal of External Therapy of Traditional Chinese Medicine 15 (3), 17.

Ma, D., 2009. Analysis of the clinical efficacy and mechanism of quadruple external therapy for the treatment of peripheral facial paralysis. Journal of Sichuan Traditional Chinese Medicine 4, 117–118.

Ma, D., 2010. One hundred and forty-eight cases of radiohumeral epicondylitis treated by combined therapy. Journal of External Therapy of Traditional Chinese Medicine 1, 6–7.

Nie, D., Peng, M., 2000. 89 cases of treatment of frozen shoulder with combination therapy. Hubei Journal of Traditional Chinese Medicine 22 (6), 461–462.

Wang, F., 2005. Du mai Gua sha cupping treatment with bloodletting in 89 cases of acute mastitis. Hebei Journal of Traditional Chinese Medicine 27 (7), 541.

Wang, L., 2004. Gua sha treatment and rehabilitation of rheumatic joint pain (366 cases). Fujian Journal of Traditional Chinese Medicine 35 (2), 48.

Wu, C.-m., 2006. Eighty-nine cases of recurrent stye treated with meridian acupuncture, gua sha and bloodletting. Mod. Hosp. 2, 53.

Xia, D., 2006. Quadruple therapy treatment of vertebral artery type of 150 cases of cervical spondylosis. Journal of External Therapy of Traditional Chinese Medicine 15 (1), 37.

Xin, X., Zhang, Y., Xie, C., et al., 2003. 56 cases of treatment of obesity with combination therapy. Jiangsu Journal of Traditional Chinese Medicine 24 (5), 37.

Yan, L., Wang, H., Wei, S., 2008. Integrative medicine for 62 cases of heat stroke. Modern Journal of Integrated Traditional Chinese and Western medicine 25, 4010.

Yang, L., 2003. Comprehensive treatment of 130 cases of cervical spondylosis: clinical experience. Journal of Traditional Chinese Orthopedics and Traumatology 15 (8), 34.

Yang, M., 2003. Treatment of children with 33 cases of food addiction. Chinese Community Doctors 19 (13), 36–37.

Yang, X., Zhang Z., Qiao, L., et al., 2007. Aerobics and other natural therapies to improve the effectiveness of sub-health status. Occupation and Health 23 (8), 651–652.

Yang, X., 2005a. Gua sha, cupping and massage in treatment of 25 cases of acute and chronic periarthritis of shoulder. Shandong Journal of Traditional Chinese Medicine 24 (4), 229–230.

Yang, X., 2005b. Twenty Patients with Rhinallergosis Treated by Comprehensive Therapy. China's Naturopathy 13 (11), 37–38.

Yue, X., Zhang, J., Lei, J., 2004. Chinese medicine treatment [acupuncture, Gua sha, and herbal Kang-San II] of eye pseudomyopia 400 cases. Chinese Journal of Information on Traditional Chinese Medicine 11 (9), 812–813.

Zhang, M., 1998. 410 cases of treatment of shoulder-neck pain with combination therapy. China's Naturopathy 2, 19–20.

Zhang, S., 1998. 104 cases of treatment of frozen shoulder with massage, cupping and Guasha therapies. Chinese Manipulation & Qigong Therapy 3, 15–16.

Zhou, L., Wang, Z., Yang, H., et al., 2006. Gua Sha Treatment with pricking for scapular neck and soft tissue shoulder disorder. Chinese Manipulation & Qi Gong Therapy 22 (5), 18.

References for Table 2.8: Gua sha *n* = 1 case studies (12 articles: 9 Chinese, 2 English, 1 German)

Chan, S., Yuen, J., Gohel, M., et al., 2011. Guasha-induced hepatoprotection in chronic active hepatitis B: A case study. Clin Chim Acta in press (May 13).

Chiu, C.-Y., Chang, C.-Y., Gau, M.-L., 2008. [An experience applying Gua-Sha to help a parturient woman with breast fullness]. Hu Li Za Zhi 55 (1) (February), 105–110.

Fang, Y., 2002. Clinical use of 'Gua sha' scraping, cupping, Tuina treatment of clinical use. Jiangxi Journal of Traditional Chinese Medicine 33 (3), 37.

Jin B.-f., Huang, Y.-f., Shao, C.-a., et al., 2005. Integrated Treatment for Priapism Caused by Circumcision: a Case Report. National Journal of Andrology 11 (7), 544–547.

Nielsen, A., 2005. Postherpetic neuralgia in the left buttock after a case of shingles. Explore (NY) 1 (1) (January), 74.

Schwickert, M.E., Saha, F.J., Braun, M., et al., 2007. [Gua Sha for migraine in inpatient withdrawal therapy of headache due to medication overuse.]. Forsch Komplementmed 14 (5) (October), 297–300.

Wang, B., Liu, Z., Duan, X., et al., 2003. Gua sha misdiagnosed as syphilis: one case of misdiagnosis. Chinese Journal of AIDS & STD 9 (3), 155.

Wei, J., 2002. 'Gua sha' back to my youth rehabilitation. Zhonghua Yangsheng Baojian Zazhi 8, 40.

Xue, X., Chen, N., 2001. Study on the effects of 'gua sha' skin-scraping therapy and foot reflexotherapy in the treatment of periarthritis of the shoulder: a case report. Chinese Journal of Natural Medicine 3 (1), 13.

Zhang, M., 2005. A conversation: the most suitable fitness for a frail person. Health Care Today 6, 10–11.

Zhang, Z., Wang, G., 2010. Case report of foot acupuncture with scraping in the cure of pelvic inflammatory disease. Journal of Clinical Acupuncture and Moxibustion 8, 25.

Zuo, J., 2005. Clinical care of Guillain–Barré syndrome with respiratory paralysis: case report. Today Nurse 5.

References for Table 2.9: Gua sha in comparative, controlled, and/or randomized controlled trials (55: 53 Chinese, 2 English)

2006. Acupuncture with Gua sha in the treatment of simple obesity clinical observation of 108 cases. Medicine Industry Information 3 (18).

Braun, M., Schwickert, M., Nielsen, A., et al., 2011 January 28. Effectiveness of Traditional Chinese 'Gua Sha' Therapy in Patients with Chronic Neck Pain; A Randomized Controlled Trial. Pain Med.

Chen, H., Chen, S., Chen, L., 2008. Gua sha treatment to improve sleep in patients with chronic obstructive pulmonary disease (COPD). Journal of Clinical Pulmonary Medicine 13 (1), 76.

Chen, M.-r., 2008. Electoacupuncture and gua sha treatment of 30 cases of breast lobular hyperplasia. Journa of Clinical Acupuncture & Moxibustion 8, 17–18.

Chiu, J.-Y., Gau, M.-L., Kuo, S.-Y., et al., 2010. Effects of Gua-Sha therapy on breast engorgement: a randomized controlled trial. J Nurs Res 18 (1) (March), 1–10.

Ji, W., Wang, Y., 2010. Observation on the effect of massage and Gua sha in treating patients with shoulder periarthritis. Chinese Nursing Research 4, 330–332.

Li, A., 2008. Gua sha and cupping treatment compared to acupuncture and Chinese herbs for 80 cases stroke sequelae (40 per group). Shaanxi Journal of Traditional Chinese Medicine 9, 1222.

Li, G., 2007. Efficacy of Treating Insomnia (Agrypnia) by Gua sha scraping on selected acupoints by differentiating symptoms and signs in combination with accommodating emotion. Journal of Nursing Science 9, 41–42.

Li, H., Huang, Q., 2003. Clinical observation of gua sha with added zhuang medical detoxification of chronic hepatitis B (added Zhuang). Guangxi Journal of Traditional Chinese Medicine 26 (5), 41–42.

Li, M., Ma, Y., Ren, Y., et al., 2006. Danggui formula and Gua sha treatment in 28 cases of dysmenorrhea. Journal of External Therapy of Traditional Chinese Medicine 15 (4), 30–31.

Li, S.-j., Wang, Y.-h., Gong, L.-l., 2008. Observation of the effect of acupuncture plus vinegar ion induction and Gua sha along channels in nerve-rooted type cervical spondylosis. Journal of Clinical Acupuncture and Moxibustion 12, 15–16.

Liao, X., Li, J., Liu, H., 2004. Meridian Gua sha with cupping treatment of 39 cases of cervical spondylosis. Shanghai Journal of Acupuncture and Moxibustion 23 (9), 28.

Lin, Q., 2009. Meridian Scraping the moxibustion treatment of 30 cases of cervical neck. Fujian Journal of Traditional Chinese Medicine 6, 31–32.

Liu, B., He, X.-w., 2008. Clinical Observation of Cough following Acute Upper Respiratory Tract Infection Treated by Zhi Sou San and Gua sha. J Modern Clin Med 34 (1), 12–13.

Liu, J., Zheng, X., Lin, H., 2002. Gua sha treatment of 72 cases if internal injuries, pain, wound wash. Fujian Journal of Traditional Chinese Medicine 33 (3), 18–19.

Liu, L., Chen, L., Zheng, S., et al., 2010. Acupoint-Injection with Guasha Treatment Efficacy of Cervical Vertigo (point injection scraping observed treatment of cervical vertigo). Journal of Clinical Acupuncture and Moxibustion 7, 24–26.

Liu, W., Yuan, H., Wang, B., et al., 2007. Gua sha with point catgut implantation TCM treatment of 100 cases of peptic ulcer. Modern Journal of Integrated Traditional Chinese and Western Medicine 16 (12), 1610–1611.

Luo, X., Liu, N., 2008. Chinese medicine external treatment of acute mastitis: clinical observation. Lishizhen Medicine and Materia Medica Research 5, 1222–1223.

Luo, X., Liu, N., 2007. Clinical observation of Gua sha scraping combined with herbal medicine in the treatment of acute mastitis. Journal of Emergency in Traditional Chinese Medicine 16 (8), 939–940.

Ma, H., Li, S., Zheng, H., 2003. Gua sha compared to point injection treatment for 83 cases of cervical spondylosis: clinical observation. J Clin Acup and Moxibust 19 (2), 27–28.

Mi, J., 2010. Observation of 60 cases of Gua sha treatment of children with stagnation of heat. Journal of Pediatrics of Traditional Chinese Medicine 1, 41–42.

Peng, Y.-l., Meng, J., Feng, D.-r., et al., 2009. Clinical observation of combined acupuncture and Gua sha therapy for improving phlegm-dampness constitution of simple obesity. Journal of Acupuncture and Tuina Science 25, 87–90.

Qiao, Q., Zuo, Q., Du Ziping, L.J., 2007. Gua sha with cupping treatment of primary dysmenorrhea. Journal of Changshi Medical College 21 (3), 230–231.

Sha, Y., 2007a. Clinical observation of acupuncture, stone gua sha and cupping therapy (baguan) for neck -type cervical spondylosis. Journal of Acupuncture and Tuina Science 6, 348–350.

Sha, Y., 2007b. Treatment of neck-type cervical spondylopathy by a composite treatment of acupuncture, stone scraping gua sha and cupping. Shanghai Journal of Acupuncture and Moxibustion 8, 19–20.

Shang, B., Zhang, J. 2009. Gua sha treatment of 176 cases of mammary glands (mastitis). Shaanxi Journal of Traditional Chinese Medicine 5, 596–597.

Shi, X., Bai, S., Xiong, D., 2000. Clinical analysis of 106 cases of shoulder myofascitis. Chinese Journal of Traditional Medical Traumatology & Orthopedics 8 (5), 51–52.

Sun, L., Wang, Y., 2010. Gua sha together athletes clear hydrolyzate children with recurrent respiratory tract infection prevention and control (heat the food product license) 79 Cases). Chinese Medical Digest (Pediatrics) 3, 201–203.

Wang, F.-r., Li, Q.-p., 2006. Clinical Study of Treatment of Acute Mastitis by Dermal Scraping on Du Channel plus Blood-letting Puncture. Shanghai Journal of Acupuncture and Moxibustion 25 (8), 22–23.

Wang, H., Wei, Q., 2009. Gua sha and massage in the treatment of headache 90. Henan Traditional Chinese Medicine 7, 704–705.

Wang, L., 2000. 'Gua sha' holographic meridian scraping for ascites due to liver cirrhosis. China's Naturopathy 8 (7), 15.

Wang, L., 2007. The clinical application of 'jingluo gua sha' holographic meridian scraping in patients with chronic hepatitis B. China's Naturopathy 15 (9), 14–15.

Wang, L.-q., 2006. Observation on therapeutic effects of Gua sha scraping therapy and warming acupuncture-moxibustion on 50 cases of fasciitis of back muscles. Chinese Acupuncture & Moxibustion 26 (7), 478–480.

Wang, M., 2009a. Acupuncture and Gua Sha treatment of acute peripheral facial paralysis. Chinese Journal of Primary Medicine and Pharmacy 7, 1315.

Wang, M., 2009b. Gua Sha Acupuncture and Traction Cervical Vertebral Artery clinical observation. Journal of Huaihai Medicine 4, 342–343.

Wang, Q., Li, X., 2004. Effect observation of scapulohumeral periarthritis treated with acupuncture and cutaneous scraping. J Clin Acup and Moxibust 10, 7–8.

Wang, Z., Tao, i., Wu, N., et al., 2004. Gua sha 'coin scraping' treatment of lumbar disc herniation. Chinese Journal of Traditional Medical Traumatology & Orthopedics 12 (6), 7–10.

Wei, L., 2008. Gua sha and cupping treatment of low back pain (120, 60 in control). Shaanxi Journal of Traditional Chinese Medicine 6, 721–722.

Wei, Q., Tu, G., Zhang, H., Zeng, M., et al., 2003. Observation of 160 cases of simple obesity treated with Gua sha and Qi gong. Gansu Journal of Traditional Chinese Medicine 16 (4), 20–22.

Xie, Z., 2000. Gua Sha Treatment of incomplete adhesions after abdominal cancer, 24 cases of intestinal obstruction – attached to conventional Western medicine treatment of 20 cases of control observation. Zhejiang Journal of Traditional Chinese Medicine 35 (8), 333.

Ya, T., 2009. (Zhuang medicine, Chinese medicine treatment of chronic colitis with clinical observation of 250 cases). Henan Traditional Chinese Medicine 10, 1002–1003.

Ya, T., 2009b. Randomized clinical study of treatment of chronic colitis with Zhuang medicine detoxification therapy together with Gua sha scraping together Bupiyichang pills). Journal of Liaoning College of Traditional Chinese Medicine 8, 143–144.

Yang, X., Lu, X., Zhang, G., 2006. Forty-nine Patients with Obstinate Sleeplessness Treated by Comprehensive Therapy. China's Naturopathy 14 (5), 54–55.

Yao, H., Guo, Z., 2009. Gua sha treatment of infantile 'autumn diarrhea.' Hebei Traditional Chinese Journal of Medicine 1, 106.

Yu, J., 2005. Gua sha treatment of rheumatoid arthritis clinical observation. Practical Clinical Journal of Integrated Chinese and Western Medicine 5 (2), 52–53.

Zhang, J., 2007. Fever point acupuncture treatment of 48 cases of cervical spondylosis. Shanghai Journal of Acupuncture and Moxibustion 26 (5), 25–26.

Zhang, J., 2006. Gua sha scraping therapy to improve sleep quality: observation in 128 patients with diabetes. Tianjin Journal of Nursing 14 (3), 159.

Zhang, L., Wang, D., 2006. Plum-blossom needle with Gua sha treatment of neurodermatitis: a comparative study. Hebei Journal of Traditional Chinese Medicine 28 (9), 682.

Zhang, X., Yang, X., 2008. Forty cases of cervical spondylosis treated by gua sha and plasters. Journal of External Therapy of Traditional Chinese Medicine 5, 20–21.

Zhang, Y., Liu, L., Zhang, Y., 2009. Efficacy in 180 cases of wind cold dampness type Bi syndrome (arthralgia) using Gua sha, and cupping with analgesic cream. Guiding Journal of Traditional Chinese Medicine and Pharmacology 6, 43–45.

Zhong, X., 2006. Acupuncture and Gua sha treatment of 45 cases of intractable hiccup. Shaanxi Journal of Traditional Chinese Medicine (TCM Shaanxi). 27 (1), 94–95.

Zhou, L., 2008. Four hundred and forty-seven cases of lumber disc herniation treated with Tongbi ointment applied after gua sha. Journal of External Therapy of Traditional Chinese Medicine 3, 24–25.

Zhou, P., Xu, Y., 2001. Holographic meridian scraping for children in prevention and treatment of influenza. China's Naturopathy 9 (1), 24.

Zhu, X., Ding, L., Yang, B., 2010. The comparative effect of Gua sha, cupping or electroacupuncture in the treatment of head cold. Lishizhen Medicine and Materia Medica Research 7, 1827.

Zou, J., 2009. Methylcobalimin (B12) treatment with Gua sha in 24 cases of postherpetic neuralgia. Journal of Shaanxi College of Traditional Chinese Medicine 5, 46.

References for Table 2.10: Gua sha reviews (5: 4 Chinese, 1 English)

Lee, M.S., Choi, T.-Y., Kim, J.-K., et al., 2010. Using 'Gua sha' to treat musculoskeletal pain: A systematic review of controlled clinical trials. Chinese Medicine 5 (5) (January), 1–5.

Liang, W., Yuan, B., 2009. Progress in Gua sha clinical research. China's Naturopathy 2, 65–66.

Luo, L.-N., 2008. Gua sha therapy research. Guiding Journal of Traditional Chinese Medicine and Pharmacology 4:84–85.

Wang, L., Dang, H., Xu, L., et al., 2006. Analysis of efficacy of Gua sha Scraping Therapy. China's Naturopathy 14 (6), 55.

Wang, Y.-Y., Yang, J.-S., 2009. [Study and prospects for clinical diseases treated with Gua sha therapy]. Chinese Acupuncture & Moxibustion (Zhongguo Zhen Jiu) 29 (2) (February), 167–171.

Glossary of terms

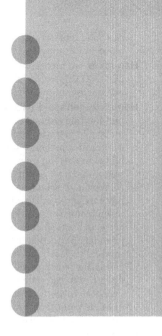

Ah Shi refers to points that are painful on palpation and may or may not represent 'trigger points'.

Anatripsis – from early Western medicine: to rub back again.

Apotherapy a term derived from Greek to describe hands-on techniques that are applied to the body to affect the outcome of a disorder.

Bloodletting a counteractive and antiphlogistic technique where the skin is pierced at specific body sites to intentionally allow blood to come out. Some bloodletting techniques extravasate blood from the vascular without letting it come out of the skin, such as Gua sha and cupping. There are many micro bloodletting techniques that should not be confused with venesection, letting blood from a vein.

Bu tong ze: tong; tong ze: bu tong means if there is no free flow (of Qi), there is pain; if there is free flow, there is 'bu tong', no pain.

Cao Gio is the Vietnamese practice of press-stroking the skin with a coin or other smooth edged instrument to alleviate various common symptoms of illness. The technique is identical to Gua sha.

Cautery is a counteractive technique involving burning small spots or areas of the skin.

Chasing the Dragon's Tail is a treatment approach that follows and treats the area of most pain. When that area is relieved the next is found and treated, and so on until the pain is completely resolved.

Classical Chinese medicine refers to various traditional East Asian medical practices based in the scholarly archive of classical medical texts as well as in oral and domestic practice and transmission. Classical practice was common before the articulation of TCM that emphasized internal organ patterns of disharmony. The oeuvre and practice of Dr James Tin Yau So was based in classical Chinese medicine.

Cou Li refers to 'pores' in much of the *Su Wen*. The Cou Li is between the skin and muscles. It serves as an entrance and outlet for the flow of Qi and Blood, as one of the routes for the excretion of Body Fluid and as a barrier against or transmitter of exogenous evils. It has been compared to the subcutaneous fascia.

Counteraction methods are physical therapies intended to counter imbalance and disease. Warmth counters cold, drying counters moisture, etc. Also, creating benign inflammation at the surface counteracts more serious internal inflammation.

Counterirritation is a term used interchangeably with counteraction. Counterirritation is, by Galenic definition, a derivation technique.

Croup tent is an adjunct therapy using steam to treat congestion or inflammation of the nasal passages, sinuses, chest and lungs.

De qi is the sensation of Ying Qi arriving at the acupuncture point as it is being needled. De qi can feel like soreness, heaviness, an ache or sharp twitch.

Derivation is a bloodletting technique involving diversion of blood from an affected part to a nearby one. Local bloodletting as well as cupping were considered derivative.

Diapedesis vasodilation and extravasation of blood cells into the tissue from the surface capillaries without necessarily damaging the capillaries.

Disperse – to scatter obstructed Qi, Blood, fluid or Phlegm.

Ebers Papyrus is the oldest, most complete and unspoiled book in existence It documents that Egyptian medical and surgical knowledge was as advanced at the time of its writing as it was 1500 years later during the time of Galen.

Ecchymosis represents the passage of blood into subcutaneous tissue, marked by red or purple discoloration of the skin. Sha petechiae readily become ecchymosis, or ecchymotic patches.

Exterior refers to the outermost tissue of the body including the Tai Yang area and the Biao or skin.

Extravasation refers to blood cells moved outside their vessels.

Frictio – Latin from *fricare*, to rub.

Galen (AD 129–200) was one of the most famous physicians in Rome during the reign of Marcus Aurelius who established direct trade with China. Galen followed Greek methods of medicine known as Hippocratic.

Gao Huang refers to the greasy membrane or Li, the lining between the Heart and diaphragm, and to acupoint BL 43 (classical BL 38).

Ga sal is Cambodian for Gua sha.

Gua sha is a traditional East Asian medicine healing technique that applies instrument-assisted unidirectional 'press-stroking' of a lubricated area of body surface to intentionally create *transitory therapeutic* *petechiae* representing extravasation of blood in the subcutis.

Han texts are medical texts written in 220–200 BC, sealed in a tomb in 165 BC and uncovered in 1975.

Heme oxygenase-1 (HO-1) is the rate-limiting enzyme of ferroheme metabolic pathway, which catalyzes the transformation of ferroheme into biliverdin, carbon monoxide (CO) and free iron. HO-1 and its catalysates (biliverdin, bilirubin and CO) exhibit not only anti-oxidative but also anti-inflammatory effects. HO-1 regulates cell cycle and anti-smooth muscle hyperplasia providing protection in many disease models, such asthma, hepatitis, organ transplant rejection, inflammatory bowel disease and experimental autoimmune encephalomyelitis, even though the immune pathological mechanisms of these diseases are dissimilar.

Hsieh is the term used to describe pathogenic aspects of illness or disease associated with factors with agency to, for example, penetrate from the Exterior and progress to the Interior. Gua sha is one technique that liberates the Exterior aspect of hsieh syndrome.

Iatralyptes from Latin means a physician who heals by anointing with oil.

Iatramea from Latin meaning a female physician who heals by anointing with oil.

Issue was a *seton* made with bulkier material such as metal.

Jin Ye are the Body Fluids, a kind of nourishing substance produced by the joint functions of the Stomach, Spleen, Lungs and San Jiao. Body Fluid is a constituent of Blood when in the blood vessels. When it is outside the blood vessels, it stays in the slit of the body Organs. Jin fluids are lighter and clearer; Ye fluids are heavier and thicker.

Jing (Ching) vessels are deep and not visible. They are the main channels associated with the Internal Organs (*Ling Shu*).

Jue Yin associates the Liver and Pericardium and is characterized by Hot and Cold symptoms complexes and delirium, reflecting illness of a serious nature.

Kerik or kerok is Indonesian for Gua sha

Khoud lam is Laotian for Gua sha

Ling Shu is the part of the *Nei Ching*, known as the *Spiritual Axis* or *Divine Pivot*, and is thought to have been written much later than the bulk of the *Su Wen*.

Lo Luo vessels are channels at the surface, visible just beneath the surface of the skin (*Ling Shu*). Lo vessels connect the *Jing* vessels to one another.

Ming Men Gate of Life, is considered the origin of the Yang aspect in the human body.

Mo Yuan refers to the membrane found between the viscera and the wall of the trunk, connected to the muscles externally and close to the Stomach internally. It is the gateway to the San Jiao or Triple Burner and, in fact, is at the half-Exterior, half-Interior level of the body. It is another term for mesentery, greater omentum, peritoneum or, broadly, the fascia of the abdominal cavity.

Moxibustion is a form of cautery using moxa, processed *Artemisia vulgaris*, at points on the skin. Direct moxa burns the herb directly on the skin, aggressively moving Qi and dispersing cold; indirect moxa burns the herb close to the skin that moves Qi and warms.

Mu points also know as alarm or front collecting points, are on the Yin or ventral aspect of the body. Each Organ's ability to be influenced is concentrated in a bilateral Mu point. The point can become tender or alarmed when the Organ is imbalanced.

Neti wash is a daily hygenic practice that uses water and salt mixed in a Neti pot and allowed to wash through the nasal passages and into the back of the throat. Neti washes are used to treat and prevent cold, flu, headaches, rhinitis and sinusitis.

Pain is defined as obstruction in the movement of Qi and or Blood.

Path of Qi refers to the horizontal emanation of Qi within the Jiao whereby Mu points on the front, Shu points on the back and stimulation at the surface affect underlying muscles and Organs.

Pathogenic factors (Hsieh) are factors able to penetrate the body causing imbalance and illness. When elements of Wind, Cold, Heat, Damp and Dryness are in excess of the body's ability to regulate, there occurs penetration, obstruction and Excess. They are also known as exogenous factors not only because they can enter from outside the body but because entry is indicated by symptoms at the body Exterior.

Petechiae are small crimson, purple, red or livid and sometimes slightly raised spots on the skin due to extravasation of blood. Sha rash appears as transitory therapeutic petechiae.

Piezoelectric effect is electricity produced by pressure on crystals. One theory hypothesizes that the fibers found in connective tissue ground substance produce piezoelectricity that is conducted within the connective tissue system.

Pneuma is the Galenic term for air as it applies to body function; it resembles the Chinese Qi.

Qi – literally air. Regarding the body Qi is substance and function. Qi is not limited to a notion of 'energy'.

Release the Exterior refers to liberating the pathogenic factor that is obstructing the surface and includes techniques like sweating and Gua sha.

Revulsion is a bloodletting technique diverting blood from an affected part to a distant one.

Rice congee is used for patients with serious illness or digestive disorder. One cup of rice is cooked with eight cups of water. The gruel is given as a warm drink. Congee can be cooked with herbs, vegetable, meat or fish.

San Jiao is the organ in Chinese medicine that regulates Fire and Water, transformation and circulation of life humors in the three burning spaces, the Upper, Middle and Lower Jiao. Also known as the Triple Burner or Triple Heater, it is said to surround and protect the Kidneys in the way that the Pericardium or Heart Protector surrounds and protects the Heart. The San Jiao is the organ associated with the Li or lining, the fascia and connective tissue.

Sedate – to calm.

Seton was the threading of strands of silk, twine or hair through the skin, leaving it in place indefinitely. The effect was to counteract an internal disease or inflammation by creating an external running sore.

Shao Yang is the lateral aspect of the body, traversed by the Gall Bladder and San Jiao channels. Shao Yang is said to be the hinge between the outside and inside of the body and corresponds to aspects of connective tissue. Pathogenesis at the Shao Yang is characterized by chills alternating with fever, body aches and mild sweating that does not result in resolution.

Shao Yin involves the Heart and Kidney Organs and channels characterized by extreme aversion to cold, lack of fever and desire to sleep, it is considered extreme Deficiency of Yang.

Shi indicates an Excess condition.

Shu points also known as associated or back transporting points, are on the Yang or dorsal aspect of the body. They are said to transport Qi to the inner Organs.

Six body areas and six stages dates to the *Shang Han Lun*, AD 220. Illness caused by external pathogenic factors progressively penetrates areas of the body. The presence of factors in an area is characterized by a particular symptom complex. The six areas are the Tai Yang, Shao Yang, Yang Ming, Tai Yin, Shao Yin and Jue Yin.

Su Wen is the part of the *Nei Ching*, known as the *Plain Questions*. It is the earliest book of Chinese medical theory and dates from the 3rd to the 1st century BC.

Tai Yang is the outermost aspect of the body including the area traversed by the Small Intestine and Bladder channels. Pathogenesis at the Tai Yang is characterized by chills, low or no fever, no sweat or change in the Tongue coat.

Tai Yin aspect of the body is the area traversed by and associated with the Lungs and the Spleen. Pathogenesis at the Tai Yin resembles the pattern of Deficient Spleen Yang with digestive problems: vomit, diarrhea or loose stool, abdominal distension.

TCM refers to traditional Chinese medicine, the official traditional medicine of China as promulgated by the postrevolutionary government, the People's Republic of China (PRC) that was articulated in the 1980s to emphasize diagnostic 'organ patterns of disharmony'.

TEAM refers to traditional East Asian medicine.

Tonify – to strengthen.

Tripsis – an Early Western medicine term, to move along the surface of a body with pressure, friction or stress, to aggravate.

Venesection is to cut a vein for the purpose of letting blood, an early Western medicine form of bloodletting that was excessive and eventually abandoned.

Wei Qi is the body's protective aspect. The Wei is greasy, slippery, cannot enter the channels or vessels, but resides in between the skin and the muscles, at the Couli. This is the superficial fascia in Western anatomy. Wei assumes form as body fat, the adipose tissue of the superficial fascia. Functionally, Wei Qi warms the muscles, fills up the skin, opens and closes the pores (Cou Li) to protect the body from penetration of Cold and Wind. Wei Qi is an espect of body resistance, circulating within the Couli, controlled by the San Jiao.

Xian biao hou li – 'first treat the Exterior, then the Interior'.

Xu indicates a Deficiency condition.

Yang Ming is the Interior aspect of the body, traversed by the Stomach and Large Intestine channels. Pathogenesis at the Yang Ming is characterized by the Four Bigs: big fever, thirst, sweat and pulse.

Yang – sunny side of the river, active, functional aspect.

Yin – shaded side of the river, quiescent, containing aspect.

Ying Qi is the nourishing Qi. Ying flows in the blood vessels and channels, suffuses the entire body through the vascular system and the meridian system. Ying and Blood are often synonymous; though the Blood carries Ying, Ying is not contained only in Blood. Ying Qi is the Qi activated when a needle is inserted in an acupuncture point.

Yuan Qi means original, primordial source Qi. It is our life force endowed by heaven, manifest through our parents, accumulated in the Kidneys and circulated by the San Jiao.

Index

Printed in the United States
By Bookmasters